2020

Nelson's Pediatric Antimicrobial Therapy

26th Edition

John S. Bradley, MD
Editor in Chief

John D. Nelson, MD
Emeritus

Elizabeth D. Barnett, MD
Joseph B. Cantey, MD
David W. Kimberlin, MD
Paul E. Palumbo, MD
Jason Sauberan, PharmD
J. Howard Smart, MD
William J. Steinbach, MD
Contributing Editors

American Academy of Pediatrics

DEDICATED TO THE HEALTH OF ALL CHILDREN®

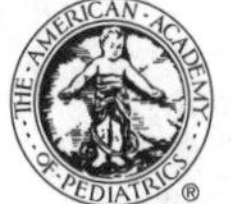

American Academy of Pediatrics Publishing Staff

Mary Lou White, *Chief Product and Services Officer/SVP, Membership, Marketing, and Publishing*
Mark Grimes, *Vice President, Publishing*
Peter Lynch, *Senior Manager, Publishing Acquisitions and Digital Strategy*
Mary Kelly, *Senior Editor, Professional and Clinical Publishing*
Shannan Martin, *Production Manager, Consumer Publications*
Jason Crase, *Manager, Editorial Services*
Linda Smessaert, MSIMC, *Senior Marketing Manager, Professional Resources*
Mary Louise Carr, MBA, *Marketing Manager, Clinical Publications*

Published by the American Academy of Pediatrics
345 Park Blvd
Itasca, IL 60143
Telephone: 630/626-6000
Facsimile: 847/434-8000
www.aap.org

The American Academy of Pediatrics is an organization of 67,000 primary care pediatricians, pediatric medical subspecialists, and pediatric surgical specialists dedicated to the health, safety, and well-being of infants, children, adolescents, and young adults.

The recommendations in this publication do not indicate an exclusive course of treatment or serve as a standard of medical care. Variations, taking into account individual circumstances, may be appropriate.

Statements and opinions expressed are those of the authors and not necessarily those of the American Academy of Pediatrics.

Any websites, brand names, products, or manufacturers are mentioned for informational and identification purposes only and do not imply an endorsement by the American Academy of Pediatrics (AAP). The AAP is not responsible for the content of external resources. Information was current at the time of publication.

The publishers have made every effort to trace the copyright holders for borrowed materials. If they have inadvertently overlooked any, they will be pleased to make the necessary arrangements at the first opportunity.

This publication has been developed by the American Academy of Pediatrics. The authors, editors, and contributors are expert authorities in the field of pediatrics. No commercial involvement of any kind has been solicited or accepted in the development of the content of this publication. Disclosures: Dr Kimberlin disclosed a consulting relationship with Slack Incorporated. Dr Palumbo disclosed a safety monitoring board relationship with Janssen Pharmaceutical Companies. Dr Steinbach disclosed an advisory board relationship with Merck & Company and Astellas Pharma, Inc.

Every effort has been made to ensure that the drug selection and dosages set forth in this text are in accordance with current recommendations and practice at the time of publication. It is the responsibility of the health care professional to check the package insert of each drug for any change in indications or dosage and for added warnings and precautions, and to review newly published, peer-reviewed data in the medical literature for current data on safety and efficacy.

Special discounts are available for bulk purchases of this publication.
Email Special Sales at aapsales@aap.org for more information.

First edition published in 1975.
Printed in the United States of America.

9-442/1219 1 2 3 4 5 6 7 8 9 10
MA0935
ISSN: 2164-9278 (print)
ISSN: 2164-9286 (electronic)
ISBN: 978-1-61002-352-8
eBook: 978-1-61002-353-5

Editor in Chief

John S. Bradley, MD, FAAP
Distinguished Professor of Pediatrics
Division of Infectious Diseases, Department of Pediatrics
University of California, San Diego, School of Medicine
Director, Division of Infectious Diseases, Rady Children's Hospital San Diego
San Diego, CA
Chapters 1, 3, 4, 6, 7, 13, and 14

Emeritus

John D. Nelson, MD
Professor Emeritus of Pediatrics
The University of Texas
Southwestern Medical Center at Dallas
Southwestern Medical School
Dallas, TX

Contributing Editors

Elizabeth D. Barnett, MD, FAAP
Professor of Pediatrics
Boston University School of Medicine
Director, International Clinic and Refugee Health Assessment Program, Boston Medical Center
GeoSentinel Surveillance Network, Boston Medical Center
Boston, MA
Chapter 10

Joseph B. Cantey, MD, FAAP
Assistant Professor of Pediatrics
Divisions of Pediatric Infectious Diseases and Neonatology/Perinatal Medicine
University of Texas Health Science Center at San Antonio
San Antonio, TX
Chapter 5

David W. Kimberlin, MD, FAAP
Editor, *Red Book: 2018–2021 Report of the Committee on Infectious Diseases*, 31st Edition
Professor of Pediatrics
Co-Director, Division of Pediatric Infectious Diseases
Sergio Stagno Endowed Chair in Pediatric Infectious Diseases
University of Alabama at Birmingham
Birmingham, AL
Chapter 9

Paul E. Palumbo, MD
Professor of Pediatrics and Medicine
Geisel School of Medicine at Dartmouth
Director, International Pediatric HIV Program
Dartmouth-Hitchcock Medical Center
Lebanon, NH
HIV treatment

Jason Sauberan, PharmD
Assistant Clinical Professor
University of California, San Diego, Skaggs School of Pharmacy and Pharmaceutical Sciences
Rady Children's Hospital San Diego
San Diego, CA
Chapters 5, 11, and 12

J. Howard Smart, MD, FAAP
Chairman, Department of Pediatrics
Sharp Rees-Stealy Medical Group
Assistant Clinical Professor of Pediatrics
University of California, San Diego, School of Medicine
San Diego, CA
App development

William J. Steinbach, MD, FAAP
Samuel L. Katz Professor of Pediatrics
Professor in Molecular Genetics and Microbiology
Chief, Division of Pediatric Infectious Diseases
Director, Duke Pediatric Immunocompromised Host Program
Director, International Pediatric Fungal Network
Duke University School of Medicine
Durham, NC
Chapters 2 and 8

Contents

Introduction

Hard to believe, but we are now in our 26th edition of *Nelson's Pediatric Antimicrobial Therapy*—and more than a decade with the American Academy of Pediatrics (AAP)! We had the incredible opportunity late last year to publicly thank John Nelson for his many contributions to the field of pediatric infectious diseases over his decades-long career, including his creation of the *Pocket Book of Pediatric Antimicrobial Therapy*, which was the predecessor of *Nelson's* and the model for the Sanford guide for adults. Clinicians did not have so many options for antibiotic therapy when he was first recruited to Dallas, where he recruited George McCracken to join him. We have trained John on the iPhone app for his book, but he still prefers the printed version. We are working with the AAP to further enhance the ability of clinicians to access treatment recommendations easily and allow us to bring important new advances in the field of pediatric anti-infective therapy more often than once yearly.

A number of new antibiotics, antivirals, and antifungals have been recently approved by the US Food and Drug Administration (FDA) for pediatric age groups and are highlighted in the Notable Changes. Some new agents only have approvals for children 12 years and older, but virtually all have federal mandates for clinical trials through all pediatric age groups, including neonates. Most of the newly approved antibacterial agents are for drug-resistant pathogens, not for pneumococcus or *Haemophilus influenzae* type b, given the spectacular success of the protein-conjugated vaccines. For the community, *Escherichia coli* is now giving us headaches with increasing resistance; for hospital pathogens, *everything* is getting more resistant.

The contributing editors, all very active in clinical work, have updates in their sections with relevant new recommendations (beyond FDA approvals) based on current published data, guidelines, and clinical experience. We believe that the reference list for each chapter provides the available evidence to support our recommendations, for those who wish to see the actual clinical trial and in vitro data.

The *Nelson's* app has made significant advances this past year thanks to the Apple programing abilities of our contributing editor, Dr Howard Smart, a full-time office-based pediatrician and the chief of pediatrics at the Sharp Rees-Stealy multispecialty medical group in San Diego, CA. With the support of the AAP (particularly Peter Lynch) and the editors, we are putting even more of Howard's enhancements in this 2020 edition. I use the app during rounds now, and we have provided the app to all our residents. There are clear advantages to the app over the printed book, but as with all software, glitches may pop up, so if your app doesn't work, please let us know at nelsonabx@aap.org so we can fix the bugs!

We always appreciate the talent and advice of our collaborators/colleagues who take the time to see if what we are sharing "makes sense." In particular, we wish to thank Drs John van den Anker and Pablo Sanchez for their valuable suggestions on antimicrobial therapy of the newborn in support of the work done by JB Cantey and Jason Sauberan in Chapter 5.

We are also fortunate to have 3 reviewers for the entire book and app this year. Returning to assist us is Dr Brian Williams, a pediatric/adult hospitalist who recently moved from San Diego to Madison, WI. Brian's suggestions are always focused and practical, traits that John Nelson specifically values and promotes. New for this year, to help us with the user experience of the app, we welcome input from Dr Juan Chapparro, who is double boarded in pediatric infectious diseases and biomedical informatics, and Dr Daniel Sklansky, a pediatric hospitalist at the University of Wisconsin.

We continue to harmonize the *Nelson's* book with *Red Book®: 2018–2021 Report of the Committee on Infectious Diseases*, 31st Edition (easy to understand, given that Dr David Kimberlin is also the editor of the *Red Book*). We are virtually always in sync but often with additional explanations (that do not necessarily represent AAP policy) to allow the reader to understand the basis for recommendations.

We continue to provide grading of our recommendations—our assessment of how strongly we feel about a recommendation and the strength of the evidence to support our recommendation (noted in the Table). This is not the GRADE method (*G*rading of *R*ecommendations *A*ssessment, *D*evelopment, and *E*valuation) but certainly uses the concepts on which GRADE is based: the strength of recommendation and level of evidence. Similar to GRADE, we review the literature (and the most important manuscripts are referenced), but importantly, we work within the context of professional society recommendations (eg, the AAP) and our experience. The data may never have been presented to or reviewed by the FDA and, therefore, are not in the package label. We all find ourselves in this situation frequently. Many of us are working closely with the FDA to try to narrow the gap in our knowledge of antimicrobial agents between adults and children; the FDA pediatric infectious diseases staff is providing an exceptional effort to shed light on the doses that are safe and effective for neonates, infants, and children, with major efforts, supported by grants from the Eunice Kennedy Shriver National Institute of Child Health and Human Development (with Dr Danny Benjamin from Duke leading the charge), to place important new data on safety and efficacy in the antibiotic package labels for all to use in clinical practice.

Strength of Recommendation	Description
A	Strongly recommended
B	Recommended as a good choice
C	One option for therapy that is adequate, perhaps among many other adequate therapies
Level of Evidence	**Description**
I	Based on well-designed, prospective, randomized, and controlled studies in an appropriate population of children
II	Based on data derived from prospectively collected, small comparative trials, or noncomparative prospective trials, or reasonable retrospective data from clinical trials in children, or data from other populations (eg, adults)
III	Based on case reports, case series, consensus statements, or expert opinion for situations in which sound data do not exist

As we state each year, many of the recommendations by the editors for specific situations have not been systematically evaluated in controlled, prospective, comparative clinical trials.

Mary Kelly, our senior editor at the AAP, has done an impressive job organizing the editors and being an outstanding advocate for us and the clinician-users of the book. She was also instrumental in helping to launch the *Nelson's Neonatal Antimicrobial Therapy* manual in spring 2019.

Peter Lynch (AAP senior manager, publishing acquisitions and digital strategy) continues to work on developing *Nelson's* online, as well as working with Howard and the editors to enhance the functionality of the app. Thanks to Mark Grimes, vice president, Publishing, and our steadfast friends and supporters in AAP Membership, Marketing, and Publishing—Jeff Mahony, director, professional and consumer publishing (who has been with us since we first joined with the AAP a decade ago); Linda Smessaert, senior marketing manager, professional resources; and the entire staff—who make certain that the considerable information in *Nelson's* makes it to those who are actually caring for children.

We continue to be very interested to learn from readers/users if there are new chapters or sections you wish for us to develop—and whether you find certain sections particularly helpful, so we don't change or delete them! Please feel free to share your suggestions with us at nelsonabx@aap.org.

John S. Bradley, MD

Notable Changes to *2020 Nelson's Pediatric Antimicrobial Therapy*, 26th Edition

References have been updated, with more than 150 *new* references. Based on comments we received, we now have the supporting references in the app that are as easily accessible as in the book; we are quite grateful to our contributing editor, Dr Howard Smart, for entering every reference by hand (nearly 400 references for Chapter 6 alone) and writing the code so that both the references *and* the abstracts from PubMed are now just a few taps away on your screen. Just amazing.

Bacterial/Mycobacterial Infections and Antibiotics

We were quite disappointed that cefotaxime is no longer being manufactured for the US market. This was one of the first of the third-generation cephalosporins that was documented to be safe and effective for many infections (including meningitis) in all pediatric age groups, including the neonate, caused by a wide variety of susceptible pathogens. Because it is not available, we have removed it from all our recommendations (including neonates), but we hope that someone will manufacture it again in the future. For older children, ceftriaxone should continue to work well, but for neonates, it is the consensus opinion of the editors that cefepime now be substituted in situations where you would have previously used cefotaxime, based on its gram-positive and enteric bacilli spectrum and pharmacokinetic profile, which is very similar to cefotaxime. Effectiveness in pediatric meningitis was demonstrated by one of John Nelson's previous pediatric infectious disease fellows, Xavier Saez-Llorens. The broader spectrum of meropenem is not needed for neonatal sepsis in 2020.

We are now shifting our recommendation for serious, invasive methicillin-resistant *Staphylococcus aureus* (MRSA) infections from vancomycin to ceftaroline for several reasons, primarily safety and more predictable efficacy for MRSA, although we are holding off recommendations for MRSA endocarditis and central nervous system infections, as the US companies that have owned the antibiotic (Cerexa/Forest/Actavis/Allergan) have not supported prospective pediatric clinical trials for these indications.

Updates for gastrointestinal pathogen infections (including traveler's diarrhea) from the new Infectious Diseases Society of America guidelines have now been incorporated.

For children with latent tuberculosis, we support once-weekly isoniazid and rifapentine for 12 weeks as the preferred regimen, given data on improved compliance.

Ceftazidime/avibactam was approved for pediatrics by the US Food and Drug Administration (FDA) in March 2019 and has activity against extended-spectrum beta-lactamase *Escherichia coli* as well as carbapenem-resistant *Klebsiella pneumoniae* carbapenemase–bearing strains of *E coli* and *Klebsiella*.

Fungal Infections and Antifungal Agents

New approaches to mucormycosis, a devastating infection, have been added, based on published data, animal models, and the extensive experience of William J. Steinbach, MD, whom we all call for advice.

New references on dosing fluconazole and anidulafungin for invasive candidiasis have been added.

Viral Infections and Antiviral Agents

Just want to remind everyone that current recommendations about HIV and antiretrovirals, including those for the management of newborns exposed to HIV, are posted on the AIDSinfo website (https://aidsinfo.nih.gov), which is continuously updated.

Baloxavir, an influenza antiviral, was approved for adults and children older than 12 years for outpatient management of uncomplicated influenza in otherwise healthy patients (just a single dose). This antiviral has a completely different mechanism of action against influenza, compared with oseltamivir, zanamivir, and peramivir, as it blocks early initiation of influenza virus nucleic acid replication. There are no data in the United States yet for younger children, although it is approved in Japan for children down to 2 years of age.

Parasitic Infections and Antiparasitic Agents

Intravenous (IV) quinidine is no longer an option for treatment for severe malaria, with IV artesunate, available from the Centers for Disease Control and Prevention, as the only remaining option.

Tafenoquine is now available for prophylaxis and treatment of malaria.

Triclabendazole is now approved by the FDA for treatment of fascioliasis in those 6 years and older.

1. Choosing Among Antibiotics Within a Class: Beta-lactams and Beta-lactamase Inhibitors, Macrolides, Aminoglycosides, and Fluoroquinolones

New drugs should be compared with others in the same class regarding (1) antimicrobial spectrum; (2) degree of antibiotic exposure (a function of the pharmacokinetics of the nonprotein-bound drug at the site of infection and the pharmacodynamic properties of the drug); (3) demonstrated efficacy in adequate and well-controlled clinical trials; (4) tolerance, toxicity, and side effects; and (5) cost. If there is no substantial benefit for efficacy or safety for one antimicrobial over another for the isolated or presumed bacterial pathogen(s), one should opt for using an older, more extensively used agent (with presumably better-defined efficacy and safety) that is usually less expensive and preferably with a narrower spectrum of activity.

Beta-lactams and Beta-lactamase Inhibitors

Beta-lactam (BL)/Beta-lactamase Inhibitor (BLI) Combinations. Increasingly studied and approved by the US Food and Drug Administration (FDA) are BL/BLI combinations that target antibiotic resistance based on the presence of a pathogen's beta-lactamase. The BL antibiotic may demonstrate activity against a pathogen, but if a beta-lactamase is present in that pathogen, it will hydrolyze the BL ring structure and inactivate the antibiotic. The BLI is usually a BL structure, which explains why it binds readily to certain beta-lactamases and can inhibit their activity; however, the BLI usually does not demonstrate direct antibiotic activity itself. As amoxicillin and ampicillin were used extensively against *Haemophilus influenzae* following their approval, resistance increased based on the presence of a beta-lactamase that hydrolyzes the BL ring of amoxicillin/ampicillin (with up to 40% of isolates demonstrating resistance in some regions). Clavulanate, a BLI that binds to and inactivates the *H influenzae* beta-lactamase, allows amoxicillin/ampicillin to "survive" and inhibit cell wall formation, leading to the death of the organism. The first oral BL/BLI combination of amoxicillin/clavulanate, originally known as Augmentin, has been very effective. Similar combinations, primarily intravenous (IV), have now been studied, pairing penicillins, cephalosporins, and carbapenems with other BLIs such as tazobactam, sulbactam, and avibactam. Under investigation in children are the IV BL/BLI combinations meropenem/vaborbactam, ceftolozane/tazobactam, and imipenem/relebactam.

Beta-lactam Antibiotics

Oral Cephalosporins (cephalexin, cefadroxil, cefaclor, cefprozil, cefuroxime, cefixime, cefdinir, cefpodoxime, cefditoren [tablet only], and ceftibuten). As a class, the oral cephalosporins have the advantage over oral penicillins of somewhat greater spectrum of activity. The serum half-lives of cefpodoxime, ceftibuten, and cefixime are greater than 2 hours. This pharmacokinetic feature accounts for the fact that they may be given in 1 or 2 doses per day for certain indications, particularly otitis media, where the middle ear fluid half-life is likely to be much longer than the serum half-life. For more resistant pathogens, twice daily is preferred (see Chapter 3). The spectrum of activity increases for gram-negative organisms as one goes from the first-generation cephalosporins (cephalexin and cefadroxil), to the second generation (cefaclor, cefprozil, and cefuroxime) that demonstrates activity against *H influenzae* (including beta-lactamase–producing strains), to the third-generation agents (cefdinir, cefixime, cefpodoxime, and ceftibuten) that have enhanced coverage of many enteric gram-negative bacilli (*Escherichia coli, Klebsiella* spp). However, ceftibuten and cefixime, in particular, have a disadvantage of less activity against *Streptococcus pneumoniae* than the others, particularly against penicillin non-susceptible strains. No oral fourth- or fifth-generation cephalosporins (see the Parenteral Cephalosporins section) currently exist (ie, no oral cephalosporins with activity against *Pseudomonas* or methicillin-resistant *Staphylococcus aureus* [MRSA]). The palatability of generic versions of these products may not have the same better-tasting characteristics as the original products.

Parenteral Cephalosporins. First-generation cephalosporins, such as cefazolin, are used mainly for treatment of gram-positive infections caused by *S aureus* (excluding MRSA) and group A streptococcus and for surgical prophylaxis; the gram-negative spectrum is limited but more extensive than ampicillin. Cefazolin is well tolerated on intramuscular or IV injection.

A second-generation cephalosporin (cefuroxime) and the cephamycins (cefoxitin and cefotetan) provide increased activity against many gram-negative organisms, particularly *H influenzae* and *E coli*. Cefoxitin has, in addition, activity against only 80% of strains of *Bacteroides fragilis* but can be considered for use in place of the more active agents like metronidazole or carbapenems when beta-lactamase–positive *Bacteroides* and *Prevotella* spp are suspected, and up to 20% treatment failure is acceptable.

Third-generation cephalosporins (cefotaxime, ceftriaxone, and ceftazidime) all have enhanced potency against many enteric gram-negative bacilli. As with all cephalosporins at readily achievable serum concentrations, they are less active against enterococci and *Listeria;* only ceftazidime has significant activity against *Pseudomonas.* Cefotaxime (currently not being manufactured) and ceftriaxone have been used very successfully to treat meningitis caused by pneumococcus (mostly penicillin-susceptible strains), *H influenzae* type b, meningococcus, and susceptible strains of *E coli* meningitis. These drugs have the greatest usefulness for treating gram-negative bacillary infections due to their safety, compared with other classes of antibiotics (including aminoglycosides). Because ceftriaxone is excreted to a large extent via the liver, it can be used with little dosage adjustment in patients with renal failure. With a serum half-life of 4 to 7 hours, it can be given once a day for all infections, including meningitis, that are caused by susceptible organisms.

Cefepime, a fourth-generation cephalosporin approved for use in children in 1999, exhibits (1) enhanced antipseudomonal activity over ceftazidime; (2) the gram-positive activity of second-generation cephalosporins; (3) better activity against gram-negative enteric bacilli; and (4) stability against the inducible ampC beta-lactamases of *Enterobacter* and *Serratia* (and some strains of *Proteus* and *Citrobacter*) that can hydrolyze third-generation cephalosporins. It can be used as single-drug antibiotic therapy against these pathogens, rather than paired with an aminoglycoside, as is commonly done with third-generation cephalosporins to decrease the emergence of ampC-resistant strains. In general, cefepime is hydrolyzed by many of the newly emergent extended-spectrum beta-lactamase (ESBL) enzymes and should not be used if an ESBL *E coli* or *Klebsiella* is suspected.

Ceftaroline is a fifth-generation cephalosporin, the first of the cephalosporins with activity against MRSA. Ceftaroline was approved by the FDA in December 2010 for adults and approved for children in June 2016 for treatment of complicated skin infections (including MRSA) and community-acquired pneumonia. The pharmacokinetics of ceftaroline have been evaluated in all pediatric age groups, including neonates and children with cystic fibrosis; clinical studies for pediatric community-acquired pneumonia and complicated skin infection are published.[1,2] Based on these published data, review by the FDA, and post-marketing experience for infants and children 2 months and older, we believe that ceftaroline should be as effective and safer than vancomycin for treatment of MRSA infections. Just as BLs like cefazolin are preferred over vancomycin for methicillin-susceptible *S aureus* infections, ceftaroline should be considered preferred treatment over vancomycin for MRSA infection. Neither renal function nor drug levels need to be followed with ceftaroline therapy. Limited pharmacokinetic and clinical data also support the use of ceftaroline in neonates.

Penicillinase-Resistant Penicillins (dicloxacillin [capsules only]; nafcillin and oxacillin [parenteral only]). "Penicillinase" refers specifically to the beta-lactamase produced by *S aureus* in this case and not those produced by gram-negative bacteria. These antibiotics are active against penicillin-resistant *S aureus* but not against MRSA. Nafcillin differs pharmacologically from the others in being excreted primarily by the liver rather than by the kidneys, which may explain the relative lack of nephrotoxicity compared with methicillin, which is no longer available in the United States. Nafcillin pharmacokinetics are erratic in persons with liver disease, and the drug is often painful with IV infusion.

Antipseudomonal and Anti-enteric Gram-negative BLs (piperacillin/tazobactam, aztreonam, ceftazidime, cefepime, meropenem, and imipenem). Piperacillin/tazobactam (Zosyn) and ceftazidime/avibactam (Avycaz) (both FDA approved for children), and still under investigation in children, ceftolozane/tazobactam (Zerbaxa) and meropenem/vaborbactam (Vabomere), represent BL/BLI combinations, as noted previously. The BLI (clavulanic acid, tazobactam, avibactam, or vaborbactam in these combinations) binds irreversibly to and neutralizes specific beta-lactamase enzymes produced by the organism. The combination only adds to the spectrum of the original antibiotic when the mechanism of resistance is a beta-lactamase enzyme and only when the BLI is capable of binding to and inhibiting that particular organism's beta-lactamase enzyme(s). The combinations extend the spectrum of activity of the primary antibiotic to include many beta-lactamase–positive bacteria, including some strains of enteric gram-negative bacilli (*E coli, Klebsiella,* and *Enterobacter*), *S aureus,* and *B fragilis.* Piperacillin/tazobactam, ceftolozane/tazobactam, and ceftazidime/avibactam may still be inactive against *Pseudomonas* because their BLIs may not effectively inhibit all of the beta-lactamases of *Pseudomonas*, and other mechanisms of resistance may also be present.

Pseudomonas has an intrinsic capacity to develop resistance following exposure to any BL, based on the activity of several inducible chromosomal beta-lactamases, upregulated efflux pumps, and changes in the permeability of the cell wall, as well as mutational changes in the antibacterial target sites. Because development of resistance during therapy is not uncommon (particularly beta-lactamase–mediated resistance against piperacillin or ceftazidime), an aminoglycoside such as tobramycin is often used in combination, assuming that the tobramycin may kill strains developing resistance to the BLs. Cefepime, meropenem, and imipenem are relatively stable to the beta-lactamases induced while on therapy and can be used as single-agent therapy for most *Pseudomonas* infections, but resistance may still develop to these agents based on other mechanisms of resistance. For *Pseudomonas* infections in compromised hosts or in life-threatening infections, these drugs, too, should be used in combination with an aminoglycoside or a second active agent. The benefits of the additional antibiotic should be weighed against the potential for additional toxicity and alteration of host flora.

Aminopenicillins (amoxicillin and amoxicillin/clavulanate [oral formulations only, in the United States], ampicillin [oral and parenteral], and ampicillin/sulbactam [parenteral only]). Amoxicillin is very well absorbed, good tasting, and associated with very few side effects. Augmentin is a combination of amoxicillin and clavulanate (as noted previously) that is available in several fixed proportions that permit amoxicillin to remain active against many beta-lactamase–producing bacteria, including *H influenzae* and *S aureus* (but not MRSA). Amoxicillin/clavulanate has undergone many changes in formulation since its introduction. The ratio of amoxicillin to clavulanate was originally 4:1, based on susceptibility data of pneumococcus and *Haemophilus* during the 1970s. With the emergence of penicillin-resistant pneumococcus, recommendations for increasing the dosage of amoxicillin, particularly for upper respiratory tract infections, were made. However, if one increases the dosage of clavulanate even slightly, the incidence of diarrhea increases dramatically. If one keeps the dosage of clavulanate constant while increasing the dosage of amoxicillin, one can treat the relatively resistant pneumococci while not increasing gastrointestinal side effects of the combination. The original 4:1 ratio is present in suspensions containing 125-mg and 250-mg amoxicillin/5 mL and the 125-mg and 250-mg chewable tablets. A higher 7:1 ratio is present in the suspensions containing 200-mg and 400-mg amoxicillin/5 mL and in the 200-mg and 400-mg chewable tablets. A still higher ratio of 14:1 is present in the suspension formulation Augmentin ES-600 that contains 600-mg amoxicillin/5 mL; this preparation is designed to deliver 90 mg/kg/day of amoxicillin, divided twice daily, for the treatment of ear (and sinus) infections. The high serum and middle ear fluid concentrations achieved with 45 mg/kg/dose, combined with the long middle ear fluid half-life (4–6 hours) of amoxicillin, allow for a therapeutic antibiotic exposure to pathogens in the middle ear with a twice-daily regimen. However, the prolonged half-life in the middle ear fluid is not necessarily found in other infection sites (eg, skin, lung tissue, joint tissue), for which dosing of amoxicillin and Augmentin should continue to be 3 times daily for most susceptible pathogens.

For older children who can swallow tablets, the amoxicillin to clavulanate ratios are as follows: 500-mg tablet (4:1); 875-mg tablet (7:1); 1,000-mg tablet (16:1).

Sulbactam, another BLI like clavulanate, is combined with ampicillin in the parenteral formulation Unasyn. The cautions regarding spectrum of activity for piperacillin/tazobactam with respect to the limitations of the BLI in increasing the spectrum of activity also apply to ampicillin/sulbactam, in which ampicillin does not even have the extended activity against the enteric bacilli seen with piperacillin or ceftazidime.

Carbapenems. Meropenem, imipenem, and ertapenem are currently available carbapenems with a broader spectrum of activity than any other class of BL currently available. Meropenem, imipenem, and ertapenem are approved by the FDA for use in children. At present, we recommend them for treatment of infections caused by bacteria resistant to standard therapy or for mixed infections involving aerobes and anaerobes. Imipenem has greater central nervous system (CNS) irritability compared with other carbapenems, leading to an increased risk of seizures in children with meningitis, but this is not clinically significant in children without underlying CNS inflammation. Meropenem was not associated with an increased rate of seizures, compared with cefotaxime in children with meningitis. Imipenem and meropenem are active against virtually all coliform bacilli, including ceftriaxone-resistant (ESBL-producing or ampC-producing) strains, against *Pseudomonas aeruginosa* (including most ceftazidime-resistant strains), and against anaerobes, including *B fragilis*. While ertapenem lacks the excellent activity against *P aeruginosa* of the other carbapenems, it has the advantage of a prolonged serum half-life, which allows for once-daily dosing in adults and children aged 13 years and older and twice-daily dosing in younger children. Newly emergent strains of *Klebsiella pneumoniae* contain *K pneumoniae* carbapenemases (KPC) that degrade and inactivate all the carbapenems. These strains, as well as strains carrying the less common New Delhi metallo-beta-lactamase, which is also active against carbapenems, have begun to spread to many parts of the world, reinforcing the need to keep track of your local antibiotic susceptibility patterns. Carbapenems that have been paired with BLIs, as noted previously, but these BLIs only inhibit KPC carbapenemase.

Macrolides

Erythromycin is the prototype of macrolide antibiotics. Almost 30 macrolides have been produced, but only 3 are FDA approved for children in the United States: erythromycin, azithromycin (also called an azalide), and clarithromycin, while a fourth, telithromycin (also called a ketolide), is approved for adults and only available in tablet form. As a class, these drugs achieve greater concentrations intracellularly than in serum, particularly with azithromycin and clarithromycin. As a result, measuring serum concentrations is usually not clinically useful. Gastrointestinal intolerance to erythromycin is caused by the breakdown products of the macrolide ring structure. This is much less of a problem with azithromycin and clarithromycin. Azithromycin, clarithromycin, and telithromycin extend the clinically relevant activity of erythromycin to include

Haemophilus; azithromycin and clarithromycin also have substantial activity against certain mycobacteria. Azithromycin is also active in vitro and effective against many enteric gram-negative pathogens, including *Salmonella* and *Shigella,* when given orally.

Aminoglycosides

Although 5 aminoglycoside antibiotics are available in the United States, only 3 are widely used for systemic therapy of aerobic gram-negative infections and for synergy in the treatment of certain gram-positive and gram-negative infections: gentamicin, tobramycin, and amikacin. Streptomycin and kanamycin have more limited utility due to increased toxicity compared with the other agents. Resistance in gram-negative bacilli to aminoglycosides is caused by bacterial enzymes that adenylate, acetylate, or phosphorylate the aminoglycoside, resulting in inactivity. The specific activities of each enzyme against each aminoglycoside in each pathogen are highly variable. As a result, antibiotic susceptibility tests must be done for each aminoglycoside drug separately. There are small differences in toxicities to the kidneys and eighth cranial nerve hearing/vestibular function, although it is uncertain whether these small differences are clinically significant. For all children receiving a full treatment course, it is advisable to monitor peak and trough serum concentrations early in the course of therapy, as the degree of drug exposure correlates with toxicity and elevated trough concentrations may predict impending drug accumulation. With amikacin, desired peak concentrations are 20 to 35 mcg/mL and trough drug concentrations are less than 10 mcg/mL; for gentamicin and tobramycin, depending on the frequency of dosing, peak concentrations should be 5 to 10 mcg/mL and trough concentrations less than 2 mcg/mL. Children with cystic fibrosis require greater dosages to achieve equivalent therapeutic serum concentrations due to enhanced clearance. Inhaled tobramycin has been very successful in children with cystic fibrosis as an adjunctive therapy of gram-negative bacillary infections. The role of inhaled aminoglycosides in other gram-negative pneumonias (eg, ventilator-associated pneumonia) has not yet been defined.

Once-Daily Dosing of Aminoglycosides. Once-daily dosing of 5 to 7.5 mg/kg gentamicin or tobramycin has been studied in adults and in some neonates and children; peak serum concentrations are greater than those achieved with dosing 3 times daily. Aminoglycosides demonstrate concentration-dependent killing of pathogens, suggesting a potential benefit to higher serum concentrations achieved with once-daily dosing. Regimens giving the daily dosage as a single infusion, rather than as traditionally split doses every 8 hours, are effective and safe for normal adult hosts and immune-compromised hosts with fever and neutropenia and may be less toxic. Experience with once-daily dosing in children is increasing, with similar encouraging results as noted for adults. A recent Cochrane review for children (and adults) with cystic fibrosis comparing once-daily with 3-times–daily administration found equal efficacy with decreased toxicity in children.[2] Once-daily dosing should be considered as effective as multiple, smaller doses per day and is likely to be safer for children; therefore, it should be the preferred regimen for treatment.

Fluoroquinolones

More than 40 years ago, fluoroquinolone (FQ) toxicity to cartilage in weight-bearing joints in experimental juvenile animals was documented to be dose and duration-of-therapy dependent. Pediatric studies were therefore not initially undertaken with ciprofloxacin or other FQs. However, with increasing antibiotic resistance in pediatric pathogens and an accumulating database in pediatrics suggesting that joint toxicity may be uncommon, the FDA allowed prospective studies to proceed in 1998. As of July 2019, no cases of FQ-attributable joint toxicity have been documented to occur in children with FQs that are approved for use in the United States. Limited published data are available from prospective, blinded studies to accurately assess this risk, although some uncontrolled retrospective published data are reassuring. A prospective, randomized, double-blind study of moxifloxacin for intra-abdominal infection, with 1-year follow-up specifically designed to assess tendon/joint toxicity, demonstrated no concern for toxicity.[3] Unblinded studies with levofloxacin for respiratory tract infections and unpublished randomized studies comparing ciprofloxacin versus other agents for complicated urinary tract infection suggest the possibility of an uncommon, reversible, FQ-attributable arthralgia, but these data should be interpreted with caution. The use of FQs in situations of antibiotic resistance where no other active agent is available is reasonable, weighing the benefits of treatment against the low risk of toxicity of this class of antibiotics. The use of an oral FQ in situations in which the only alternative is parenteral therapy is also justified.[4] For clinicians reading this book, a well-documented case of FQ joint toxicity in a child is publishable (and reportable to the FDA).

Ciprofloxacin usually has very good gram-negative activity (with great regional variation in susceptibility) against enteric bacilli (*E coli, Klebsiella, Enterobacter, Salmonella,* and *Shigella*) and against *P aeruginosa*. However, it lacks substantial gram-positive coverage and should not be used to treat streptococcal, staphylococcal, or pneumococcal infections. Newer-generation FQs are more active against these pathogens; levofloxacin has documented efficacy and safety in pediatric clinical trials for respiratory tract infections, acute otitis media, and community-acquired pneumonia. Children with any question of joint/tendon/bone toxicity in the levofloxacin studies were followed up to 5 years after treatment, with no difference in joint/tendon outcomes in these randomized studies, compared with the standard FDA-approved antibiotics used in these studies.[5] None of the newer-generation FQs are significantly more active against gram-negative pathogens than ciprofloxacin. Quinolone antibiotics are bitter tasting. Ciprofloxacin and levofloxacin are currently available in a suspension form; ciprofloxacin is FDA approved in pediatrics for complicated urinary tract infections and inhalation anthrax, while levofloxacin is approved for inhalation anthrax only, as the sponsor chose not to apply for approval for pediatric respiratory tract infections. For reasons of safety and to prevent the emergence of widespread resistance, FQs should still not be used for primary therapy of pediatric infections and should be limited to situations in which safe and effective oral therapy with other classes of antibiotics does not exist.

2. Choosing Among Antifungal Agents: Polyenes, Azoles, and Echinocandins

Separating antifungal agents by class, much like navigating the myriad of antibacterial agents, allows one to best understand the underlying mechanisms of action and then appropriately choose which agent would be optimal for empirical therapy or a targeted approach. There are certain helpful generalizations that should be considered; for example, echinocandins are fungicidal against yeasts and fungistatic against molds, while azoles are the opposite. Coupled with these concepts is the need for continued surveillance for fungal epidemiology and resistance patterns. While some fungal species are inherently or very often resistant to specific agents or even classes, there are also an increasing number of fungal isolates that are developing resistance due to environmental pressure or chronic use in individual patients. Additionally, new (often resistant) fungal species emerge that deserve special attention, such as *Candida auris,* which can be multidrug resistant. In 2020, there are 14 individual antifungal agents approved by the US Food and Drug Administration (FDA) for systemic use, and several more in development, including entirely new classes. This chapter will focus only on the most commonly used systemic agents and will not highlight the many anticipated new agents until they are approved for use in patients. For each agent, there are sometimes several formulations, each with unique pharmacokinetics that one must understand to optimize the agent, particularly in patients who are critically ill. Therefore, it is more important than ever to establish a firm foundation in understanding how these antifungal agents work to optimize pharmacokinetics and where they work best to target fungal pathogens most appropriately.

Polyenes

Amphotericin B (AmB) is a polyene antifungal antibiotic that has been available since 1958. A *Streptomyces* species, isolated from the soil in Venezuela, produced 2 antifungals whose names originated from the drug's amphoteric property of reacting as an acid as well as a base. Amphotericin A was not as active as AmB, so only AmB is used clinically. Nystatin is another polyene antifungal, but, due to systemic toxicity, it is only used in topical preparations. Nystatin was named after the New York State Department of Health, where the discoverers were working at the time. AmB remains the most broad-spectrum antifungal available for clinical use. This lipophilic drug binds to ergosterol, the major sterol in the fungal cell membrane, and for years it was thought to create transmembrane pores that compromise the integrity of the cell membrane and create a rapid fungicidal effect through osmotic lysis. However, new biochemical studies suggest a mechanism of action more related to inhibiting ergosterol synthesis. Toxicity is likely due to cross-reactivity with the human cholesterol bi-lipid membrane, which resembles fungal ergosterol. The toxicity of the conventional formulation, AmB deoxycholate (AmB-D)—the parent molecule coupled with an ionic detergent for clinical use—can be substantial from the standpoints of systemic reactions (fever, rigors) and acute and chronic renal toxicity. Premedication with acetaminophen, diphenhydramine, and meperidine has historically been used to prevent systemic reactions during infusion. Renal dysfunction manifests primarily as decreased glomerular filtration with a rising serum creatinine concentration, but substantial tubular nephropathy is associated with potassium and magnesium wasting, requiring supplemental potassium for many neonates and children, regardless of clinical symptoms associated with infusion. Fluid loading with saline pre- and post-AmB-D infusion seems to somewhat mitigate renal toxicity.

Three lipid preparations approved in the mid-1990s decrease toxicity with no apparent decrease in clinical efficacy. Decisions on which lipid AmB preparation to use should, therefore, largely focus on side effects and costs. Two clinically useful lipid formulations exist: one in which ribbonlike lipid complexes of AmB are created (amphotericin B lipid complex [ABLC]), Abelcet, and one in which AmB is incorporated into true liposomes (liposomal amphotericin B [L-AmB]), AmBisome. The classic clinical dosage used of these preparations is 5 mg/kg/day, in contrast to the 1 mg/kg/day of AmB-D. In most studies, the side effects of L-AmB were somewhat less than those of ABLC, but both have significantly fewer side effects than AmB-D. The advantage of the lipid preparations is the ability to safely deliver a greater overall dose of the parent AmB drug. The cost of conventional AmB-D is substantially less than either lipid formulation. A colloidal dispersion of AmB in cholesteryl sulfate, Amphotec, which is no longer available in the United States, with decreased nephrotoxicity but infusion-related side effects, is closer to AmB-D than to the lipid formulations and precludes recommendation for its use. The decreased nephrotoxicity of the 3 lipid preparations is thought to be due to the preferential binding of its AmB to high-density lipoproteins, compared with AmB-D binding to low-density lipoproteins. Despite in vitro concentration-dependent killing, a clinical trial comparing L-AmB at doses of 3 mg/kg/day versus 10 mg/kg/day found no efficacy benefit for the higher dose and only greater toxicity.[1] Recent pharmacokinetic analyses of L-AmB found that while children receiving L-AmB at lower doses exhibit linear pharmacokinetics, a significant proportion of children receiving L-AmB at daily doses greater than 5 mg/kg/day exhibit nonlinear pharmacokinetics with significantly higher peak concentrations and some toxicity.[2,3] Therefore, it is generally not recommended to use any lipid AmB preparations at very high dosages (>5 mg/kg/day), as it will likely only incur greater toxicity with no real therapeutic advantage. There are reports of using higher dosing in very difficult infections where a lipid AmB formulation is the first-line therapy (eg, mucormycosis), and while experts remain divided on this practice, it is clear that at least 5 mg/kg/day of a lipid AmB formulation should be used in such a setting. AmB has a long terminal half-life and, coupled with the concentration-dependent killing, the agent is best used as single daily doses. These pharmacokinetics explain the use in some studies of once-weekly, or even once every 2 weeks,[4] AmB for antifungal prophylaxis or preemptive therapy, albeit with mixed clinical results. If the overall AmB exposure needs to be decreased due to toxicity, it is best to increase the dosing interval (eg, 3 times weekly) but retain the full mg/kg dose for optimal pharmacokinetics.

AmB-D has been used for nonsystemic purposes, such as in bladder washes, intraventricular instillation, intrapleural instillation, and other modalities, but there are no firm data supporting those clinical indications, and it is likely that the local toxicities outweigh the theoretic benefits. One exception is aerosolized AmB for antifungal prophylaxis (not treatment) in lung transplant recipients due to the different pathophysiology of invasive aspergillosis (often originating at the bronchial anastomotic site, more so than parenchymal disease) in that specific patient population. This aerosolized prophylaxis approach, while indicated for lung transplant recipients, has not been shown to be effective in other patient populations. Due to the lipid chemistry, the L-AmB does not interact well with renal tubules and L-AmB is recovered from the urine at lower levels than AmB-D, so there is a theoretic concern with using a lipid formulation, as opposed to AmB-D, when treating isolated urinary fungal disease. This theoretic concern is likely outweighed by the real concern of toxicity with AmB-D. Most experts believe AmB-D should be reserved for use in resource-limited settings in which no alternative agents (eg, lipid formulations) are available. An exception is in neonates, where limited retrospective data suggest that the AmB-D formulation had better efficacy for invasive candidiasis.[5] Importantly, there are several pathogens that are inherently or functionally resistant to AmB, including *Candida lusitaniae, Trichosporon* spp, *Aspergillus terreus, Fusarium* spp, and *Pseudallescheria boydii* (*Scedosporium apiospermum*) or *Scedosporium prolificans*.

Azoles

This class of systemic agents was first approved in 1981 and is divided into imidazoles (ketoconazole), triazoles (fluconazole, itraconazole), and second-generation triazoles (voriconazole, posaconazole, and isavuconazole) based on the number of nitrogen atoms in the azole ring. All the azoles work by inhibition of ergosterol synthesis (fungal cytochrome P450 [CYP] sterol 14-demethylation) that is required for fungal cell membrane integrity. While the polyenes are rapidly fungicidal, the azoles are fungistatic against yeasts and fungicidal against molds. However, it is important to note that ketoconazole and fluconazole have no mold activity. The only systemic imidazole is ketoconazole, which is primarily active against *Candida* spp and is available in an oral formulation. Three azoles (itraconazole, voriconazole, posaconazole) need therapeutic drug monitoring with trough levels within the first 4 to 7 days (when patient is at pharmacokinetic steady state); it is unclear at present if isavuconazole will require drug-level monitoring. It is less clear if therapeutic drug monitoring is required during primary azole prophylaxis, although low levels have been associated with a higher probability of breakthrough infection.

Fluconazole is active against a broader range of fungi than ketoconazole and includes clinically relevant activity against *Cryptococcus, Coccidioides,* and *Histoplasma.* The pediatric treatment dose is 12 mg/kg/day, which targets exposures that are observed in critically ill adults who receive 800 mg of fluconazole per day. Like most other azoles, fluconazole requires a loading dose on the first day, and this approach is routinely used in adult patients. A loading dose of 25 mg/kg on the first day has been nicely studied in infants[6,7] but has not been definitively studied in all children; yet it is likely also beneficial and the patient will reach steady-state concentrations quicker based on adult and neonatal studies. The exception where it has been formally studied is children of all ages on extracorporeal membrane oxygenation, for whom, because of the higher volume of distribution, a higher loading dose (35 mg/kg) is required to achieve comparable exposure.[8,9] Fluconazole achieves relatively high concentrations in urine and cerebrospinal fluid (CSF) compared with AmB due to its low lipophilicity, with urinary concentrations often so high that treatment against even "resistant" pathogens that are isolated only in the urine is possible. Fluconazole remains one of the most active and, so far, one of the safest systemic antifungal agents for the treatment of most *Candida* infections. *Candida albicans* remains generally sensitive to fluconazole, although resistance is increasingly present in many non-*albicans Candida* spp as well as in *C albicans* in children repeatedly exposed to fluconazole. For instance, *Candida krusei* is considered inherently resistant to fluconazole, *Candida glabrata* demonstrates dose-dependent resistance to fluconazole (and usually voriconazole), *Candida tropicalis* is developing more resistant strains, and the newly identified *Candida auris* is generally fluconazole resistant. Fluconazole is available in parenteral and oral (with >90% bioavailability) formulations and toxicity is unusual and primarily hepatic.

Itraconazole is active against an even broader range of fungi and, unlike fluconazole, includes molds such as *Aspergillus*. It is currently available as a capsule or oral solution (the intravenous [IV] form was discontinued); the oral solution provides approximately 30% higher and more consistent serum concentrations than capsules and should be used preferentially. Absorption using itraconazole oral solution is improved on an empty stomach and not influenced by gastric pH (unlike the capsule form, which is best administered under fed conditions or with a more acidic cola beverage to increase absorption), and monitoring itraconazole serum concentrations, like most azole antifungals, is a key principal in management (generally, itraconazole serum trough levels should be 1–2 mcg/mL, >1 mcg/mL for treatment, and >0.5 mcg/mL for prophylaxis; trough levels >5 mcg/mL may be associated with increased toxicity). Concentrations should be checked after 5 days of therapy to ensure adequate drug exposure. When measured by high-pressure liquid chromatography, itraconazole and its bioactive hydroxy-itraconazole metabolite are reported, the sum of which should be considered in assessing drug levels. In adult patients, itraconazole is recommended to be loaded at 200 mg twice daily for 2 days, followed by 200 mg daily starting on the third day. Loading dose studies have not been performed in children. Dosing itraconazole in children requires twice-daily dosing throughout treatment, compared with once-daily maintenance dosing in adults, and the key to treatment success is following drug levels. Limited pharmacokinetic data are available in children; itraconazole has not been approved by the FDA for pediatric indications. Itraconazole is indicated in adults for therapy of mild/moderate disease with blastomycosis, histoplasmosis, and others. Although it possesses antifungal activity, itraconazole is not indicated as primary therapy against invasive aspergillosis, as voriconazole is a far superior option. Itraconazole is not active against *Zygomycetes* (eg, mucormycosis). Toxicity in adults is primarily hepatic.

Voriconazole was approved in 2002 and is FDA approved for children 2 years and older.[10] Voriconazole is a fluconazole derivative, so think of it as having the greater tissue and CSF penetration of fluconazole but the added antifungal spectrum like itraconazole to include molds. While the bioavailability of voriconazole in adults is approximately 96%, multiple studies have shown that it is only approximately 50% to 60% in children, requiring clinicians to carefully monitor voriconazole trough concentrations in patients taking the oral formulation, further complicated by great inter-patient variability in clearance. Voriconazole serum concentrations are tricky to interpret, but monitoring concentrations is essential to using this drug, like all azole antifungals, and especially important in circumstances of suspected treatment failure or possible toxicity. Most experts suggest voriconazole trough concentrations of 2 mcg/mL (at a minimum, 1 mcg/mL) or greater, which would generally exceed the pathogen's minimum inhibitory concentration, but, generally, toxicity will not be seen until concentrations of approximately 6 mcg/mL or greater. Trough levels should be monitored 2 to 5 days after initiation of therapy and repeated the following week to confirm the patient remains in the therapeutic range or repeated 4 days after change of dose. One important point is the acquisition of an accurate trough concentration, one obtained just before the next dose is due and not obtained through a catheter infusing the drug. These simple trough parameters will make interpretation possible. The fundamental voriconazole pharmacokinetics are different in adults versus children; in adults, voriconazole is metabolized in a nonlinear fashion, whereas in children, the drug is metabolized in a linear fashion. This explains the increased pediatric loading dosing for voriconazole at 9 mg/kg/dose versus loading with 6 mg/kg/dose in adult patients. Younger children, especially those younger than 3 years, require even higher dosages of voriconazole and also have a larger therapeutic window for dosing. However, many studies have shown an inconsistent relationship, on a population level, between dosing and levels, highlighting the need for close monitoring after the initial dosing scheme and then dose adjustment as needed in the individual patient. For children younger than 2 years, some have proposed 3-times–daily dosing to achieve sufficient serum levels.[11] Given the poor clinical and microbiological response of *Aspergillus* infections to AmB, voriconazole is now the treatment of choice for invasive aspergillosis and many other invasive mold infections (eg, pseudallescheriasis, fusariosis). Importantly, infections with *Zygomycetes* (eg, mucormycosis) are resistant to voriconazole. Voriconazole retains activity against most *Candida* spp, including some that are fluconazole resistant, but it is unlikely to replace fluconazole for treatment of fluconazole-susceptible *Candida* infections. Importantly, there are increasing reports of *C glabrata* resistance to voriconazole. Voriconazole produces some unique transient visual field abnormalities in about 10% of adults and children. There are an increasing number of reports, seen in as high as 20% of patients, of a photosensitive sunburn-like erythema that is not aided by sunscreen (only sun avoidance). In some rare long-term (mean of 3 years of therapy) cases, this voriconazole phototoxicity has developed into cutaneous squamous cell carcinoma. Discontinuing voriconazole is recommended in patients experiencing chronic phototoxicity. The rash is the most common indication for switching from voriconazole to posaconazole/isavuconazole if a triazole antifungal is required. Hepatotoxicity is uncommon, occurring only in 2% to 5% of patients. Voriconazole is CYP metabolized (CYP2C19), and allelic polymorphisms in the population could lead to personalized dosing.[12] Results have shown that some Asian patients will achieve higher toxic serum concentrations than other patients. Voriconazole also interacts with many similarly P450 metabolized drugs to produce some profound changes in serum concentrations of many concurrently administered drugs.

Posaconazole, an itraconazole derivative, was FDA approved in 2006 as an oral suspension for adolescents 13 years and older. An extended-release tablet formulation was approved in November 2013, also for adolescents 13 years and older, and an IV formulation was approved in March 2014 for patients 18 years and older. Effective absorption of the oral suspension strongly requires taking the medication with food, ideally a high-fat meal; taking posaconazole on an empty stomach will result in approximately one-fourth of the absorption as in the fed state. The tablet formulation has significantly better absorption due to its delayed release in the small intestine, but absorption will still be slightly increased with food. If the patient can take the (relatively large) tablets, the extended-release tablet is the much-preferred form due to the ability to easily obtain higher and more consistent drug levels. Due to the low pH (<5) of IV posaconazole, a central venous catheter is required for administration. The IV formulation contains only slightly lower amounts of the cyclodextrin vehicle than voriconazole, so similar theoretic renal accumulation concerns exist. The exact pediatric dosing for posaconazole has not been completely determined and requires consultation with a pediatric infectious diseases expert. The pediatric oral suspension dose recommended by some experts for treating invasive disease is estimated to be at least 18 mg/kg/day divided 3 times daily, but the true answer is likely higher and serum trough level monitoring is recommended. A study with a new pediatric formulation for suspension, essentially the tablet form that is able to be suspended, has recently been completed, and results are pending. Importantly, the current tablet cannot be broken for use due to its chemical coating. Pediatric dosing with the current IV or extended-release tablet dosing is completely unknown, but adolescents can likely follow the adult dosing schemes. In adult patients, IV posaconazole is loaded at 300 mg twice daily on the first day, and then 300 mg once daily starting on the second day. Similarly, in adult patients, the extended-release tablet is dosed as 300 mg twice daily on the first day, and then 300 mg once daily starting on the second day. In adult patients, the maximum amount of posaconazole oral suspension given is 800 mg per day due to its excretion, and that has been given as 400 mg twice daily or 200 mg 4 times a day in severely ill patients due to saturable absorption and findings of a marginal increase in exposure with more frequent dosing. Greater than 800 mg per day is not indicated in any patient. Like voriconazole and itraconazole, trough levels should be monitored, and most experts feel that posaconazole levels for treatment should be greater than or equal to 1 mcg/mL (and greater than 0.7 mcg/mL for prophylaxis). Monitor posaconazole trough levels on day 5 of therapy or soon after. The in vitro activity of posaconazole against *Candida* spp is better than that of fluconazole and similar to voriconazole. Overall in vitro antifungal activity against *Aspergillus* is also equivalent to voriconazole, but, notably, it is the first triazole with substantial activity against some *Zygomycetes,* including *Rhizopus* spp and *Mucor* spp, as well as activity against *Coccidioides, Histoplasma,* and *Blastomyces* and the pathogens of phaeohyphomycosis. Posaconazole treatment of invasive aspergillosis in patients with chronic granulomatous disease appears to be superior to voriconazole in this specific patient population for an unknown reason. Posaconazole is eliminated by hepatic glucuronidation but does demonstrate inhibition of the CYP3A4 enzyme system, leading to many drug interactions with other P450 metabolized drugs. It is currently approved for prophylaxis of *Candida* and *Aspergillus* infections in high-risk adults and for treatment of *Candida* oropharyngeal disease or esophagitis in adults. Posaconazole, like itraconazole, has generally poor CSF penetration.

Isavuconazole is a new triazole that was FDA approved in March 2015 for treatment of invasive aspergillosis and invasive mucormycosis with oral (capsules only) and IV formulations. Isavuconazole has a similar antifungal spectrum as voriconazole and some activity against *Zygomycetes* (yet, potentially, not as potent against *Zygomycetes* as posaconazole). A phase 3 clinical trial in adult patients demonstrated non-inferiority versus voriconazole against invasive aspergillosis and other mold infections,[13] and an open-label study showed activity against mucormycosis.[14] Isavuconazole is actually dispensed as the prodrug isavuconazonium sulfate. Dosing in adult patients is loading with isavuconazole 200 mg (equivalent to 372-mg isavuconazonium sulfate) every 8 hours for 2 days (6 doses), followed by 200 mg once daily for maintenance dosing. The half-life is long (>5 days), there is 98% bioavailability in adults, and there is no reported food effect with oral isavuconazole. The manufacturer suggests no need for therapeutic drug monitoring, but some experts suggest trough levels may be needed in difficult-to-treat infections and, absent well-defined therapeutic targets, the mean concentrations from phase II/III studies suggest a range of 2 to 3 mcg/mL after day 5 is adequate exposure. The IV formulation does not contain the vehicle cyclodextrin, unlike voriconazole, which could make it more attractive in patients with renal failure. Early experience suggests a much lower rate of photosensitivity and skin disorders as well as visual disturbances compared with voriconazole. No specific pediatric dosing data exist for isavuconazole yet, but pharmacokinetic studies have recently completed and efficacy studies are underway.

Echinocandins

This class of systemic antifungal agents was first approved in 2001. The echinocandins inhibit cell wall formation (in contrast to acting on the cell membrane by the polyenes and azoles) by noncompetitively inhibiting beta-1,3-glucan synthase, an enzyme present in fungi but absent in mammalian cells. These agents are generally very safe, as there is no beta-1,3-glucan in humans. The echinocandins are not metabolized through the CYP system, so fewer drug interactions are problematic, compared with the azoles. There is no need to dose-adjust in renal failure, but one needs a lower dosage in the setting of very severe hepatic dysfunction. As a class, these antifungals generally have poor CSF penetration, although animal studies have shown adequate brain parenchyma levels, and do not penetrate the urine well. While the 3 clinically available echinocandins each individually have some unique and important dosing and pharmacokinetic parameters, especially in children, efficacy is generally equivalent. Opposite the azole class, the echinocandins are fungicidal against yeasts but fungistatic against molds. The fungicidal activity against yeasts has elevated the echinocandins to the preferred therapy against invasive candidiasis. Echinocandins are thought to be best utilized against invasive aspergillosis only as salvage therapy if a triazole fails or in a patient with suspected triazole resistance, but never as primary monotherapy against invasive aspergillosis or any other invasive mold infection. Improved efficacy with combination therapy with the echinocandins and triazoles against *Aspergillus* infections is unclear, with disparate results in multiple smaller studies and a definitive clinical trial demonstrating minimal benefit over voriconazole monotherapy in only certain patient populations. Some experts have used combination therapy in invasive aspergillosis with a triazole plus echinocandin only during the initial phase of waiting for triazole drug levels to be appropriately high. There are reports of echinocandin resistance in *Candida* spp, as high as 12% in *C glabrata* in some studies, and the echinocandins as a class have previously been shown to be somewhat less active against *Candida parapsilosis* isolates (approximately 10%–15% respond poorly, but most are still susceptible, and guidelines still recommend echinocandin empiric therapy for invasive candidiasis). There is no therapeutic drug monitoring required for the echinocandins.

Caspofungin received FDA approval for children aged 3 months to 17 years in 2008 for empiric therapy of presumed fungal infections in febrile, neutropenic children; treatment of candidemia as well as *Candida* esophagitis, peritonitis, and empyema; and salvage therapy of invasive aspergillosis. Due to its earlier approval, there are generally more reports with caspofungin than the other echinocandins. Caspofungin dosing in children is calculated according to body surface area, with a loading dose on the first day of 70 mg/m^2, followed by daily maintenance dosing of 50 mg/m^2, and not to exceed 70 mg regardless of the calculated dose. Significantly higher doses of caspofungin have been studied in adult patients without any clear added benefit in efficacy, but if the 50 mg/m^2 dose is tolerated and does not provide adequate clinical response, the daily dose can be increased to 70 mg/m^2. Dosing for caspofungin in neonates is 25 mg/m^2/day.

Micafungin was approved in adults in 2005 for treatment of candidemia, *Candida* esophagitis and peritonitis, and prophylaxis of *Candida* infections in stem cell transplant recipients, and in 2013 for pediatric patients aged 4 months and older. Micafungin has the most pediatric and neonatal data available of all 3 echinocandins, including more extensive pharmacokinetic studies surrounding dosing and several efficacy studies.[15–17] Micafungin dosing in children is age dependent, as clearance increases dramatically in the younger age groups (especially neonates), necessitating higher doses for younger children. Doses in children are generally thought to be 2 mg/kg/day, with higher doses likely needed for younger patients, and preterm neonates dosed at 10 mg/kg/day. Adult micafungin dosing (100 or 150 mg once daily) is to be used in patients who weigh more than 40 kg. Unlike the other echinocandins, a loading dose is not required for micafungin.

Anidulafungin was approved for adults for candidemia and *Candida* esophagitis in 2006 and is not officially approved for pediatric patients. Like the other echinocandins, anidulafungin is not P450 metabolized and has not demonstrated significant drug interactions. Limited pediatric pharmacokinetic data suggest weight-based dosing

(3 mg/kg/day loading dose, followed by 1.5 mg/kg/day maintenance dosing).[18] This dosing achieves similar exposure levels in neonates and infants.[18] The adult dose for invasive candidiasis is a loading dose of 200 mg on the first day, followed by 100 mg daily. An open-label study of pediatric invasive candidiasis in children showed similar efficacy and minimal toxicity, comparable to the other echinocandins.[19]

3. How Antibiotic Dosages Are Determined Using Susceptibility Data, Pharmacodynamics, and Treatment Outcomes

Factors Involved in Dosing Recommendations

Our view of the optimal use of antimicrobials is continually changing. As the published literature and our experience with each drug increases, our recommendations for specific dosages evolve as we compare the efficacy, safety, and cost of each drug in the context of current and previous data from adults and children. Virtually every new antibiotic that treats infections that occur in both adults and children must demonstrate some degree of efficacy and safety in adults with antibiotic exposures that occur at specific dosages, which we duplicate in children as closely as possible. We keep track of reported toxicities and unanticipated clinical failures and on occasion may end up modifying our initial recommendations for an antibiotic.

Important considerations in any recommendations we make include (1) the susceptibilities of pathogens to antibiotics, which are constantly changing, are different from region to region, and are often hospital- and unit-specific; (2) the antibiotic concentrations achieved at the site of infection over a 24-hour dosing interval; (3) the mechanism of how antibiotics kill bacteria; (4) how often the dose we select produces a clinical and microbiological cure; (5) how often we encounter toxicity; (6) how likely the antibiotic exposure will lead to antibiotic resistance in the treated child and in the population in general; and (7) the effect on the child's microbiome.

Susceptibility

Susceptibility data for each bacterial pathogen against a wide range of antibiotics are available from the microbiology laboratory of virtually every hospital. This antibiogram can help guide you in antibiotic selection for empiric therapy while you wait for specific susceptibilities to come back from your cultures. Many hospitals can separate the inpatient culture results from outpatient results, and many can give you the data by hospital ward (eg, pediatric ward vs neonatal intensive care unit vs adult intensive care unit). Susceptibility data are also available by region and by country from reference laboratories or public health laboratories. The recommendations made in *Nelson's Pediatric Antimicrobial Therapy* reflect overall susceptibility patterns present in the United States. Tables A and B in Chapter 7 provide some overall guidance on susceptibility of gram-positive and gram-negative pathogens, respectively. Wide variations may exist for certain pathogens in different regions of the United States and the world. New techniques for rapid molecular diagnosis of a bacterial, mycobacterial, fungal, or viral pathogen based on polymerase chain reaction or next-generation sequencing may quickly give you the name of the pathogen, but with current molecular technology, susceptibility data are usually not available.

Drug Concentrations at the Site of Infection

With every antibiotic, we can measure the concentration of antibiotic present in the serum. We can also directly measure the concentrations in specific tissue sites, such as spinal fluid or middle ear fluid. Because "free," nonprotein-bound antibiotic is required to inhibit and kill pathogens, it is also important to calculate the amount of free drug available at the site of infection. While traditional methods of measuring antibiotics focused on the peak concentrations in serum and how rapidly the drugs were excreted, complex models of drug distribution in plasma and tissue sites (eg, cerebrospinal fluid, urine, peritoneal fluid) and elimination from plasma and tissue compartments now exist. Antibiotic exposure to pathogens at the site of infection can be described mathematically in many ways: (1) the percentage of time in a 24-hour dosing interval that the antibiotic concentrations are above the minimum inhibitory concentration (MIC; the antibiotic concentration required for inhibition of growth of an organism) at the site of infection (%T>MIC); (2) the mathematically calculated area below the serum concentration-versus-time curve (area under the curve [AUC]); and (3) the maximal concentration of drug achieved at the tissue site (Cmax). For each of these 3 values, a ratio of that value to the MIC of the pathogen in question can be calculated and provides more useful information on specific drug activity against a specific pathogen, rather than simply looking at the MIC. It allows us to compare the exposure of different antibiotics (that achieve quite different concentrations in tissues) to a pathogen (where the MIC for each drug may be different) and to assess the activity of a single antibiotic that may be used for empiric therapy against the many different pathogens (potentially with many different MICs) that may be causing an infection at that tissue site.

Pharmacodynamics

Pharmacodynamic (PD) descriptions provide the clinician with information on *how* the bacterial pathogens are killed (see Suggested Reading). Beta-lactam antibiotics tend to eradicate bacteria following prolonged exposure of relatively low concentrations of the antibiotic to the pathogen at the site of infection, usually expressed as the percent of time over a dosing interval that the antibiotic is present at the site of infection in concentrations greater than the MIC (%T>MIC). For example, amoxicillin needs to be present at the site of pneumococcal infection (such as the middle ear) at a concentration above the MIC for only 40% of a 24-hour dosing interval. Remarkably, neither higher concentrations of amoxicillin nor a more prolonged exposure will substantially increase the cure rate. On the other hand, gentamicin's activity against *Escherichia coli* is based primarily on the absolute concentration of free antibiotic at the site of infection, in the context of the MIC of the pathogen (Cmax:MIC). The more antibiotic you can deliver to the site of infection, the more rapidly you can sterilize the tissue; we are only limited by the toxicities of gentamicin. For fluoroquinolones like ciprofloxacin, the antibiotic exposure best linked to clinical and microbiologic success is, like aminoglycosides, concentration-dependent. However, the best mathematical correlate to microbiologic (and clinical) outcomes for fluoroquinolones is the AUC:MIC, rather than Cmax:MIC. All 3 PD metrics of antibiotic exposure should be linked to the MIC of the pathogen to best understand how well the antibiotic will eradicate the pathogen causing the infection.

Assessment of Clinical and Microbiological Outcomes

In clinical trials of anti-infective agents, most adults and children will hopefully be cured, but a few will fail therapy. For those few, we may note unanticipated inadequate drug exposure (eg, more rapid drug elimination in a particular patient; the inability of a particular antibiotic to penetrate to the site of infection in its active form, not bound to salts or proteins) or infection caused by a pathogen with a particularly high MIC. By analyzing the successes and the failures based on the appropriate exposure parameters outlined previously (%T>MIC, AUC:MIC, or Cmax:MIC), we can often observe a particular value of exposure, above which we observe a higher rate of cure and below which the cure rate drops quickly. Knowing this target value in adults (the "antibiotic exposure break point") allows us to calculate the dosage that will create treatment success in most children. We do not evaluate antibiotics in children with study designs that have failure rates sufficient to calculate a pediatric exposure break point. It is the adult *exposure value* that leads to success that we all (including the US Food and Drug Administration [FDA] and pharmaceutical companies) subsequently share with you, a pediatric health care practitioner, as one likely to cure your patient. US FDA-approved break points that are reported by microbiology laboratories (S, I, and R) are now determined by outcomes linked to drug pharmacokinetics and exposure, the MIC, and the PD parameter for that agent. Recommendations to the FDA for break points for the United States often come from "break point organizations," such as the US Committee on Antimicrobial Susceptibility Testing (www.uscast.org) or the Clinical and Laboratory Standards Institute Subcommittee on Antimicrobial Susceptibility Testing (https://clsi.org).

Suggested Reading

Bradley JS, et al. *Pediatr Infect Dis J.* 2010;29(11):1043–1046 PMID: 20975453

Onufrak NJ, et al. *Clin Ther.* 2016;38(9):1930–1947 PMID: 27449411

Sy SK, et al. *Expert Opin Drug Metab Toxicol.* 2016;12(1):93–114 PMID: 26652832

4. Approach to Antibiotic Therapy of Drug-Resistant Gram-negative Bacilli and Methicillin-Resistant *Staphylococcus aureus*

Multidrug-Resistant Gram-negative Bacilli

Increasing antibiotic resistance in gram-negative bacilli, primarily the enteric bacilli, *Pseudomonas aeruginosa* and *Acinetobacter* spp, has caused profound difficulties in management of patients around the world; some of the pathogens are now resistant to all available agents. At this time, a limited number of pediatric tertiary care centers in North America have reported outbreaks, but sustained transmission of completely resistant organisms has not yet been reported in children, likely due to the critical infection control strategies in place to prevent spread within pediatric health care institutions. However, for complicated hospitalized neonates, infants, and children, multiple treatment courses of antibiotics for documented or suspected infections can create substantial resistance to many classes of agents, particularly in *P aeruginosa.* These pathogens have the genetic capability to express resistance to virtually any antibiotic used, as a result of more than one hundred million years of exposure to antibiotics elaborated by other organisms in their environment. Inducible enzymes to cleave antibiotics and modify binding sites, efflux pumps, and gram-negative cell wall alterations to prevent antibiotic penetration (and combinations of mechanisms) all may be present. Some mechanisms of resistance, if not intrinsic, can be acquired from other bacilli. By using antibiotics, we "awaken" resistance; therefore, only using antibiotics when appropriate limits the selection, or induction, of resistance for both that child and for all children. Community prevalence, as well as health care institution prevalence of resistant organisms, such as extended-spectrum beta-lactamase (ESBL)-containing *Escherichia coli,* is increasing.

In Figure 4-1, we assume that the clinician has the antibiotic susceptibility report in hand (or at least a local antibiogram). Each tier provides increasingly broader spectrum activity, from the narrowest of the gram-negative agents to the broadest (and most toxic), colistin. Tier 1 is ampicillin, safe and widely available but not active against *Klebsiella, Enterobacter,* or *Pseudomonas* and only active against about half of *E coli* in the community setting. Tier 2 contains antibiotics that have a broader spectrum but are also very safe and effective (trimethoprim/sulfamethoxazole [TMP/SMX] and cephalosporins), with decades of experience. In general, use an antibiotic from tier 2 before going to broader spectrum agents. Please be aware that many enteric bacilli (the SPICE bacteria, *Enterobacter, Citrobacter, Serratia,* and indole-positive *Proteus*) have inducible beta-lactam resistance (active against third-generation cephalosporins cefotaxime, ceftriaxone, and ceftazidime, as well as the fifth-generation cephalosporin ceftaroline), which may manifest only after exposure of the pathogen to the antibiotic. Tier 3 is made up of very broad-spectrum antibiotics (carbapenems, piperacillin/tazobactam) and aminoglycosides (with significantly more toxicity than beta-lactam antibacterial agents, although we have used them safely for decades). Use any antibiotic from tier 3 before going to broader spectrum agents. Tier 4 is fluoroquinolones, to be used only when lower-tier antibiotics cannot be used due to potential (and not yet verified in children) toxicities. Tier 5 is represented by a new

Figure 4-1. Enteric Bacilli: Bacilli and *Pseudomonas* With Known Susceptibilities (See Text for Interpretation)

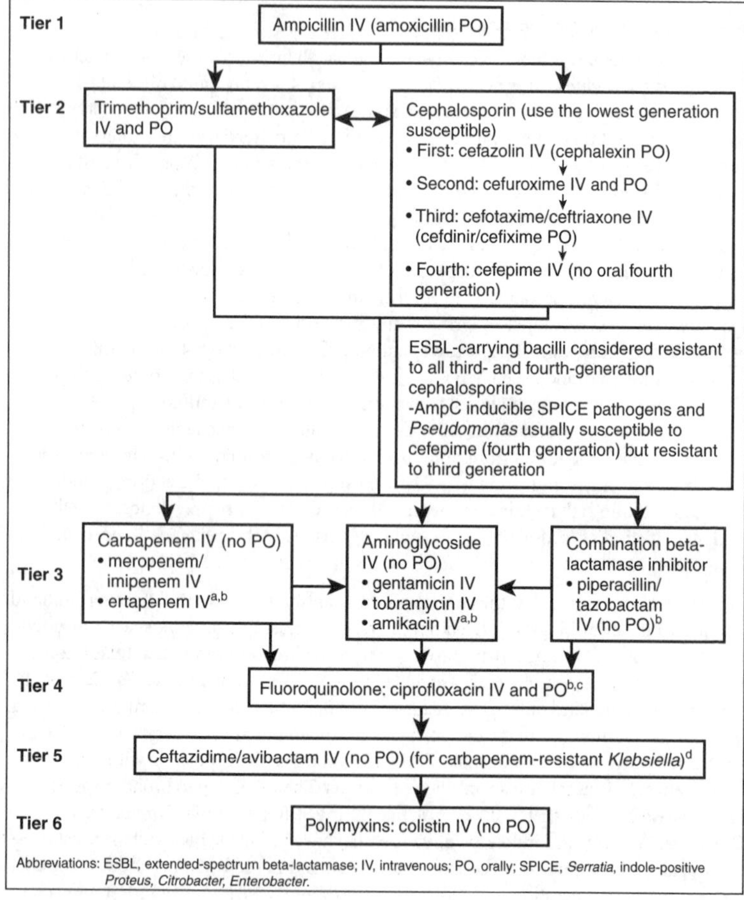

[a] Ertapenem is the only carbapenem *not* active against *Pseudomonas*. Ertapenem and amikacin can be given once daily as outpatient IV/intramuscular (IM) therapy for infections where these drugs achieve therapeutic concentrations (eg, urinary tract). Some use once-daily gentamicin or tobramycin.

[b] For mild to moderate ESBL infections caused by organisms susceptible only to IV/IM beta-lactam or aminoglycoside therapy but also susceptible to fluoroquinolones, oral fluoroquinolone therapy is preferred over IV/IM therapy for infections amenable to treatment by oral therapy.

[c] If you have susceptibility to only a few remaining agents, consider combination therapy to prevent the emergence of resistance to your last-resort antibiotics (no prospective, controlled data in these situations).

[d] Active against carbapenem-resistant *Klebsiella pneumoniae* strains; US Food and Drug Administration approved for adults and children.

set of beta-lactam/beta-lactamase inhibitor combinations, represented by ceftazidime/avibactam, that demonstrate activity against ESBL-producing enteric bacilli and against the *Klebsiella pneumoniae* serine carbapenemase (KPC) but not metallo-carbapenemases (NDM). Tier 6 is colistin, one of the broadest-spectrum agents available. Colistin was US Food and Drug Administration (FDA) approved in 1962 with significant toxicity and limited clinical experience in children. Many newer drugs for multidrug-resistant gram-negative organisms are currently investigational for adults and children.

Investigational Agents Recently Approved for Adults That Are Being Studied in Children

Ceftolozane and tazobactam. Ceftolozane represents a more active cephalosporin agent against *Pseudomonas aeruginosa,* paired with tazobactam allowing for activity again ESBL-producing enteric bacilli.

Meropenem and vaborbactam. Meropenem, a familiar broad-spectrum aerobic/anaerobic coverage carbapenem that is already stable to ESBL beta-lactamases, is now paired with vaborbactam allowing for activity against the KPC but not metallo-carbapenemases.

Plazomicin. A new aminoglycoside antibiotic that is active against many of the gentamicin-, tobramycin-, and amikacin-resistant enteric bacilli and *Pseudomonas.*

Community-Associated Methicillin-Resistant *Staphylococcus aureus*

Community-associated methicillin-resistant *Staphylococcus aureus* (CA-MRSA) is a community pathogen for children (that can also spread from child to child in hospitals) that first appeared in the United States in the mid-1990s and currently represents 30% to 80% of all community isolates in various regions of the United States (check your hospital microbiology laboratory for your local rate); it is present in many areas of the world, with some strain variation documented. Notably, we have begun to see a decrease in invasive MRSA infections in some institutions, as documented in Houston, TX, by Hultén and Mason.[1] CA-MRSA is resistant to beta-lactam antibiotics, with the notable exception of ceftaroline, a fifth-generation cephalosporin antibiotic FDA approved for pediatrics in June 2016 (see Chapter 1).

There are an undetermined number of pathogenicity factors that make CA-MRSA more aggressive than methicillin-susceptible *S aureus* (MSSA) strains. CA-MRSA seems to cause greater tissue necrosis, an increased host inflammatory response, an increased rate of complications, and an increased rate of recurrent infections compared with MSSA. Response to therapy with non–beta-lactam antibiotics (eg, vancomycin, clindamycin) seems to be inferior compared with the response of MSSA to oxacillin/nafcillin or cefazolin, but it is unknown whether poorer outcomes are due to a hardier, better-adapted, more aggressive strain of *S aureus*, or whether these alternative agents are just not as effective against MRSA as beta-lactam agents are against MSSA. Studies in children using ceftaroline to treat skin infections (many caused by MRSA) were conducted using a non-inferiority clinical trial design, compared with vancomycin, with the finding that ceftaroline was equivalent to vancomycin. Guidelines for management of MRSA infections (2011) and management of skin and soft tissue infections (2014) have been published by the Infectious Diseases Society of America[2] and are available at www.idsociety.org, as well as in *Red Book: 2018–2021 Report of the Committee on Infectious Diseases.*

Antimicrobials for CA-MRSA

Vancomycin (intravenous [IV]) has been the mainstay of parenteral therapy of MRSA infections for the past 4 decades and continues to have activity against more than 98% of strains isolated from children. A few cases of intermediate resistance and "hetero-resistance" (transient moderately increased resistance likely to be based on thickened staphylococcal cell walls) have been reported, most commonly in adults who are receiving long-term therapy or who have received multiple exposures to vancomycin. Unfortunately, the response to therapy using standard vancomycin dosing of 40 mg/kg/day in the treatment of many CA-MRSA strains has not been as predictably successful as in the past with MSSA. For vancomycin efficacy, the ratio of the area under the serum concentration curve to minimum inhibitory concentration (AUC:MIC) appears to be the best exposure metric to predict a successful outcome. Better outcomes are likely to be achieved with an AUC:MIC of about 400 or greater, rather than trying to achieve a serum trough value in the range of 15 to 20 mcg/mL (see Chapter 3 for more on the AUC:MIC), which is associated with greater renal toxicity. This ratio of 400:1 is achievable for CA-MRSA strains with in vitro MIC values of 1 mcg/mL or less but difficult to achieve for strains with 2 mcg/mL or greater.[3] Recent data suggest that vancomycin MICs may actually be decreasing in children for MRSA, causing bloodstream infections as they increase for MSSA.[4] Strains with MIC values of 4 mcg/mL or greater should be considered resistant to vancomycin. When using these higher "meningitis" treatment dosages of 60 mg/kg/day or higher to achieve a 400:1 vancomycin exposure, one needs to follow renal function carefully for the development of toxicity and subsequent possible need to switch classes of antibiotics.

Clindamycin (oral [PO] or IV) is active against approximately 70% to 90% of strains of either MRSA or MSSA, with great geographic variability (again, check with your hospital laboratory).[5] The dosage for moderate to severe infections is 30 to 40 mg/kg/day, in 3 divided doses, using the same mg/kg dose PO or IV. Clindamycin is not as bactericidal as vancomycin but achieves higher concentrations in abscesses (based on high intracellular concentrations in neutrophils). Some CA-MRSA strains are susceptible to clindamycin on testing but have inducible clindamycin resistance (methylase-mediated) that is usually assessed by the "D-test" and now can be assessed in multi-well microtiter plates. Within each population of CA-MRSA organisms, a rare organism (between 1 in 10^9 and 10^{11} organisms) will have a mutation that allows for constant (rather than induced) resistance.[6] Although still somewhat controversial, clindamycin should be effective therapy for infections that have a relatively low organism load (cellulitis, small or drained abscesses) and are unlikely to contain a significant population of these constitutive methylase-producing mutants that are truly resistant (in contrast to the strains that are not already producing methylase; in fact, methylase is poorly induced by clindamycin). Infections with a high organism load (empyema) may have a greater risk of failure (as a large population is more likely to have a significant number of truly resistant organisms), and clindamycin should not be used as the preferred agent for these infections. Many laboratories no longer report D-test results but simply call the organism "resistant," prompting the use of alternative therapy that may not be needed.

Clindamycin is used to treat most CA-MRSA infections that are not life-threatening, and, if the child responds, therapy can be switched from IV to PO (although the oral solution is not very well tolerated). *Clostridium difficile* enterocolitis is a concern; however, despite a great increase in the use of clindamycin in children during the past decade, recent published data do not document a clinically significant increase in the rate of this complication in children.

Trimethoprim/sulfamethoxazole (TMP/SMX) (PO, IV), Bactrim/Septra, is active against CA-MRSA in vitro. Prospective comparative data on treatment of skin or skin structure infections in adults and children document efficacy equivalent to clindamycin.[7] Given our current lack of prospective, comparative information in MRSA bacteremia, pneumonia, and osteomyelitis (in contrast to skin infections), TMP/SMX should not be used routinely to treat these more serious infections at this time.

Linezolid (PO, IV), active against virtually 100% of CA-MRSA strains, is another reasonable alternative but is considered bacteriostatic and has relatively frequent hematologic toxicity in adults (neutropenia, thrombocytopenia) and some infrequent neurologic toxicity (peripheral neuropathy, optic neuritis), particularly when used for courses of 2 weeks or longer (a complete blood cell count should be checked every week or 2 in children receiving prolonged linezolid therapy). The cost of generic linezolid is still substantially more than clindamycin or vancomycin.

Daptomycin (IV), FDA approved for adults for skin infections in 2003 and, subsequently, for bacteremia/endocarditis, was approved for use for children with skin infections in April 2017. It is a unique class of antibiotic, a lipopeptide, and is highly bactericidal. Daptomycin became generic in 2017 and should be considered for treatment of skin infection and bacteremia in failures with other, better studied antibiotics. **Daptomycin should not be used to treat pneumonia,** as it is inactivated by pulmonary surfactant. Pediatric studies for skin infections and bacteremia have been completed and published,[8,9] and those for osteomyelitis have concluded but have not been presented. Some newborn animal neurologic toxicity data suggest additional **caution for the use of daptomycin in infants younger than 1 year,** prompting a warning in the package label. Routine pediatric clinical trial investigations in young infants were not pursued due to these concerns.

Tigecycline and fluoroquinolones, both of which may show in vitro activity, are not generally recommended for children if other agents are available and are tolerated due to potential toxicity issues for children with tetracyclines and fluoroquinolones and rapid emergence of resistance with fluoroquinolones (with the exception of delafloxacin, which is only investigated and approved in adults at this time).

Ceftaroline, a fifth-generation cephalosporin antibiotic, the first FDA-approved beta-lactam antibiotic to be active against MRSA, was approved for children in June 2016. The gram-negative coverage is similar to cefotaxime, with no activity against *Pseudomonas*.

Published data are available for pediatric pharmacokinetics, as well as for prospective, randomized comparative treatment trials of skin and skin structure infections[10] and community-acquired pneumonia.[11,12] The efficacy and toxicity profile in adults is what one would expect from most cephalosporins. Based on these published data and review by the FDA, for infants and children 2 months and older, ceftaroline should be effective and safer than vancomycin for treatment of MRSA infections. Just as beta-lactams are preferred over vancomycin for MSSA infections, ceftaroline is now considered by the editors to be the preferred treatment for MRSA infections over vancomycin, with the exception of central nervous system infections/endocarditis only due to lack of clinical data for these infections. Neither renal function nor drug levels need to be followed with ceftaroline therapy. Since pediatric approval in mid-2016, there have been no reported post-marketing adverse experiences in children; recommendations may change if unexpected clinical data on lack of efficacy or unexpected toxicity (beyond what may be expected with beta-lactams) should be presented.

Combination therapy for serious infections, with vancomycin and rifampin (for deep abscesses) or vancomycin and gentamicin (for bacteremia), is often used, but no prospective, controlled human clinical data exist on improved efficacy over single antibiotic therapy. Some experts use vancomycin and clindamycin in combination, particularly for children with a toxic-shock clinical presentation. Ceftaroline has also been used in combination therapy with other agents in adults, but no prospective, controlled clinical data exist to assess benefits.

Investigational Gram-positive Agents Recently Approved for Adults That Are Being Studied in Children

Dalbavancin and Oritavancin. Both antibiotics are IV glycopeptides, structurally very similar to vancomycin but with enhanced in vitro activity against MRSA and a much longer serum half-life, allowing once-weekly dosing or even just a single dose to treat skin infections.

Telavancin. A glycolipopeptide with mechanisms of activity that include cell wall inhibition and cell membrane depolarization, telavancin is administered once daily.

Tedizolid. A second-generation oxazolidinone like linezolid, tedizolid is more potent in vitro against MRSA than linezolid, with somewhat decreased toxicity to bone marrow in adult clinical studies.

Recommendations for Empiric Therapy of Suspected MRSA Infections

Life-threatening and Serious Infections. If any CA-MRSA is present in your community, empiric therapy for presumed staphylococcal infections that are life-threatening or infections for which any risk of failure is unacceptable should follow the recommendations for CA-MRSA and include ceftaroline OR *high-dose* vancomycin, clindamycin, or linezolid, *in addition to nafcillin or oxacillin* (beta-lactam antibiotics are considered better than vancomycin or clindamycin for MSSA).

Moderate Infections. If you live in a location with greater than 10% methicillin resistance, consider using the CA-MRSA recommendations for hospitalized children with presumed staphylococcal infections of any severity, and start empiric therapy with clindamycin (usually active against >80% of CA-MRSA), ceftaroline, vancomycin, or linezolid IV.

In skin and skin structure abscess treatment, antibiotics may not be necessary following incision and drainage, which may be curative.

Mild Infections. For nonserious, presumed staphylococcal infections in regions with significant CA-MRSA, empiric topical therapy with mupirocin (Bactroban) or retapamulin (Altabax) ointment, or oral therapy with TMP/SMX or clindamycin, is preferred. For older children, doxycycline and minocycline are also options based on data in adults.

Prevention of Recurrent Infections

For children with problematic, recurrent infections, no well-studied, prospectively collected data provide a solution. Bleach baths (one-half cup of bleach in a full bathtub)[13] seems to be able to transiently decrease the numbers of colonizing organisms but was not shown to decrease the number of infections in a prospective, controlled study in children with eczema. Similarly, a regimen to decolonize with twice-weekly bleach baths in an attempt to prevent recurrent infection did not lead to a statistically significant decrease.[14,15] Bathing with chlorhexidine (Hibiclens, a preoperative antibacterial skin disinfectant) daily or 2 to 3 times each week should provide topical anti-MRSA activity for several hours following a bath. Treating the entire family with decolonization regimens will provide an additional decrease in risk of recurrence for the index child.[16] Nasal mupirocin ointment (Bactroban) designed to eradicate colonization may also be used. All these measures have advantages and disadvantages and need to be used together with environmental measures (eg, washing towels frequently, using hand sanitizers, not sharing items of clothing). Helpful advice can be found on the Centers for Disease Control and Prevention website at www.cdc.gov/mrsa (accessed September 26, 2019).

Vaccines are being investigated but are not likely to be available for several years.

5. Antimicrobial Therapy for Newborns

NOTES

- Prospectively collected data in newborns continue to become available, thanks in large part to federal legislation (including the US Food and Drug Administration [FDA] Safety and Innovation Act of 2012 that mandates neonatal studies). In situations of inadequate data, suggested doses are based on efficacy, safety, and pharmacological data from older children or adults. These may not account for the effect of developmental changes (effect of ontogeny) on drug metabolism that occur during early infancy and among preterm and full-term newborns.[1] These values may vary widely, particularly for the unstable preterm newborn. Oral convalescent therapy for neonatal infections has not been well studied but may be used cautiously in non–life-threatening infections in adherent families with ready access to medical care.[2]
- The recommended antibiotic dosages and intervals of administration are given in the tables in this chapter.
- **Substitution for cefotaxime in neonates and very young infants:** As of 2019, US pharmaceutical companies no longer supply this antibiotic. We have removed cefotaxime for recommendations in this 2020 edition *only* because we know that some hospitals will no longer have cefotaxime available, although we understand that some hospitals are still able to procure cefotaxime. For those who do not have cefotaxime, we are recommending the following other agents for neonates and infants requiring extended spectrum cephalosporins:

  Cefepime has been available for 23 years, with many pediatric studies published, including those in neonates. The original manufacturer did not seek approval from the FDA for neonates and infants younger than 2 months, so the FDA has not evaluated data or approved cefepime for neonates. Doses are provided in Table 5B in this chapter.

  Ceftriaxone is FDA approved for neonates with the following qualifications:

  1) *Neonates with hyperbilirubinemia should not be treated with ceftriaxone,* particularly those who are unstable or acidotic, and particularly preterm neonates and infants up to a postmenstrual age of 41 weeks (gestational + chronologic age). Term neonates and infants with total bilirubin concentrations less than 10 and falling (usually older than 1 week) may be considered for treatment, but no prospective data exist to support this bilirubin cutoff.

  2) Ceftriaxone is *contraindicated in neonates younger than 28 days if they require treatment with calcium-containing intravenous (IV) solutions.*

- **Adverse drug reaction:** Neonates should not receive IV ceftriaxone while receiving IV calcium-containing products, including parenteral nutrition, by the same or different infusion lines, as fatal reactions with ceftriaxone-calcium precipitates in lungs and kidneys in neonates have occurred. There are no data on interactions between IV ceftriaxone and oral calcium-containing products or between intramuscular ceftriaxone and IV or oral calcium-containing products.[3] Ceftazidime, cefepime, or other cephalosporins with similar microbiologic activity are preferred over ceftriaxone for neonates.[4]

- **Abbreviations:** 3TC, lamivudine; ABLC, lipid complex amphotericin; ABR, auditory brainstem response; ALT, alanine transaminase; AmB, amphotericin B; AmB-D, AmB deoxycholate; amox/clav, amoxicillin/clavulanate; AOM, acute otitis media; AUC, area under the curve; bid, twice daily; CBC, complete blood cell count; CDC, Centers for Disease Control and Prevention; CLD, chronic lung disease; CMV, cytomegalovirus; CNS, central nervous system; CSF, cerebrospinal fluid; CT, computed tomography; div, divided; ECMO, extracorporeal membrane oxygenation; ESBL, extended spectrum beta-lactamase; FDA, US Food and Drug Administration; GA, gestational age; GBS, group B streptococcus; G-CSF, granulocyte colony stimulating factor; GNR, gram-negative rods (bacilli); HIV, human immunodeficiency virus; HSV, herpes simplex virus; IAI, intra-abdominal infection; ID, infectious diseases; IM, intramuscular; IUGR, intrauterine growth restriction; IV, intravenous; IVIG, intravenous immune globulin; L-AmB, liposomal AmB; MIC, minimal inhibitory concentration; MRSA, methicillin-resistant *Staphylococcus aureus;* MSSA, methicillin-susceptible *S aureus;* NEC, necrotizing enterocolitis; NICU, neonatal intensive care unit; NVP, nevirapine; PCR, polymerase chain reaction; pip/tazo, piperacillin/tazobactam; PMA, post-menstrual age; PNA, postnatal age; PO, orally; RAL, raltegravir; RSV, respiratory syncytial virus; SCr, serum creatinine; spp, species; tab, tablet; tid, 3 times daily; TIG, tetanus immune globulin; TMP/SMX, trimethoprim/sulfamethoxazole; UCSF, University of California, San Francisco; UTI, urinary tract infection; VCUG, voiding cystourethrogram; VDRL, Venereal Disease Research Laboratories; ZDV, zidovudine.

A. RECOMMENDED THERAPY FOR SELECTED NEWBORN CONDITIONS

Condition	**Therapy (evidence grade)** *See Tables 5B–D for neonatal dosages.*	Comments
Conjunctivitis		
– Chlamydial[5–8]	Azithromycin 10 mg/kg/day PO for 1 day, then 5 mg/kg/day PO for 4 days (AII), or erythromycin ethylsuccinate PO for 10–14 days (AII)	Macrolides PO preferred to topical eye drops to prevent development of pneumonia; association of erythromycin and pyloric stenosis in young neonates.[9] Alternative: 3-day course of higher-dose azithromycin at 10 mg/kg/dose once daily, although safety not well defined in neonates (CIII). Oral sulfonamides may be used after the immediate neonatal period for infants who do not tolerate erythromycin.
– Gonococcal[10–14]	Ceftriaxone 50 mg/kg (max 125 mg) IV, IM once, AND azithromycin 10 mg/kg PO q24h for 5 days (AIII)	Cephalosporins no longer recommended as single agent therapy due to increasing resistance; therefore, addition of azithromycin recommended (no data in neonates; azithromycin dose given is that recommended for pertussis). Ceftriaxone is an alternative to cefotaxime for neonates not at risk for hyperbilirubinemia[4] or IV calcium-drug interactions.[3] Saline irrigation of eyes. Evaluate for chlamydial infection. All neonates born to mothers with untreated gonococcal infection (regardless of symptoms) require therapy. Cefixime and ciprofloxacin no longer recommended for empiric maternal therapy.
– *Staphylococcus aureus*[15–17]	Topical therapy sufficient for mild *S aureus* cases (AII), but oral or IV therapy may be considered for moderate to severe conjunctivitis. MSSA: oxacillin/nafcillin IV or cefazolin (for non-CNS infections) IM, IV for 7 days. MRSA: vancomycin IV or ceftaroline IV.	Aminoglycoside ophthalmic drops or ointment, polymyxin/trimethoprim drops No prospective data for MRSA conjunctivitis (BIII) Cephalexin PO for mild to moderate disease caused by MSSA Increased *S aureus* resistance with ciprofloxacin/levofloxacin ophthalmic formulations (AII)

A. RECOMMENDED THERAPY FOR SELECTED NEWBORN CONDITIONS (continued)

Condition	**Therapy (evidence grade)** *See Tables 5B–D for neonatal dosages.*	Comments
– *Pseudomonas aeruginosa*[18–20]	Ceftazidime IM, IV AND tobramycin IM, IV for 7–10 days (alternatives: meropenem, cefepime, pip/tazo) (BIII)	Aminoglycoside or polymyxin B–containing ophthalmic drops or ointment as adjunctive therapy
– Other gram-negative	Aminoglycoside or polymyxin B–containing ophthalmic drops or ointment if mild (AII) Systemic therapy if moderate to severe or unresponsive to topical therapy (AIII)	Duration of therapy is dependent on clinical course and may be as short as 5 days if clinically resolved.
Cytomegalovirus		
– Congenital[21–25]	For moderately to severely symptomatic neonates with congenital CMV disease: oral valganciclovir at 16 mg/kg/dose PO bid for 6 mo[24] (AI); IV ganciclovir 6 mg/kg/dose IV q12h can be used for some of or all the first 6 wk of therapy if oral therapy not advised but provides no added benefit over oral valganciclovir (AII).[26] An "induction period" starting with IV ganciclovir is not recommended if oral valganciclovir can be tolerated.	Benefit for hearing loss and neurodevelopmental outcomes (AI). Treatment recommended for neonates with moderate or severe symptomatic congenital CMV disease, with or without CNS involvement. Treatment is not routinely recommended for "mildly symptomatic" neonates congenitally infected with CMV (eg, only 1 or perhaps 2 manifestations of congenital CMV infection, which are mild in scope [eg, isolated IUGR, mild hepatomegaly] or transient and mild in nature [eg, a single platelet count of 80,000 or an ALT of 130, with these numbers serving only as examples]), as the risks of treatment may not be balanced by benefits in mild disease.[25] This includes neonates who are asymptomatic except for sensorineural hearing loss. Treatment for asymptomatic neonates congenitally infected with CMV should not be given. Neutropenia develops in 20% (oral valganciclovir) to 68% (IV ganciclovir) of neonates on long-term therapy (responds to G-CSF or temporary discontinuation of therapy). Treatment for congenital CMV should start within the first month after birth. There are no data currently on starting therapy beyond the first month after birth. CMV-IVIG not recommended for infants.

– Perinatally or postnatally acquired[23]	Ganciclovir 12 mg/kg/day IV div q12h for 14–21 days (AIII)	Antiviral treatment has not been studied in this population but can be considered in patients with acute, severe, visceral (end-organ) disease, such as pneumonitis, hepatitis, encephalitis, necrotizing enterocolitis, or persistent thrombocytopenia. If such patients are treated with parenteral ganciclovir, a reasonable approach is to treat for 2 wk and then reassess responsiveness to therapy. If clinical and laboratory data suggest benefit of treatment, an additional 1 wk of parenteral ganciclovir can be considered if symptoms and signs have not fully resolved. Oral valganciclovir is not recommended in these more severe disease presentations. Observe for possible relapse after completion of therapy (AIII).

A. RECOMMENDED THERAPY FOR SELECTED NEWBORN CONDITIONS (continued)

Condition	**Therapy (evidence grade)** *See Tables 5B–D for neonatal dosages.*	Comments
Fungal infections (See also Chapter 8.)		
– Candidiasis[27–36]	**Treatment** AmB-D (1 mg/kg/day) is recommended therapy (AII). Fluconazole (25 mg/kg on day 1, then 12 mg/kg q24h) is an alternative if patient has not been on fluconazole prophylaxis (AII).[37] For treatment of neonates and young infants (<120 days) on ECMO, fluconazole loading dose is 35 mg/kg on day 1, then 12 mg/kg q24h (BII).[38] Lipid formulation AmB is an alternative but carries a theoretical risk of decreased urinary tract penetration compared with AmB-D (CIII).[39] Duration of therapy for candidemia without obvious metastatic complications is for 2 wk after documented clearance and resolution of symptoms (therefore generally 3 wk total). **Prophylaxis** In nurseries with high rates of candidiasis (>10%),[40] IV or oral fluconazole prophylaxis (AI) (3–6 mg/kg twice weekly for 6 wk) in high-risk neonates (birth weight <1,000 g) is recommended. Oral nystatin, 100,000 units tid for 6 wk, is an alternative to fluconazole in neonates with birth weights <1,500 g if availability or resistance preclude fluconazole use (CII).	Neonates are at high risk of urinary tract and CNS infection, problematic for echinocandins with poor penetration at those sites; therefore, AmB-D is preferred, followed by fluconazole, and echinocandins discouraged, despite their fungicidal activity. Infants with invasive candidiasis should be evaluated for other sites of infection: CSF analysis, echocardiogram, abdominal ultrasound to include bladder; retinal eye examination (AIII). CT or ultrasound imaging of genitourinary tract, liver, and spleen should be performed if blood culture results are persistently positive (AIII). Meningoencephalitis in the neonate occurs at a higher rate than in older children/adults. Central venous catheter removal strongly recommended. Infected CNS devices, including ventriculostomy drains and shunts, should be removed, if possible. Length of therapy dependent on disease (BIII), usually 2 wk after all clearance. Antifungal susceptibility testing is suggested with persistent disease. *Candida krusei* inherently resistant to fluconazole; *Candida parapsilosis* may be less susceptible to echinocandins; increasing resistance of *Candida glabrata* to fluconazole and echinocandins. No proven benefit for combination antifungal therapy in candidiasis. Change from AmB or fluconazole to echinocandin if cultures persistently positive (BIII). Although fluconazole prophylaxis has been shown to reduce colonization, it has not reduced mortality.[30] Echinocandins should be used with caution and generally limited to salvage therapy or situations in which resistance or toxicity preclude use of AmB-D or fluconazole (CIII).

	Prophylaxis of neonates and children on ECMO: fluconazole 12 mg/kg on day 1, followed by 6 mg/kg/day (BII).	Role of flucytosine in neonates with meningitis is questionable and not routinely recommended due to toxicity concerns. The addition of flucytosine (100 mg/kg/day div q6h) may be considered as salvage therapy in patients who have not had a clinical response to initial AmB therapy, but adverse effects are frequent (CIII). Serum flucytosine concentrations should be obtained after 3–5 days to achieve a 2-h post-dose peak <100 mcg/mL (ideally 30–80 mcg/mL) to prevent neutropenia. See Skin and soft tissues later in this Table for management of congenital cutaneous candidiasis.

A. RECOMMENDED THERAPY FOR SELECTED NEWBORN CONDITIONS (continued)

Condition	**Therapy (evidence grade)** *See Tables 5B–D for neonatal dosages.*	Comments
– Aspergillosis (usually cutaneous infection with systemic dissemination)[24,41–43]	Voriconazole dosing never studied in neonates but likely initial dosing same or higher as pediatric ≥2 y: 18 mg/kg/day IV div q12h for a loading dose on the first day, then 16 mg/kg/day IV div q12h as a maintenance dose. Continued dosing is guided by monitoring of trough serum concentrations (AII). When stable, may switch from voriconazole IV to voriconazole PO 18 mg/kg/day div bid (AII). Unlike in adults, PO bioavailability in children is only approximately 60%. PO bioavailability in neonates has never been studied. Trough monitoring is crucial after switch.[23] Alternatives for primary therapy when voriconazole cannot be administered: L-AmB 5 mg/kg/day (AII). ABLC is another possible alternative. Echinocandin primary monotherapy should not be used for treating invasive aspergillosis (CII). AmB-D should be used only in resource-limited settings in which no alternative agent is available (AII).	Aggressive antifungal therapy and early debridement of skin lesions, which are a common presenting finding in neonatal aspergillosis (AIII). Voriconazole is preferred primary antifungal therapy for all clinical forms of aspergillosis (AI). Early initiation of therapy in patients with strong suspicion of disease is important while a diagnostic evaluation is conducted. Therapeutic voriconazole trough serum concentrations of 2–5 mg/L are important for success. It is critical to monitor trough concentrations to guide therapy due to high inter-patient variability.[25] Low voriconazole concentrations are a leading cause of clinical failure. Neonatal and infant voriconazole dosing is not well defined, but doses required to achieve therapeutic troughs are generally higher than in children >2 y (AIII). No experience with posaconazole or isavuconazole in neonates. Total treatment course is for a minimum of 6–12 wk, largely dependent on the degree and duration of immunosuppression and evidence of disease improvement. Salvage antifungal therapy options after failed primary therapy include a change of antifungal class (using L-AmB or an echinocandin), switching to posaconazole (trough concentrations >1 mcg/mL (see Chapter 11 for pediatric dosing), or using combination antifungal therapy. Combination therapy with voriconazole + an echinocandin may be considered in select patients. In vitro data suggest some synergy with 2 (but not 3) drug combinations: an azole + an echinocandin is the most well studied. If combination therapy is employed, this is likely best done initially when voriconazole trough concentrations may not yet be therapeutic.

		Routine susceptibility testing is not recommended but is suggested for patients suspected of having an azole-resistant isolate or who are unresponsive to therapy. Azole-resistant *Aspergillus fumigatus* is increasing. If local epidemiology suggests >10% azole resistance, empiric initial therapy should be voriconazole + echinocandin OR + L-AmB, and subsequent therapy guided based on antifungal susceptibilities.[44] Micafungin likely has equal efficacy to caspofungin against aspergillosis.[28]
Gastrointestinal infections		
– NEC or peritonitis secondary to bowel rupture[45–50]	Ampicillin IV AND gentamicin AND metronidazole IV for ≥10 days (AII). Clindamycin may be used in place of metronidazole (AII). Alternatives: meropenem (BI); pip/tazo ± gentamicin (AII). ADD fluconazole if known to have gastrointestinal colonization with susceptible *Candida* species (BIII).	Surgical drainage (AII). Definitive antibiotic therapy based on blood-culture results (aerobic, anaerobic, and fungal); meropenem for ESBL-positive GNR or cefepime for ampC-positive (inducible cephalosporinase) GNR. Vancomycin rather than ampicillin if MRSA prevalent. *Bacteroides* colonization may occur as early as the first week after birth (AIII).[49] Duration of therapy dependent on clinical response and risk of persisting intra-abdominal abscess (AIII). Probiotics may prevent NEC in preterm neonates born 1–1.5 kg, but the optimal strain(s), dose, and safety are not fully known.[47,50,51]
– *Salmonella* (non-typhi and typhi)[52]	Ampicillin IM, IV (if susceptible) OR ceftriaxone or cefepime IM, IV for 7–10 days (AII)	Observe for focal complications (eg, meningitis, arthritis) (AIII). TMP/SMX for focal gastrointestinal infection and low risk for unconjugated hyperbilirubinemia due to interaction between sulfa and bilirubin-albumin binding.

A. RECOMMENDED THERAPY FOR SELECTED NEWBORN CONDITIONS (continued)

Condition	Therapy (evidence grade) *See Tables 5B–D for neonatal dosages.*	Comments
Herpes simplex infection		
– CNS and disseminated disease[53–55]	Acyclovir 60 mg/kg/day div q8h IV for 21 days (AII) (if eye disease present, ADD topical 1% trifluridine or 0.15% ganciclovir ophthalmic gel) (AII). Infuse IV doses over 1 h in a well-hydrated infant to decrease risk of renal toxicity.	For babies with CNS involvement, perform CSF HSV PCR near end of 21 days of therapy and continue acyclovir until PCR negative. Serum ALT may help identify early disseminated infection. An ophthalmologist should be involved in management and treatment of acute neonatal ocular HSV disease. Foscarnet for acyclovir-resistant disease. Acyclovir PO (300 mg/m^2/dose tid) suppression for 6 mo recommended following parenteral therapy (AI).[56] Monitor for neutropenia during suppressive therapy. Different dosages than those listed in Table 5B have been modeled, but there are no safety or efficacy data in humans to support them.[57]
– Skin, eye, or mouth disease[53–55]	Acyclovir 60 mg/kg/day div q8h IV for 14 days (AII) (if eye disease present, ADD topical 1% trifluridine or 0.15% ganciclovir ophthalmic gel) (AII). Obtain CSF PCR for HSV to assess for CNS infection.	An ophthalmologist should be involved in management and treatment of acute neonatal ocular HSV disease. Acyclovir PO (300 mg/m^2/dose tid) suppression for 6 mo recommended following parenteral therapy (AI).[56] Monitor for neutropenia during suppressive therapy. Different dosages than those listed in Table 5B have been modeled, but there are no safety or efficacy data in humans to support them.[57]
Human immunodeficiency virus prophylaxis following perinatal exposure[58,59]		
– Prophylaxis following low-risk exposure (mother received antiretroviral therapy during pregnancy and had sustained viral suppression near delivery)	ZDV for the first 4 wk of age (AI). GA ≥35 wk: ZDV 8 mg/kg/day PO div q12h OR 6 mg/kg/day IV div q8h. GA 30–34 wk: ZDV 4 mg/kg/day PO (OR 3 mg/kg/day IV) div q12h. Increase at 2 wk of age to 6 mg/kg/day PO (OR 4.5 mg/kg/day IV) div q12h.	For detailed information: https://aidsinfo.nih.gov/guidelines/html/3/perinatal-guidelines/0/# (accessed September 30, 2019). UCSF Clinician Consultation Center (888/448-8765) provides free clinical consultation. Start prevention therapy as soon after delivery as possible but by 6–8 h of age for best effectiveness (AII). Monitor CBC at birth and 4 wk (AII). Perform HIV-1 DNA PCR or RNA assays at 14–21 days, 1–2 mo, and 4–6 mo (AI).

	GA ≤29 wk: ZDV 4 mg/kg/day PO (OR 3 mg/kg/day IV) div q12h. Increase at 4 wk of age to 6 mg/kg/day PO (OR 4.5 mg/kg/day IV) div q12h. The preventive ZDV doses listed herein for neonates are also treatment doses for infants with diagnosed HIV infection. Treatment of HIV-infected neonates should be considered only with expert consultation.	Initiate TMP/SMX prophylaxis for pneumocystis pneumonia at 6 wk of age if HIV infection not yet excluded (AII). TMP/SMX dosing is 2.5–5 mg/kg/dose of TMP component PO q12h.
– Prophylaxis following higher risk perinatal exposure (mothers who were not treated before delivery or who were treated but did not achieve undetectable viral load before delivery, especially if delivery was vaginal)	ZDV for 6 wk AND 3 doses of NVP (first dose at 0–48 h; second dose 48 h later; third dose 96 h after second dose [AI]). NVP dose (not per kg): birth weight 1.5–2 kg: 8 mg/dose PO; birth weight >2 kg: 12 mg/dose PO (AI).[60] OR Empiric treatment with ZDV AND NVP AND 3TC (BII). Consider the addition of RAL in consultation with a pediatric ID specialist (CIII).	Delivery management of women with HIV who are receiving antiretroviral therapy and have viral loads between 50 and 999 copies/mL varies. Data do not show a clear benefit to IV ZDV and cesarean delivery for these women. Decisions about the addition of NVP, 3TC, or RAL for infants born to these mothers should be made in consultation with a pediatric ID specialist. NVP dosing and safety not established for infants whose birth weight <1.5 kg. There has been recent interest in using "treatment" antiretroviral regimens for high-risk, exposed neonates to achieve a remission or possibly even a cure. This was initially stimulated by the experience of a baby from Mississippi: high-risk neonate treated within the first 2 days after birth with subsequent infection documentation; off therapy at 18 mo of age without evidence of circulating virus until 4 y of age, at which point HIV became detectable.[61] A clinical trial is ongoing to study issues further. When empiric treatment is used for high-risk infants and HIV infection is subsequently excluded, NVP, 3TC, and/or RAL can be discontinued and ZDV can be continued for 6 total wk. If HIV infection is confirmed, see Chapter 9 for treatment recommendations.

A. RECOMMENDED THERAPY FOR SELECTED NEWBORN CONDITIONS (continued)

Condition	Therapy (evidence grade) *See Tables 5B–D for neonatal dosages.*	Comments
Influenza A and B viruses[62–65]		
Treatment	Oseltamivir: Preterm, <38 wk PMA: 1 mg/kg/dose PO bid Preterm, 38–40 wk PMA: 1.5 mg/kg/dose PO bid Preterm, >40 wk PMA: 3 mg/kg/dose PO bid[63] Term, birth–8 mo: 3 mg/kg/dose PO bid[63,66]	Oseltamivir chemoprophylaxis not recommended for infants <3 mo unless the situation is judged critical because of limited safety and efficacy data in this age group. Parenteral peramivir is approved in the United States for use in children ≥2 y; no pharmacokinetic or safety data exist in neonates.[67] Oral baloxavir is approved in the United States for use in persons ≥12 y; no pharmacokinetic or safety data exist in neonates.[68]
Omphalitis and funisitis		
– Empiric therapy for omphalitis and necrotizing funisitis direct therapy against coliform bacilli, *S aureus* (consider MRSA), and anaerobes[69–71]	Cefepime OR gentamicin, AND clindamycin for ≥10 days (AII)	Need to culture to direct therapy. Alternatives for coliform coverage if resistance likely: cefepime, meropenem. For suspect MRSA: ADD vancomycin. Alternative for combined MSSA and anaerobic coverage: pip/tazo. Appropriate wound management for infected cord and necrotic tissue (AIII).
– Group A or B streptococci[72]	Penicillin G IV for ≥7–14 days (shorter course for superficial funisitis without invasive infection) (AII)	Group A streptococcus usually causes "wet cord" without pus and with minimal erythema; single dose of benzathine penicillin IM adequate. Consultation with pediatric ID specialist is recommended for necrotizing fasciitis (AII).
– *S aureus*[71]	MSSA: oxacillin/nafcillin IV, IM for ≥5–7 days (shorter course for superficial funisitis without invasive infection) (AIII) MRSA: vancomycin (AIII)	Assess for bacteremia and other focus of infection. Alternatives for MRSA: linezolid, clindamycin (if susceptible), or ceftaroline.

– *Clostridium* spp[73]	Clindamycin OR penicillin G IV for ≥10 days, with additional agents based on culture results (AII)	Crepitation and rapidly spreading cellulitis around umbilicus Mixed infection with other gram-positive and gram-negative bacteria common
Osteomyelitis, suppurative arthritis[73–76] Obtain cultures (aerobic; fungal if NICU) of bone or joint fluid before antibiotic therapy. Duration of therapy dependent on causative organism and normalization of erythrocyte sedimentation rate and C-reactive protein; minimum for osteomyelitis 3 wk and arthritis therapy 2–3 wk if no organism identified (AIII). Surgical drainage of pus (AIII); physical therapy may be needed (BIII).		
– Empiric therapy	Nafcillin/oxacillin IV (or vancomycin if MRSA is a concern) AND cefepime OR gentamicin IV, IM (AIII)	
– Coliform bacteria (eg, *Escherichia coli*, *Klebsiella* spp, *Enterobacter* spp)	For *E coli* and *Klebsiella:* ceftriaxone OR cefepime OR gentamicin OR ampicillin (if susceptible) (AIII). For *Enterobacter, Serratia,* or *Citrobacter:* ADD gentamicin IV, IM to ceftriaxone OR use cefepime or meropenem alone (AIII).	Meropenem for ESBL-producing coliforms (AIII)
– Gonococcal arthritis and tenosynovitis[11–14]	Ceftriaxone IV, IM AND azithromycin 10 mg/kg PO q24h for 5 days (AIII)	Ceftriaxone no longer recommended as single agent therapy due to increasing cephalosporin resistance; therefore, addition of azithromycin recommended (no data in neonates; azithromycin dose is that recommended for pertussis). Cefepime is preferred for neonates with hyperbilirubinemia[4] and those at risk for calcium drug interactions (see Notes).
– *S aureus*	MSSA: oxacillin/nafcillin IV (AII) MRSA: vancomycin IV (AIII)	Alternative for MSSA: cefazolin (AIII) Alternatives for MRSA: linezolid, clindamycin (if susceptible), ceftaroline IV (AIII) (BIII) Addition of rifampin if persistently positive cultures
– Group B streptococcus	Ampicillin or penicillin G IV (AII)	
– *Haemophilus influenzae*	Ampicillin IV OR ceftriaxone/cefepime IV, IM if ampicillin resistant	Start with IV therapy and switch to oral therapy when clinically stable. Amox/clav PO OR amoxicillin PO if susceptible (AIII).

A. RECOMMENDED THERAPY FOR SELECTED NEWBORN CONDITIONS (continued)

Condition	**Therapy (evidence grade)** *See Tables 5B–D for neonatal dosages.*	Comments
Otitis media[77] No controlled treatment trials in newborns; if no response, obtain middle ear fluid for culture.		
– Empiric therapy[78]	Ceftriaxone/cefepime OR oxacillin/nafcillin AND gentamicin	Start with IV therapy and switch to amox/clav PO when clinically stable (AIII).
– *E coli* (therapy of other coliforms based on susceptibility testing)	Ceftriaxone/cefepime	Start with IV therapy and switch to oral therapy when clinically stable. In addition to pneumococcus and *Haemophilus*, coliforms and *S aureus* may also cause AOM in neonates (AIII). For ESBL-producing strains, use meropenem (AII). Amox/clav if susceptible (AIII).
– *S aureus*	MSSA: oxacillin/nafcillin IV MRSA: vancomycin IV, clindamycin IV (if susceptible), or ceftaroline IV	Start with IV therapy and switch to oral therapy when clinically stable. MSSA: cephalexin PO for 10 days or cloxacillin PO (AIII). MRSA: linezolid PO or clindamycin PO (BIII).
– Group A or B streptococci	Penicillin G or ampicillin IV, IM	Start with IV therapy and switch to oral therapy when clinically stable. Amoxicillin 30–40 mg/kg/day PO div q8h for 10 days.
Parotitis, suppurative[79]	Oxacillin/nafcillin IV AND gentamicin IV, IM for 10 days; consider vancomycin if MRSA suspected (AIII).	Usually staphylococcal but occasionally coliform. Antimicrobial regimen without incision/drainage is adequate in $>$75% of cases.[80]
Pulmonary infections		
– Empiric therapy of the neonate with early onset of pulmonary infiltrates (within the first 48–72 h after birth)	Ampicillin IV, IM AND gentamicin or ceftriaxone/cefepime for 7–10 days; consider treating low-risk neonates for $<$7 days (see Comments).	For newborns with no additional risk factors for bacterial infection (eg, maternal chorioamnionitis) who (1) have negative blood cultures, (2) have no need for $>$8 h of oxygen, and (3) are asymptomatic at 48 h into therapy, 4 days may be sufficient therapy, based on babies with clinical pneumonia, none of whom had positive cultures.[81]

– Aspiration pneumonia[82]	Ampicillin IV, IM AND gentamicin IV, IM for 7–10 days (AIII)	Early onset neonatal pneumonia may represent aspiration of amniotic fluid, particularly if fluid is not sterile. Mild aspiration episodes may not require antibiotic therapy.
– *Chlamydia trachomatis*[83]	Azithromycin PO, IV q24h for 5 days OR erythromycin ethylsuccinate PO for 14 days (AII)	Association of erythromycin and azithromycin with pyloric stenosis in infants treated <6 wk of age[84]
– *Mycoplasma hominis*[85,86]	Clindamycin PO, IV for 10 days (Organisms are resistant to macrolides.)	Pathogenic role in pneumonia not well defined and clinical efficacy unknown; no association with bronchopulmonary dysplasia (BIII)
– Pertussis[87]	Azithromycin 10 mg/kg PO, IV q24h for 5 days OR erythromycin ethylsuccinate PO for 14 days (AII)	Association of erythromycin and azithromycin with pyloric stenosis in infants treated <6 wk of age[84] Alternatives: for >1 mo of age, clarithromycin for 7 days; for >2 mo of age, TMP/SMX for 14 days
– *P aeruginosa*[88]	Ceftazidime IV, IM AND tobramycin IV, IM for 10–14 days (AIII)	Alternatives: cefepime or meropenem, OR pip/tazo AND tobramycin

A. RECOMMENDED THERAPY FOR SELECTED NEWBORN CONDITIONS (continued)

Condition	Therapy (evidence grade) *See Tables 5B–D for neonatal dosages.*	Comments
– Respiratory syncytial virus[89]	Treatment: see Comments. Prophylaxis: palivizumab (a monoclonal antibody) 15 mg/kg IM monthly (maximum: 5 doses) for the following high-risk infants (AI): In first year after birth, palivizumab prophylaxis is recommended for infants born before 29 wk 0 days' gestation. Palivizumab prophylaxis is not recommended for otherwise healthy infants born at ≥29 wk 0 days' gestation. In first year after birth, palivizumab prophylaxis is recommended for preterm infants with CLD of prematurity, defined as birth at <32 wk 0 days' gestation and a requirement for >21% oxygen for at least 28 days after birth or at 36 wk PMA. Clinicians may administer palivizumab prophylaxis in the first year after birth to certain infants with hemodynamically significant heart disease.	Aerosol ribavirin (6-g vial to make 20-mg/mL solution in sterile water), aerosolized over 18–20 h daily for 3–5 days (BII), provides little benefit and should only be considered for use in life-threatening RSV infection. Difficulties in administration, complications with airway reactivity, concern for potential toxicities to health care workers, and lack of definitive evidence of benefit preclude routine use. Palivizumab does not provide benefit in the treatment of an active RSV infection. Palivizumab prophylaxis may be considered for children <24 mo who will be profoundly immunocompromised during the RSV season. Palivizumab prophylaxis is not recommended in the second year after birth except for children who required at least 28 days of supplemental oxygen after birth and who continue to require medical support (supplemental oxygen, chronic corticosteroid therapy, or diuretic therapy) during the 6-mo period before the start of the second RSV season. Monthly prophylaxis should be discontinued in any child who experiences a breakthrough RSV hospitalization. Children with pulmonary abnormality or neuromuscular disease that impairs the ability to clear secretions from the upper airways may be considered for prophylaxis in the first year after birth. Insufficient data are available to recommend palivizumab prophylaxis for children with cystic fibrosis or Down syndrome. The burden of RSV disease and costs associated with transport from remote locations may result in a broader use of palivizumab for RSV prevention in Alaska Native populations and possibly in selected other American Indian populations.[90,91] Palivizumab prophylaxis is not recommended for prevention of health care–associated RSV disease.

– *S aureus*[17,92–94]	MSSA: oxacillin/nafcillin IV (AIII). MRSA: vancomycin IV OR clindamycin IV if susceptible, or ceftaroline IV (AIII). Duration of therapy depends on extent of disease (pneumonia vs pulmonary abscesses vs empyema) and should be individualized with therapy up to 21 days or longer.	Alternative for MSSA: cefazolin IV Addition of rifampin or linezolid if persistently positive cultures (AIII) Thoracostomy drainage of empyema
– Group B streptococcus[95,96]	Penicillin G IV OR ampicillin IV, IM for 10 days (AIII)	For serious infections, ADD gentamicin for synergy until clinically improved. No prospective, randomized data on the efficacy of a 7-day treatment course.
– *Ureaplasma* spp (*urealyticum* or *parvum*)[97,98]	Azithromycin[99] PO, IV 20 mg/kg once daily for 3 days (BII)	Pathogenic role of *Ureaplasma* not well defined and no prophylaxis recommended for CLD Many *Ureaplasma* spp resistant to erythromycin Association of erythromycin and pyloric stenosis in young infants

Sepsis and meningitis[94,100,101]

Duration of therapy: 10 days for sepsis without a focus (AIII); minimum of 21 days for gram-negative meningitis (or at least 14 days after CSF is sterile) and 14–21 days for GBS meningitis and other gram-positive bacteria (AIII).

There are no prospective, controlled studies on 5- or 7-day courses for mild or presumed sepsis.

A. RECOMMENDED THERAPY FOR SELECTED NEWBORN CONDITIONS (continued)

Condition	**Therapy (evidence grade)** *See Tables 5B–D for neonatal dosages.*	Comments
– Initial therapy, organism unknown	Ampicillin IV AND a second agent, either ceftriaxone/cefepime IV or gentamicin IV, IM (AII)	Gentamicin is preferred over cephalosporins for empiric therapy of sepsis when meningitis has been ruled out. Cephalosporin preferred if meningitis suspected or cannot be excluded clinically or by lumbar puncture (AIII). For locations with a high rate (≥10%) of ESBL-producing *E coli,* and meningitis is suspected, empiric therapy with meropenem is preferred over cephalosporins. Initial empiric therapy of nosocomial infection should be based on each hospital's pathogens and susceptibilities. **Essential:** Always narrow antibiotic coverage once susceptibility data are available.
– *Bacteroides fragilis*	Metronidazole or meropenem IV, IM (AIII)	Alternative: clindamycin, but increasing resistance reported
– *Enterococcus* spp	Ampicillin IV, IM AND gentamicin IV, IM (AIII); for ampicillin-resistant organisms: vancomycin AND gentamicin IV (AIII)	Gentamicin needed with ampicillin or vancomycin for bactericidal activity; continue until clinical and microbiological response documented (AIII). For vancomycin-resistant enterococci that are also ampicillin resistant: linezolid (AIII).
– Enterovirus	Supportive therapy; no antivirals currently FDA approved	Pocapavir PO is currently under investigation for enterovirus (poliovirus). See Chapter 9. As of November 2019, pocapavir may be available for compassionate use. Pleconaril PO is currently under consideration for submission to FDA for approval for treatment of neonatal enteroviral sepsis syndrome.[102] As of November 2019, it is not available for compassionate use.
– *E coli*[100,101]	Ceftriaxone/cefepime IV or gentamicin IV, IM (AII)	Cephalosporins preferred if meningitis suspected or cannot be excluded clinically or by lumbar puncture (AIII). For locations with a high rate (≥10%) of ESBL-producing *E coli,* and meningitis is suspected, empiric therapy with meropenem is preferred over cephalosporins.

– Gonococcal[11–14]	Ceftriaxone IV, IM OR cefepime IV, IM, AND azithromycin 10 mg/kg PO q24h for 5 days (AIII)	Cephalosporins no longer recommended as single agent therapy due to increasing resistance; therefore, addition of azithromycin recommended (no data in neonates; azithromycin dose is that recommended for pertussis). Cefepime is preferred for neonates with hyperbilirubinemia[4] and those at risk for calcium drug interactions (see Notes).
– *Listeria monocytogenes*[103]	Ampicillin IV, IM AND gentamicin IV, IM (AIII)	Gentamicin is synergistic in vitro with ampicillin. Continue until clinical and microbiological response documented (AIII).
– *P aeruginosa*	Ceftazidime IV, IM AND tobramycin IV, IM (AIII)	Meropenem, cefepime, and tobramycin are suitable alternatives (AIII). Pip/tazo should not be used for CNS infection.
– *S aureus*[17,92–94,104–106]	MSSA: oxacillin/nafcillin IV, IM or cefazolin IV, IM (AII) MRSA: vancomycin IV (AIII)	Alternatives for MRSA: clindamycin, linezolid, ceftaroline
– *Staphylococcus epidermidis* (or any coagulase-negative staphylococci)	Vancomycin IV (AIII)	Oxacillin/nafcillin or cefazolin are alternatives for methicillin-susceptible strains. Cefazolin does not enter CNS. Add rifampin if cultures persistently positive.[107] Alternatives: linezolid, ceftaroline.
– Group A streptococcus	Penicillin G or ampicillin IV (AII)	
– Group B streptococcus[95]	Ampicillin or penicillin G IV AND gentamicin IV, IM (AI)	Continue gentamicin until clinical and microbiological response documented (AIII). Duration of therapy: 10 days for bacteremia/sepsis (AII); minimum of 14 days for meningitis (AII).
Skin and soft tissues		
– Breast abscess[108]	Oxacillin/nafcillin IV, IM (for MSSA) OR vancomycin IV or ceftaroline IV (for MRSA). ADD ceftriaxone/cefepime OR gentamicin if gram-negative rods seen on Gram stain (AIII).	Gram stain of expressed pus guides empiric therapy; vancomycin or ceftaroline if MRSA prevalent in community; other alternatives: clindamycin, linezolid; may need surgical drainage to minimize damage to breast tissue. Treatment duration individualized until clinical findings have completely resolved (AIII).

A. RECOMMENDED THERAPY FOR SELECTED NEWBORN CONDITIONS (continued)

Condition	**Therapy (evidence grade)** *See Tables 5B–D for neonatal dosages.*	Comments
– Congenital cutaneous candidiasis[109]	AmB for 14 days, or 10 days if CSF culture negative (AII). Alternative: fluconazole if *Candida albicans* or other *Candida* spp with known fluconazole susceptibility.	Treat promptly when rash presents with full IV dose, not prophylactic dosing or topical therapy. Diagnostic workup includes aerobic cultures of skin lesions, blood, and CSF. Pathology examination of placenta and umbilical cord if possible.
– Erysipelas (and other group A streptococcal infections)	Penicillin G IV for 5–7 days, followed by oral therapy (if bacteremia not present) to complete a 10-day course (AIII).	Alternative: ampicillin. GBS may produce similar cellulitis or nodular lesions.
– Impetigo neonatorum	MSSA: oxacillin/nafcillin IV, IM OR cephalexin (AIII) MRSA: vancomycin IV or ceftaroline IV for 5 days (AIII)	Systemic antibiotic therapy usually not required for superficial impetigo; local chlorhexidine cleansing may help with or without topical mupirocin (MRSA) or bacitracin (MSSA). Alternatives for MRSA: clindamycin IV, PO or linezolid IV, PO.
– *S aureus*[17,92,94,110]	MSSA: oxacillin/nafcillin IV, IM (AII) MRSA: vancomycin IV or ceftaroline IV (AIII)	Surgical drainage may be required. MRSA may cause necrotizing fasciitis. Alternatives for MRSA: clindamycin IV, linezolid IV. Convalescent oral therapy if infection responds quickly to IV therapy.
– Group B streptococcus[95]	Penicillin G IV OR ampicillin IV, IM	Usually no pus formed Treatment course dependent on extent of infection, 7–14 days

Syphilis, congenital (<1 mo of age)[111]

During periods when availability of penicillin is compromised, contact CDC.

Evaluation and treatment do not depend on mother's HIV status.

Obtain follow-up serology every 2–3 mo until nontreponemal test nonreactive or decreased 4-fold.

– Proven or highly probable disease: (1) abnormal physical examination; (2) serum quantitative nontreponemal serologic titer 4-fold higher than mother's titer; or (3) positive dark field or fluorescent antibody test of body fluid(s)	Aqueous penicillin G 50,000 U/kg/dose q12h (day after birth 1–7), q8h (>7 days) IV OR procaine penicillin G 50,000 U/kg IM q24h for 10 days (AII)	Evaluation to determine type and duration of therapy: CSF analysis (VDRL, cell count, protein), CBC, and platelet count. Other tests, as clinically indicated, including long-bone radiographs, chest radiograph, liver function tests, cranial ultrasound, ophthalmologic examination, and hearing test (ABR). If CSF positive, repeat spinal tap with CSF VDRL at 6 mo and, if abnormal, re-treat. If >1 day of therapy is missed, entire course is restarted.
– Normal physical examination, serum quantitative nontreponemal serologic titer ≤ maternal titer, and maternal treatment was (1) none, inadequate, or undocumented; (2) erythromycin, azithromycin, or other non-penicillin regimen; or (3) <4 wk before delivery.	Evaluation abnormal or not done completely: aqueous penicillin G 50,000 U/kg/dose q12h (day after birth 1–7), q8h (>7 days) IV OR procaine penicillin G 50,000 U/kg IM q24h for 10 days (AII) Evaluation normal: aqueous penicillin G 50,000 U/kg/dose q12h (day after birth 1–7), q8h (>7 days) IV OR procaine penicillin G 50,000 U/kg IM q24h for 10 days; OR benzathine penicillin G 50,000 units/kg/dose IM in a single dose (AIII)	Evaluation: CSF analysis, CBC with platelets, long-bone radiographs. If >1 day of therapy is missed, entire course is restarted. Reliable follow-up important if only a single dose of benzathine penicillin given.

A. RECOMMENDED THERAPY FOR SELECTED NEWBORN CONDITIONS (continued)

Condition	**Therapy (evidence grade)** *See Tables 5B–D for neonatal dosages.*	Comments
– Normal physical examination, serum quantitative nontreponemal serologic titer ≤ maternal titer, mother treated adequately during pregnancy and >4 wk before delivery; no evidence of reinfection or relapse in mother	Benzathine penicillin G 50,000 units/kg/dose IM in a single dose (AIII)	No evaluation required. Some experts would not treat but provide close serologic follow-up.
– Normal physical examination, serum quantitative nontreponemal serologic titer ≤ maternal titer, mother's treatment adequate before pregnancy	No treatment	No evaluation required. Some experts would treat with benzathine penicillin G 50,000 U/kg as a single IM injection, particularly if follow-up is uncertain.
Syphilis, congenital (>1 mo of age)[111]	Aqueous crystalline penicillin G 200,000–300,000 U/kg/day IV div q4–6h for 10 days (AII)	Evaluation to determine type and duration of therapy: CSF analysis (VDRL, cell count, protein), CBC and platelet count. Other tests as clinically indicated, including long-bone radiographs, chest radiograph, liver function tests, neuroimaging, ophthalmologic examination, and hearing evaluation. If no clinical manifestations of disease, CSF examination is normal, and CSF VDRL test result is nonreactive, some specialists would treat with up to 3 weekly doses of benzathine penicillin G 50,000 U/kg IM.

		Some experts would provide a single dose of benzathine penicillin G 50,000 U/kg IM after 10 days of parenteral treatment, but value of this additional therapy is not well documented.
Tetanus neonatorum[112]	Metronidazole IV, PO (alternative: penicillin G IV) for 10–14 days (AIII) Human TIG 3,000–6,000 U IM for 1 dose (AIII)	Wound cleaning and debridement vital; IVIG (200–400 mg/kg) is an alternative if TIG not available; equine tetanus antitoxin not available in the United States but is alternative to TIG.
Toxoplasmosis, congenital[113,114]	Sulfadiazine 100 mg/kg/day PO div q12h AND pyrimethamine 2 mg/kg PO daily for 2 days (loading dose), then 1 mg/kg PO q24h for 2–6 mo, then 3 times weekly (M-W-F) up to 1 y (AII) Folinic acid (leucovorin) 10 mg 3 times weekly (AII)	Corticosteroids (1 mg/kg/day div q12h) if active chorioretinitis or CSF protein >1 g/dL (AIII). Round sulfadiazine dose to 125 or 250 mg (¼ or ½ of 500-mg tab); round pyrimethamine dose to 6.25 or 1.25 mg (¼ or ½ of 25-mg tab). OK to crush tabs to give with feeding. Start sulfadiazine after neonatal jaundice has resolved. Therapy is only effective against active trophozoites, not cysts.
Urinary tract infection[115] No prophylaxis for grades 1–3 reflux.[116,117] In neonates with reflux, prophylaxis reduces recurrences but increases likelihood of recurrences being due to resistant organisms. Prophylaxis does not affect renal scarring.[116]		
– Initial therapy, organism unknown	Ampicillin AND gentamicin; OR ampicillin AND ceftriaxone/cefepime pending culture and susceptibility test results for 7–10 days	Renal ultrasound and VCUG indicated after first UTI to identify abnormalities of urinary tract Oral therapy acceptable once neonate asymptomatic and culture sterile
– Coliform bacteria (eg, *E coli, Klebsiella, Enterobacter, Serratia*)	Ceftriaxone/cefepime IV, IM OR, in absence of renal or perinephric abscess, gentamicin IV, IM for 7–10 days (AII)	Ampicillin used for susceptible organisms
– *Enterococcus*	Ampicillin IV, IM for 7 days for cystitis, may need 10–14 days for pyelonephritis, add gentamicin until cultures are sterile (AIII); for ampicillin resistance, use vancomycin, add gentamicin until cultures are sterile.	Aminoglycoside needed with ampicillin or vancomycin for synergistic bactericidal activity (assuming organisms is susceptible to an aminoglycoside)

A. RECOMMENDED THERAPY FOR SELECTED NEWBORN CONDITIONS (continued)

Condition	**Therapy (evidence grade)** *See Tables 5B–D for neonatal dosages.*	Comments
– *P aeruginosa*	Ceftazidime IV, IM OR, in absence of renal or perinephric abscess, tobramycin IV, IM for 7–10 days (AIII)	Meropenem or cefepime are alternatives.
– *Candida* spp[32–34]	See Fungal infections, Candidiasis, earlier in this Table.	

B. ANTIMICROBIAL DOSAGES FOR NEONATES—Lead author Jason Sauberan, assisted by the editors and John Van Den Anker

		Dosages (mg/kg/day) and Intervals of Administration				
		Chronologic Age ≤28 days				Chronologic Age 29–60 days
		Body Weight ≤2,000 g		Body Weight >2,000 g		
Antimicrobial	**Route**	**0–7 days old**	**8–28 days old**	**0–7 days old**	**8–28 days old**	
NOTE: This table contains empiric dosage recommendations for each agent listed. See Table 5A (Recommended Therapy for Selected Newborn Conditions) for more details of dosages for specific pathogens in specific tissue sites and for information on anti-influenza and antiretroviral drug dosages.						
Acyclovir (treatment of acute disease)	IV	40 div q12h	60 div q8h	60 div q8h	60 div q8h	60 div q8h
Acyclovir (suppression following treatment for acute disease)	PO	—	900/m²/day div q8h	—	900/m²/day div q8h	900/m²/day div q8h
Only parenteral acyclovir should be used for the treatment of acute neonatal HSV disease. Oral suppression therapy for 6 mo duration after completion of initial neonatal HSV treatment. See text in Table 5A, Herpes simplex infection.						
Amoxicillin-clavulanate[a]	PO	—	—	30 div q12h	30 div q12h	30 div q12h
Amphotericin B						
– deoxycholate	IV	1 q24h	1 q24h	1 q24h	1 q24h	1 q24h
– lipid complex	IV	5 q24h	5 q24h	5 q24h	5 q24h	5 q24h
– liposomal	IV	5 q24h	5 q24h	5 q24h	5 q24h	5 q24h
Ampicillin	IV, IM	100 div q12h	150 div q12h	150 div q8h	150 div q8h	200 div q6h
Ampicillin (GBS meningitis)	IV	300 div q8h	300 div q6h	300 div q8h	300 div q6h	300 div q6h
Anidulafungin[b]	IV	1.5 q24h	1.5 q24h	1.5 q24h	1.5 q24h	1.5 q24h
Azithromycin[c]	PO	10 q24h	10 q24h	10 q24h	10 q24h	10 q24h
	IV	10 q24h	10 q24h	10 q24h	10 q24h	10 q24h

B. ANTIMICROBIAL DOSAGES FOR NEONATES (continued)—Lead author Jason Sauberan, assisted by the editors and John Van Den Anker

		Dosages (mg/kg/day) and Intervals of Administration				
		Chronologic Age ≤28 days				Chronologic Age 29–60 days
		Body Weight ≤2,000 g		Body Weight >2,000 g		
Antimicrobial	**Route**	**0–7 days old**	**8–28 days old**	**0–7 days old**	**8–28 days old**	
Aztreonam	IV, IM	60 div q12h	90 div q8h[d]	90 div q8h	120 div q6h	120 div q6h
Cefazolin (Enterobacteriaceae)[e]	IV, IM	50 div q12h	75 div q8h	100 div q12h	150 div q8h	100–150 div q6–8h
Cefazolin (MSSA)	IV, IM	50 div q12h	50 div q12h	75 div q8h	75 div q8h	75 div q8h
Cefepime	IV, IM	60 div q12h	60 div q12h	100 div q12h	100 div q12h	150 div q8h[f]
Cefotaxime	IV, IM	100 div q12h	150 div q8h	100 div q12h	150 div q6h	200 div q6h
Ceftaroline	IV, IM	12 div q12h	18 div q8h	18 div q8h	18 div q8h	18 div q8h
Ceftazidime	IV, IM	100 div q12h	150 div q8h[d]	100 div q12h	150 div q8h	150 div q8h
Ceftriaxone[g]	IV, IM	—	—	50 q24h	50 q24h	50 q24h
Ciprofloxacin	IV	15 div q12h	15 div q12h	25 div q12h	25 div q12h	25 div q12h
Clindamycin	IV, IM, PO	15 div q8h	15 div q8h	21 div q8h	27 div q8h	30 div q8h
Daptomycin (Potential neurotoxicity; use cautiously if no other options.)	IV	12 div q12h	12 div q12h	12 div q12h	12 div q12h	12 div q12h
Erythromycin	IV, PO	40 div q6h	40 div q6h	40 div q6h	40 div q6h	40 div q6h
Fluconazole						
– treatment[h]	IV, PO	12 q24h	12 q24h	12 q24h	12 q24h	12 q24h
– prophylaxis	IV, PO	6 mg/kg/dose twice weekly	6 mg/kg/dose twice weekly	6 mg/kg/dose twice weekly	6 mg/kg/dose twice weekly	6 mg/kg/dose twice weekly

Flucytosine[i]	PO	75 div q8h	100 div q6h[d]	100 div q6h	100 div q6h	100 div q6h
Ganciclovir	IV	Insufficient data	Insufficient data	12 div q12h	12 div q12h	12 div q12h
Linezolid	IV, PO	20 div q12h	30 div q8h	30 div q8h	30 div q8h	30 div q8h
Meropenem						
– sepsis, IAI[j]	IV	40 div q12h	60 div q8h[j]	60 div q8h	90 div q8h[j]	90 div q8h
– meningitis	IV	80 div q12h	120 div q8h[j]	120 div q8h	120 div q8h	120 div q8h
Metronidazole[k]	IV, PO	15 div q12h	15 div q12h	22.5 div q8h	30 div q8h	30 div q8h
Micafungin	IV	10 q24h	10 q24h	10 q24h	10 q24h	10 q24h
Nafcillin,[l] oxacillin[l]	IV, IM	50 div q12h	75 div q8h[d]	75 div q8h	100 div q6h	150 div q6h
Penicillin G benzathine	IM	50,000 U	50,000 U	50,000 U	50,000 U	50,000 U
Penicillin G crystalline (GBS sepsis, congenital syphilis)	IV	100,000 U div q12h	150,000 U div q8h	100,000 U div q12h	150,000 U div q8h	200,000 U div q6h
Penicillin G crystalline (GBS meningitis)	IV	450,000 U div q8h	500,000 U div q6h	450,000 U div q8h	500,000 U div q6h	500,000 U div q6h
Penicillin G procaine	IM	50,000 U q24h	50,000 U q24h	50,000 U q24h	50,000 U q24h	50,000 U q24h
Piperacillin/tazobactam	IV	300 div q8h	320 div q6h[m]	320 div q6h	320 div q6h	320 div q6h
Rifampin	IV, PO	10 q24h	10 q24h	10 q24h	10 q24h	10 q24h
Valganciclovir	PO	Insufficient data	Insufficient data	32 div q12h	32 div q12h	32 div q12h
Voriconazole[n]	IV	16 div q12h	16 div q12h	16 div q12h	16 div q12h	16 div q12h

B. ANTIMICROBIAL DOSAGES FOR NEONATES (continued)—Lead author Jason Sauberan, assisted by the editors and John Van Den Anker

		Dosages (mg/kg/day) and Intervals of Administration				
		Chronologic Age ≤28 days				Chronologic Age 29–60 days
		Body Weight ≤2,000 g		Body Weight >2,000 g		
Antimicrobial	**Route**	**0–7 days old**	**8–28 days old**	**0–7 days old**	**8–28 days old**	
Zidovudine	IV	3 div q12h[o]	3 div q12h[o]	6 div q12h	6 div q12h	See Table 5A, Human immunodeficiency virus prophylaxis.
	PO	4 div q12h[o]	4 div q12h[o]	8 div q12h	8 div q12h	See Table 5A, Human immunodeficiency virus prophylaxis.

[a] 25- or 50-mg/mL formulation.

[b] Loading dose 3 mg/kg followed 24 h later by maintenance dose listed.

[c] See Table 5A for pathogen-specific dosing.

[d] Use 0–7 days old dosing until 14 days old if birth weight <1,000 g.

[e] If isolate susceptible and no CNS focus.

[f] May require infusion over 3 h, or 200 mg/kg/day div q6h, to treat organisms with MIC ≥8 mg/L.

[g] Usually avoided in neonates. Can be considered for transitioning to outpatient treatment of GBS bacteremia in well-appearing neonates at low risk for hyperbilirubinemia. Contraindicated if concomitant IV calcium; see Notes section at beginning of chapter.

[h] Loading dose 25 mg/kg followed 24 h later by maintenance dose listed.

[i] Desired serum concentrations peak 60–80 mg/L, trough 5–10 mg/L to achieve time-above-MIC of >40% for invasive candidiasis (trough 10–20 mg/L acceptable for *Cryptococcus*). Dose range 50–100 mg/kg/day. Always use in combination with other agents; be alert to development of resistance. Time-above-MIC of >40% for invasive candidiasis is our target.

[j] Adjust dosage after 14 days of age instead of after 7 days of age.

[k] Loading dose 15 mg/kg.

[l] Double the dose for meningitis.

[m] When PMA reaches >30 wk.

[n] Initial loading dose of 18 mg/kg div q12h on day 1. Desired serum concentrations, trough 2–5 mg/L. See text in Table 5A, Aspergillosis.

[o] Starting dose if GA <35+0 wk and PNA ≤14 days. See Table 5A, Human immunodeficiency virus prophylaxis, for ZDV dosage after 2 wk of age and for NVP and 3TC recommendations.

C. AMINOGLYCOSIDES

		Empiric Dosage (mg/kg/dose) by Gestational and Postnatal Age					
		<30 wk		30–34 wk		≥35 wk	
Medication	**Route**	**0–14 days**	**>14 days**	**0–10 days**	**>10 days[a]**	**0–7 days**	**>7 days[a]**
Amikacin[b]	IV, IM	15 q48h	15 q24h	15 q24h	15 q24h	15 q24h	17.5 q24h
Gentamicin[c]	IV, IM	5 q48h	5 q36h	5 q36h	5 q24h	4 q24h	5 q24h
Tobramycin[c]	IV, IM	5 q48h	5 q36h	5 q36h	5 q24h	4 q24h	5 q24h

[a] If >60 days of age, see Chapter 11.

[b] Desired serum concentrations: 20–35 mg/L or >10 × MIC (peak), <7 mg/L (trough).

[c] Desired serum concentrations: 6–12 mg/L or 10 × MIC (peak), <2 mg/L (trough). A 7.5 mg/kg dose q48h, or q36h if ≥30 wk GA and >7 days PNA, more likely to achieve desired concentrations if pathogen MIC = 1 mg/L.[118]

D. VANCOMYCIN[a]

Empiric Dosage by Gestational Age and SCr
Begin with a 20 mg/kg loading dose.

≤28 wk GA			>28 wk GA		
SCr (mg/dL)	**Dose (mg/kg)**	**Frequency**	**SCr (mg/dL)**	**Dose (mg/kg)**	**Frequency**
<0.5	15	q12h	<0.7	15	q12h
0.5–0.7	20	q24h	0.7–0.9	20	q24h
0.8–1.0	15	q24h	1.0–1.2	15	q24h
1.1–1.4	10	q24h	1.3–1.6	10	q24h
>1.4	15	q48h	>1.6	15	q48h

[a] SCr concentrations normally fluctuate and are partly influenced by transplacental maternal creatinine in the first wk after birth. Cautious use of creatinine-based dosing strategy with frequent reassessment of renal function and vancomycin serum concentrations are recommended in neonates ≤7 days old.

Desired serum concentrations: A 24-h AUC:MIC of at least 400 mg·h/L is recommended based on adult studies of invasive MRSA infections. The AUC is best calculated from 2 concentrations (ie, peak and trough) rather than 1 trough serum concentration measurement. In situations in which AUC calculation is not feasible, a trough concentration ≥10 mg/L is very highly likely (>90%) to achieve the goal AUC target in neonates when the MIC is 1 mg/L. However, troughs as low as 7 mg/L can still achieve an AUC ≥400 in some preterm neonates due to their slower clearance. Thus, AUC is preferred over trough monitoring to prevent unnecessary overexposure.

For centers where invasive MRSA infection is relatively common or where MRSA with MIC of 1 mg/L is common, an online dosing tool is available that may improve the likelihood of empirically achieving AUC ≥400 compared with Table 5D (http://neovanco.insight-rx.com/neo-vanco; accessed September 30, 2019).

If >60 days of age, see Chapter 11.

E. Use of Antimicrobials During Pregnancy or Breastfeeding

The use of antimicrobials during pregnancy and lactation should balance benefit to the mother with the risk of fetal and infant toxicity (including anatomic anomalies with fetal exposure). A number of factors determine the degree of transfer of antibiotics across the placenta: lipid solubility, degree of ionization, molecular weight, protein binding, placental maturation, and placental and fetal blood flow. The previous FDA labeling of 5 categories of risk will be phased out, replaced by narrative summaries of risks associated with the use of a drug during pregnancy and lactation for the mother, the fetus, and the breastfeeding child. The risk categories from A to X were felt to be too simplistic and are to be phased out by 2020. Risks are now all clearly noted, and for drugs with high fetal risk, black box warnings are included (eg, ribavirin).[119]

Fetal serum antibiotic concentrations (or cord blood concentrations) following maternal administration have not been systematically studied, but new pharmacokinetic models of transplacental drug transfer and fetal metabolism have recently been developed to provide some insight into fetal drug exposure.[120–122] The following commonly used drugs appear to achieve fetal concentrations that are equal to or only slightly less than those in the mother: penicillin G, amoxicillin, ampicillin, sulfonamides, trimethoprim, tetracyclines, and oseltamivir. The aminoglycoside concentrations in fetal serum are 20% to 50% of those in maternal serum. Cephalosporins, carbapenems, nafcillin, oxacillin, clindamycin, and vancomycin penetrate poorly (10%–30%), and fetal concentrations of erythromycin and azithromycin are less than 10% of those in the mother.

The most current, updated information on the pharmacokinetics and safety of antimicrobials and other agents in human milk can be found at the National Library of Medicine LactMed website (www.ncbi.nlm.nih.gov/books/NBK501922; accessed November 12, 2019).[123]

In general, neonatal exposure to antimicrobials in human milk is minimal or insignificant. Aminoglycosides, beta-lactams, ciprofloxacin, clindamycin, macrolides, fluconazole, and agents for tuberculosis are considered safe for the mother to take during breastfeeding.[124,125] The most common reported neonatal side effect of maternal antimicrobial use during breastfeeding is increased stool output.[126] Clinicians should recommend mothers alert their pediatric health care professional if stool output changes occur. Maternal treatment with sulfa-containing antibiotics should be approached with caution in the breastfed infant who is jaundiced or ill.

6. Antimicrobial Therapy According to Clinical Syndromes

NOTES

- This chapter should be considered a rough guidance for a typical patient. Dosage recommendations are for patients with relatively normal hydration, renal function, and hepatic function. Because the dose required is based on the exposure of the antibiotic to the pathogen at the site of infection, higher dosages may be necessary if the antibiotic does not penetrate well into the infected tissue (eg, meningitis) or if the child eliminates the antibiotic from the body more quickly than average. Higher dosages/longer courses may also be needed if the child is immunocompromised and the immune system cannot help resolve the infection, as it is becoming clearer that the host contributes significantly to microbiologic and clinical cure above and beyond the antimicrobial-attributable effect. Most of the doses reviewed and approved by the US Food and Drug Administration (FDA) are from the original clinical trials for drug registration unless a safety issue becomes apparent when the label is modified. The original sponsor of the drug may not have studied all pathogens at all sites of infection in neonates, infants, and children. The FDA carefully reviews data presented to it but does not have a federal mandate or the funding to review the entire literature on each antibiotic and update the package labels annually (or at some predetermined interval). If the FDA has not reviewed data for a specific indication (eg, ampicillin for group A streptococcal cellulitis), there is usually no opinion about whether the drug may or may not work. In fact, ampicillin is not "approved" for skin and soft tissue infections caused by any bacteria. The editors will provide suggestions for clinical situations that may not have been reviewed and approved by the FDA. These recommendations are considered *off-label,* which does not mean that they are incorrect; they have just not been reviewed by the FDA at its level of rigor.
- Duration of treatment should be individualized. Those recommended are based on the literature, common practice, and general experience. Critical evaluations of duration of therapy have been carried out in very few infectious diseases. In general, a longer duration of therapy should be used (1) for tissues in which antibiotic concentrations may be relatively low (eg, undrained abscess, central nervous system [CNS] infection); (2) for tissues in which repair following infection-mediated damage is slow (eg, bone); (3) when the organisms are less susceptible; (4) when a relapse of infection is unacceptable (eg, CNS infections); or (5) when the host is immunocompromised in some way. An assessment after therapy will ensure that your selection of antibiotic, dose, and duration of therapy were appropriate. Until prospective, comparative studies are performed for different durations, we cannot assign a specific increased risk of failure for shorter courses. We support the need for these studies in a controlled clinical research setting, either outpatient or inpatient.
- Our approach to therapy is continuing to move away from the concept that "one dose fits all," as noted previously. In addition to the dose that provides antibiotic exposure and host immune competence, the concept of *target attainment* is being better defined.

The severity of illness and the willingness of the practitioner to accept a certain rate of failure needs to be considered. Hence the use of broad-spectrum, high-dose treatment for a child in florid septic shock (where you need to be right virtually 100% of the time), compared with the child with impetigo where a treatment that is approximately 80% effective is acceptable, as you can just see the child back in the office in a few days and alter therapy as necessary.

- Diseases in this chapter are arranged by body systems. Please consult the index for the alphabetized listing of diseases and chapters 7 through 10 for the alphabetized listing of pathogens and for uncommon organisms not included in this chapter.
- A more detailed description of treatment options for methicillin-resistant *Staphylococcus aureus* (MRSA) infections and multidrug-resistant gram-negative bacilli infections, including a stepwise approach to increasingly broad-spectrum agents, is provided in Chapter 4. Although in the past, vancomycin has been the mainstay of therapy for invasive MRSA, it is nephrotoxic and ototoxic, and it requires monitoring renal function and serum drug concentrations. Its use in organisms with a minimal inhibitory concentration of 2 or greater may not provide adequate exposure for a cure with realistic pediatric doses. Ceftaroline, the first MRSA-active beta-lactam antibiotic approved by the FDA for adults in 2010 and children in 2016, is as effective for most staphylococcal tissue site infections (no controlled data on CNS infections) as vancomycin, but safer, and should be considered as preferred therapy over vancomycin.
- Therapy of *Pseudomonas aeruginosa* systemic infections has evolved from intravenous (IV) ceftazidime plus tobramycin to single-drug IV therapy with cefepime for most infections in immune-competent and immune-compromised children, due to the relative stability of cefepime to beta-lactamases, compared with ceftazidime. Oral therapy with ciprofloxacin has replaced IV therapy in children who are compliant and able to take oral therapy, particularly for "step-down" therapy of invasive infections.
- **Abbreviations:** AAP, American Academy of Pediatrics; ACOG, American College of Obstetricians and Gynecologists; ADH, antidiuretic hormone; AFB, acid-fast bacilli; AHA, American Heart Association; ALT, alanine transaminase; AmB, amphotericin B; amox/clav, amoxicillin/clavulanate; AOM, acute otitis media; ARF, acute rheumatic fever; AST, aspartate transaminase; AUC:MIC, area under the serum concentration vs time curve: minimum inhibitory concentration; bid, twice daily; CA-MRSA, community-associated methicillin-resistant *Staphylococcus aureus;* cap, capsule; CDC, Centers for Disease Control and Prevention; CMV, cytomegalovirus; CNS, central nervous system; CRP, C-reactive protein; CSD, cat-scratch disease; CSF, cerebrospinal fluid; CT, computed tomography; DAT, diphtheria antitoxin; div, divided; DOT, directly observed therapy; EBV, Epstein-Barr virus; ESBL, extended spectrum beta-lactamase; ESR, erythrocyte sedimentation rate; ETEC, enterotoxin-producing *Escherichia coli;* FDA, US Food and Drug Administration; GI, gastrointestinal; HACEK, *Haemophilus aphrophilus, Aggregatibacter* (formerly *Actinobacillus*) *actinomycetemcomitans, Cardiobacterium hominis, Eikenella corrodens, Kingella* spp; HIV,

human immunodeficiency virus; HSV, herpes simplex virus; HUS, hemolytic uremic syndrome; I&D, incision and drainage; IDSA, Infectious Diseases Society of America; IM, intramuscular; INH, isoniazid; IV, intravenous; IVIG, intravenous immune globulin; KPC, *Klebsiella pneumoniae* carbapenemase; L-AmB, liposomal amphotericin B; LFT, liver function test; LP, lumbar puncture; MDR, multidrug resistant; MRI, magnetic resonance imaging; MRSA, methicillin-resistant *S aureus;* MRSE, methicillin-resistant *Staphylococcus epidermidis;* MSSA, methicillin-susceptible *S aureus;* MSSE, methicillin-sensitive *S epidermidis;* ophth, ophthalmic; PCR, polymerase chain reaction; PCV7, pneumococcal 7-valent conjugate vaccine; PCV13, Prevnar 13-valent pneumococcal conjugate vaccine; pen-R, penicillin-resistant; pen-S, penicillin-susceptible; PIDS, Pediatric Infectious Diseases Society; pip/tazo, piperacillin/tazobactam; PMA, post-menstrual age; PO, oral; PPD, purified protein derivative; PZA, pyrazinamide; qd, once daily; qid, 4 times daily; qod, every other day; RIVUR, Randomized Intervention for Children with Vesicoureteral Reflux; RSV, respiratory syncytial virus; soln, solution; SPAG-2, small particle aerosol generator-2; spp, species; STEC, Shiga toxin-producing *E coli;* STI, sexually transmitted infection; tab, tablet; TB, tuberculosis; Td, tetanus, diphtheria; Tdap, tetanus, diphtheria, acellular pertussis; tid, 3 times daily; TIG, tetanus immune globulin; TMP/SMX, trimethoprim/sulfamethoxazole; ULN, upper limit of normal; UTI, urinary tract infection; VDRL, Venereal Disease Research Laboratories; WBC, white blood cell.

A. SKIN AND SOFT TISSUE INFECTIONS

Clinical Diagnosis	Therapy (evidence grade)	Comments
NOTE: CA-MRSA (see Chapter 4) is prevalent in most areas of the world but may now be decreasing, rather than increasing.[1,2] Recommendations for staphylococcal infections are given for 2 scenarios: standard MSSA and CA-MRSA. Antibiotic recommendations "for CA-MRSA" should be used for empiric therapy in regions with greater than 5% to 10% of invasive staphylococcal infections caused by MRSA, in situations where CA-MRSA is suspected, and for documented CA-MRSA infections, while "standard recommendations" refer to treatment of MSSA. During the past few years, clindamycin resistance in MRSA has increased to 40% in some areas but remained stable at 5% in others, although this increase may be an artifact of changes in reporting, with many laboratories now reporting all clindamycin-susceptible but D-test–positive strains as resistant. Please check your local susceptibility data for *Staphylococcus aureus* before using clindamycin for empiric therapy. For MSSA, oxacillin/nafcillin are considered equivalent agents.		
Adenitis, acute bacterial[3–9] (*S aureus,* including CA-MRSA, and group A streptococcus; consider *Bartonella* [CSD] for subacute adenitis.)[10]	Empiric therapy Standard: oxacillin/nafcillin 150 mg/kg/day IV div q6h OR cefazolin 100 mg/kg/day IV div q8h (AI), OR cephalexin 50–75 mg/kg/day PO div tid CA-MRSA: clindamycin 30 mg/kg/day IV or PO (AI) div q8h OR ceftaroline: 2 mo–<2 y, 24 mg/kg/day IV div q8h; ≥2 y, 36 mg/kg/day IV div q8h (max single dose 400 mg); >33 kg, either 400 mg/dose IV q8h or 600 mg/dose IV q12h (BI), OR vancomycin 40 mg/kg/day IV q8h (BII), OR daptomycin: 1–<2 y, 10 mg/kg IV qd; 2–6 y, 9 mg/kg IV qd; 7–11 y, 7 mg/kg qd; 12–17 y, 5 mg/kg qd (BI) CSD: azithromycin 12 mg/kg qd (max 500 mg) for 5 days (BIII)	May need surgical drainage for staph/strep infection; not usually needed for CSD. Following drainage of mild to moderate suppurative adenitis caused by staph or strep, additional antibiotics may not be required. For oral therapy for MSSA: cephalexin or amox/clav. For CA-MRSA: clindamycin, TMP/SMX, or linezolid. For oral therapy of group A strep: amoxicillin or penicillin V. Avoid daptomycin in infants until 1 y due to potential toxicity. Total IV plus PO therapy for 7–10 days. For CSD: this is the same high dose of azithromycin that is recommended routinely for strep pharyngitis.
Adenitis, nontuberculous (atypical) mycobacterial[11–14]	Excision usually curative (BII); azithromycin PO OR clarithromycin PO for 6–12 wk (with or without rifampin) if susceptible (BII)	Antibiotic susceptibility patterns are quite variable; cultures should guide therapy: excision >97% effective; medical therapy 60%–70% effective. No well-controlled trials available.

Adenitis, tuberculous[15,16] (*Mycobacterium tuberculosis* and *Mycobacterium bovis*)	INH 10–15 mg/kg/day (max 300 mg) PO, IV qd, for 6 mo AND rifampin 10–20 mg/kg/day (max 600 mg) PO, IV qd, for 6 mo AND PZA 20–40 mg/kg/day PO qd for first 2 mo therapy (BI); if suspected multidrug resistance, add ethambutol 20 mg/kg/day PO qd.	Surgical excision usually not indicated because organisms are treatable. Adenitis caused by *M bovis* (unpasteurized dairy product ingestion) is uniformly resistant to PZA. Treat 9–12 mo with INH and rifampin, if susceptible (BII). No contraindication to fine needle aspirate of node for diagnosis.
Anthrax, cutaneous[17]	Empiric therapy: ciprofloxacin 20–30 mg/kg/day PO div bid OR doxycycline 4.4 mg/kg/day (max 200 mg) PO div bid (regardless of age) (AIII)	If susceptible, amoxicillin or clindamycin (BIII). Ciprofloxacin and levofloxacin are FDA approved for inhalational anthrax for children $>$ 6 mo and should be effective for skin infection (BIII).
Bites, dog and cat[3,18–23] (*Pasteurella multocida; S aureus,* including CA-MRSA; *Streptococcus* spp, anaerobes; *Capnocytophaga canimorsus,* particularly in asplenic hosts)	Amox/clav 45 mg/kg/day PO div tid (amox/clav 7:1; see Chapter 1, Aminopenicillins) for 5–10 days (AII). For hospitalized children, use ampicillin AND clindamycin (BII) OR ceftriaxone AND clindamycin (BII) OR ceftaroline: 2 mo–$<$2 y, 24 mg/kg/day IV div q8h; $\geq$2 y, 36 mg/kg/day IV div q8h (max single dose 400 mg); $>$33 kg, either 400 mg/dose IV q8h or 600 mg/dose IV q12h (BIII).	Amox/clav has good *Pasteurella,* MSSA, and anaerobic coverage but lacks MRSA coverage. Ampicillin/amox plus clindamycin has good *Pasteurella,* MSSA, MRSA, and anaerobic coverage. Ceftaroline has good *Pasteurella,* MSSA, and MRSA coverage but lacks *Bacteroides fragilis* anaerobic coverage.[23] Ampicillin/sulbactam also lacks MRSA coverage. Consider rabies prophylaxis[24] for bites from at-risk animals that were not provoked (observe animal for 10 days, if possible) (AI); CDC can provide advice on risk and management (www.cdc.gov/rabies/resources/contacts.html); consider tetanus prophylaxis. For penicillin allergy, ciprofloxacin (for *Pasteurella*) plus clindamycin (BIII). Doxycycline may be considered for *Pasteurella* coverage.

A. SKIN AND SOFT TISSUE INFECTIONS (continued)

Clinical Diagnosis	Therapy (evidence grade)	Comments
Bites, human[3,20,21,25] (*Eikenella corrodens; S aureus,* including CA-MRSA; *Streptococcus* spp, anaerobes)	Amox/clav 45 mg/kg/day PO div tid (amox/clav 7:1; see Chapter 1, Aminopenicillins) for 5–10 days (AII). For hospitalized children, use ampicillin and clindamycin (BII) OR ceftriaxone and clindamycin (BII).	Human bites have a very high rate of infection (do not routinely close open wounds). Amox/clav has good *Eikenella,* MSSA, and anaerobic coverage but lacks MRSA coverage. Ampicillin/sulbactam also lacks MRSA coverage. For penicillin allergy, moxifloxacin can be used.[25]
Bullous impetigo[3,4,8,26] (usually *S aureus,* including CA-MRSA)	Standard: cephalexin 50–75 mg/kg/day PO div tid OR amox/clav 45 mg/kg/day PO div tid (CII) CA-MRSA: clindamycin 30 mg/kg/day PO div tid OR TMP/SMX 8 mg/kg/day of TMP PO div bid; for 5–7 days (CI)	For topical therapy if mild infection: mupirocin or retapamulin ointment
Cellulitis of unknown etiology (usually *S aureus,* including CA-MRSA, or group A streptococcus)[3–5,8,9,26–28]	Empiric IV therapy Standard: oxacillin/nafcillin 150 mg/kg/day IV div q6h OR cefazolin 100 mg/kg/day IV div q8h (BII) CA-MRSA: clindamycin 30 mg/kg/day IV div q8h OR ceftaroline: 2 mo–$<$2 y, 24 mg/kg/day IV div q8h; $\geq$2 y, 36 mg/kg/day IV div q8h (max single dose 400 mg); $>$33 kg, either 400 mg/dose IV q8h or 600 mg/dose IV q12h (BI) OR vancomycin 40 mg/kg/day IV q8h (BII) OR daptomycin: 1–$<$2 y, 10 mg/kg IV qd; 2–6 y, 9 mg/kg IV qd; 7–11 y, 7 mg/kg qd; 12–17 y, 5 mg/kg qd (BI) For oral therapy for MSSA: cephalexin (AII) OR amox/clav 45 mg/kg/day PO div tid (BII); for CA-MRSA: clindamycin (BII), TMP/SMX (AII), or linezolid (BII)	For periorbital or buccal cellulitis, also consider *Streptococcus pneumoniae* or *Haemophilus influenzae* type b in unimmunized infants. Total IV plus PO therapy for 7–10 days. Because nonsuppurative cellulitis is most often caused by group A streptococcus, cephalexin alone is usually effective. In adults, a prospective, randomized study of non-purulent cellulitis did not find that the addition of TMP/SMX improved outcomes over cephalexin alone.[28]

Cellulitis, buccal (for unimmunized infants and preschool-aged children, *H influenzae* type b)[29]	Ceftriaxone 50 mg/kg/day (AI) IV, IM q24h, for 2–7 days parenteral therapy before switch to oral (BII)	Rule out meningitis (larger dosages may then be needed). For penicillin allergy, levofloxacin IV/PO covers pathogens, but no clinical data available. Oral therapy: amoxicillin if beta-lactamase negative; amox/clav or oral 2nd- or 3rd-generation cephalosporin if beta-lactamase positive.
Cellulitis, erysipelas (streptococcal)[3,4,9,30]	Penicillin G 100,000–200,000 U/kg/day IV div q4–6h (BII) initially, then penicillin V 100 mg/kg/day PO div qid (BIII) OR amoxicillin 50 mg/kg/day PO div tid (BIII) for 10 days	Clindamycin and macrolides are also effective for most strains of group A streptococcus.
Gas gangrene (See Necrotizing fasciitis.)		
Impetigo (*S aureus*, including CA-MRSA; occasionally group A streptococcus)[3,4,8,9,31,32]	Mupirocin OR retapamulin topically (BII) to lesions tid; OR for more extensive lesions, oral therapy Standard: cephalexin 50–75 mg/kg/day PO div tid OR amox/clav 45 mg/kg/day PO div tid (AII) CA-MRSA: clindamycin 30 mg/kg/day (CII) PO div tid OR TMP/SMX 8 mg/kg/day TMP PO div bid (AI); for 5–7 days	Bacitracin ointment, widely available to treat skin infections, is inferior to cephalexin and mupirocin.[32]
Ludwig angina[33] (mixed oral aerobes/anaerobes)	Penicillin G 200,000–250,000 U/kg/day IV div q6h AND clindamycin 40 mg/kg/day IV div q8h (CIII)	Alternatives: ceftriaxone/clindamycin; meropenem, imipenem or pip/tazo if gram-negative aerobic bacilli also suspected (CIII); high risk of respiratory tract obstruction from inflammatory edema
Lymphadenitis (See Adenitis, acute bacterial.)		

A. SKIN AND SOFT TISSUE INFECTIONS (continued)

Clinical Diagnosis	Therapy (evidence grade)	Comments
Lymphangitis (usually group A streptococcus)[3,4,9]	Penicillin G 200,000 U/kg/day IV div q6h (BII) initially, then penicillin V 100 mg/kg/day PO div qid OR amoxicillin 50 mg/kg/day PO div tid for 10 days	Cefazolin IV (for group A strep or MSSA) or clindamycin IV (for group A strep, most MSSA and MRSA) For mild disease, penicillin V 50 mg/kg/day PO div qid for 10 days Some recent reports of *S aureus* as a cause
Myositis, suppurative[34] (*S aureus*, including CA-MRSA; synonyms: tropical myositis, pyomyositis)	Standard: oxacillin/nafcillin 150 mg/kg/day IV div q6h OR cefazolin 100 mg/kg/day IV div q8h (CII) CA-MRSA: clindamycin 40 mg/kg/day IV div q8h OR ceftaroline: 2 mo–<2 y, 24 mg/kg/day IV div q8h; ≥2 y, 36 mg/kg/day IV div q8h (max single dose 400 mg); >33 kg, either 400 mg/dose IV q8h or 600 mg/dose IV q12h (BI) OR vancomycin 40 mg/kg/day IV q8h (CIII) OR daptomycin: 1–<2 y, 10 mg/kg IV qd; 2–6 y, 9 mg/kg IV qd; 7–11 y, 7 mg/kg qd; 12–17 y, 5 mg/kg qd (BIII)	Surgical debridement is usually necessary. For disseminated MRSA infection, may require aggressive, emergent debridement; use clindamycin to help decrease toxin production (BIII); consider IVIG to bind bacterial toxins for life-threatening disease (CIII); abscesses may develop with CA-MRSA while on therapy. Highly associated with Panton-Valentine leukocidin.[35]
Necrotizing fasciitis (Pathogens vary depending on the age of the child and location of infection. Single pathogen: group A streptococcus; *Clostridia* spp, *S aureus* [including CA-MRSA], *Pseudomonas aeruginosa, Vibrio* spp, *Aeromonas*. Multiple pathogen, mixed aerobic/anaerobic synergistic fasciitis: any organism[s] above, plus gram-negative bacilli, plus *Bacteroides* spp, and other anaerobes.)[3,36–38]	Empiric therapy: ceftazidime 150 mg/kg/day IV div q8h, or cefepime 150 mg/kg/day IV div q8h or cefotaxime 200 mg/kg/day IV div q6h AND clindamycin 40 mg/kg/day IV div q8h (BIII); OR meropenem 60 mg/kg/day IV div q8h; OR pip/tazo 400 mg/kg/day pip component IV div q6h (AIII). ADD vancomycin OR ceftaroline for suspect CA-MRSA, pending culture results (AIII). Group A streptococcal: penicillin G 200,000–250,000 U/kg/day div q6h AND clindamycin 40 mg/kg/day div q8h (AIII). Mixed aerobic/anaerobic/gram-negative: meropenem or pip/tazo AND clindamycin (AIII).	Aggressive emergent wound debridement (AII). ADD clindamycin to inhibit synthesis of toxins during the first few days of therapy (AIII). If CA-MRSA identified and susceptible to clindamycin, additional vancomycin is not required. Consider IVIG to bind bacterial toxins for life-threatening disease (BIII). Value of hyperbaric oxygen is not established (CIII).[39] Focus definitive antimicrobial therapy based on culture results.

Pyoderma, cutaneous abscesses (*S aureus,* including CA-MRSA; group A streptococcus)[4,5,8,9,26,27,40–42]	Standard: cephalexin 50–75 mg/kg/day PO div tid OR amox/clav 45 mg/kg/day PO div tid (BII) CA-MRSA: clindamycin 30 mg/kg/day PO div tid (BII) OR TMP/SMX 8 mg/kg/day of TMP PO div bid (AI)	I&D when indicated; IV for serious infections. For prevention of recurrent CA-MRSA infection, use bleach baths twice weekly (½ cup of bleach per full bathtub) (BII), OR bathe with chlorhexidine soap daily or qod (BIII). Decolonization with nasal mupirocin may also be helpful, as is decolonization of the entire family.[43]
Rat-bite fever (*Streptobacillus moniliformis, Spirillum minus*)[44]	Penicillin G 100,000–200,000 U/kg/day IV div q6h (BII) for 7–10 days; for endocarditis, ADD gentamicin for 4–6 wk (CIII). For mild disease, oral therapy with amox/clav (CIII).	Organisms are normal oral flora for rodents. One does not require a bite to get infected. High rate of associated endocarditis. Alternatives: doxycycline; 2nd- and 3rd-generation cephalosporins (CIII).
Staphylococcal scalded skin syndrome[8,45,46]	Standard: oxacillin 150 mg/kg/day IV div q6h OR cefazolin 100 mg/kg/day IV div q8h (CII) CA-MRSA: clindamycin 30 mg/kg/day IV div q8h (CIII) OR ceftaroline: 2 mo–$<$2 y, 24 mg/kg/day IV div q8h; $\geq$2 y, 36 mg/kg/day IV div q8h (max single dose 400 mg); $>$33 kg, either 400 mg/dose IV q8h or 600 mg/dose IV q12h (BI), OR vancomycin 40 mg/kg/day IV q8h (CIII) OR daptomycin: 1–$<$2 y, 10 mg/kg IV qd; 2–6 y, 9 mg/kg IV qd; 7–11 y, 7 mg/kg qd; 12–17 y, 5 mg/kg qd (BI)	Burow or Zephiran compresses for oozing skin and intertriginous areas. Corticosteroids are contraindicated.

B. SKELETAL INFECTIONS

Clinical Diagnosis	Therapy (evidence grade)	Comments
NOTE: CA-MRSA (see Chapter 4) is prevalent in most areas of the world, although epidemiologic data suggest that MRSA infections are less common in skeletal infections than in skin infections. Recommendations are given for CA-MRSA and MSSA. Antibiotic recommendations for empiric therapy should include CA-MRSA when it is suspected or documented, while treatment for MSSA with beta-lactam antibiotics (eg, cephalexin) is preferred over clindamycin. During the past few years, clindamycin resistance in MRSA has increased to 40% in some areas but remained stable at 5% in others, although this increase may be an artifact of changes in reporting, with many laboratories now reporting all clindamycin-susceptible but D-test–positive strains as resistant. Please check your local susceptibility data for *Staphylococcus aureus* before using clindamycin for empiric therapy. For MSSA, oxacillin/nafcillin are considered equivalent agents. The first pediatric-specific PIDS/IDSA guidelines for bacterial osteomyelitis and bacterial arthritis are currently being written.		
Arthritis, bacterial[47–52]	Switch to appropriate high-dose oral therapy when clinically improved, CRP decreasing (see Chapter 13).[49,53,54]	
– Newborns	See Chapter 5.	
– Infants (*S aureus,* including CA-MRSA; group A streptococcus; *Kingella kingae*) – Children (*S aureus,* including CA-MRSA; group A streptococcus; *K kingae*) In unimmunized or immunocompromised children: pneumococcus, *H influenzae* type b For Lyme disease and brucellosis, see Table L, Miscellaneous Systemic Infections.	Empiric therapy: clindamycin 30 mg/kg/day IV div q8h (to cover CA-MRSA unless clindamycin resistance locally is >10%, then use vancomycin or ceftaroline). For serious, disseminated infections, ADD cefazolin 100 mg/kg/day IV div q8h if your primary antibiotic is clindamycin or vancomycin to provide better MSSA coverage. See Comments for discussion of dexamethasone adjunctive therapy. For documented CA-MRSA: clindamycin 30 mg/kg/day IV div q8h (AI) OR ceftaroline: 2 mo–<2 y, 24 mg/kg/day IV div q8h; ≥2 y, 36 mg/kg/day IV div q8h (max single dose 400 mg); >33 kg, either 400 mg/dose IV q8h or 600 mg/dose IV q12h (BI) OR vancomycin 40 mg/kg/day IV q8h (BI) For MSSA: oxacillin/nafcillin 150 mg/kg/day IV div q6h OR cefazolin 100 mg/kg/day IV div q8h (AI).	Dexamethasone adjunctive therapy (0.15 mg/kg/dose every 6 h for 4 days in one study) demonstrated significant benefit in decreasing symptoms and earlier hospital discharge (but with some "rebound" symptoms).[55,56] **NOTE:** children with rheumatologic, postinfectious, fungal/mycobacterial infections or malignancy are also likely to improve with steroid therapy despite ineffective antibiotics. Oral step-down therapy options: For CA-MRSA: clindamycin OR linezolid[51] For MSSA: cephalexin OR dicloxacillin caps for older children For *Kingella:* most penicillins or cephalosporins (but not clindamycin)

	For *Kingella:* cefazolin 100 mg/kg/day IV div q8h OR ampicillin 150 mg/kg/day IV div q6h, OR ceftriaxone 50 mg/kg/day IV, IM q24h (AII). For pen-S pneumococci or group A streptococcus: penicillin G 200,000 U/kg/day IV div q6h (BII). For pen-R pneumococci or *Haemophilus:* ceftriaxone 50–75 mg/kg/day IV, IM q24h, OR cefotaxime (BII). Total therapy (IV plus PO) for up to 21 days with normal ESR; low-risk, non-hip MSSA arthritis may respond to a 10-day course (AII).[51]	
– Gonococcal arthritis or tenosynovitis[57,58]	Ceftriaxone 50 mg/kg IV, IM q24h (BII) for 7 days AND azithromycin 20 mg/kg PO as a single dose	Combination therapy with azithromycin to decrease risk of development of resistance. Cefixime 8 mg/kg/day PO as a single daily dose may not be effective due to increasing resistance. Ceftriaxone IV, IM is preferred over cefixime PO.
– Other bacteria	See Chapter 7 for preferred antibiotics.	
Osteomyelitis[47–54,59–64]	Step down to appropriate high-dose oral therapy when clinically improved (see Chapter 13).[49,51,53,62]	
– Newborns	See Chapter 5.	

B. SKELETAL INFECTIONS (continued)

Clinical Diagnosis	Therapy (evidence grade)	Comments
– Infants and children, acute infection (usually *S aureus,* including CA-MRSA; group A streptococcus; *K kingae*[64])	Empiric therapy: clindamycin (for coverage of MSSA and MRSA in most locations). For serious infections, ADD cefazolin to provide better MSSA and *Kingella* coverage (CIII). For CA-MRSA: clindamycin 30 mg/kg/day IV div q8h OR vancomycin 40 mg/kg/day IV q8h (BII), OR ceftaroline: 2 mo–<2 y, 24 mg/kg/day IV div q8h; ≥2 y, 36 mg/kg/day IV div q8h (max single dose 400 mg); >33 kg, either 400 mg/dose IV q8h or 600 mg/dose IV q12h (BI). For MSSA: oxacillin/nafcillin 150 mg/kg/day IV div q6h OR cefazolin 100 mg/kg/day IV div q8h (AII). For *Kingella:* cefazolin 100 mg/kg/day IV div q8h OR ampicillin 150 mg/kg/day IV div q6h, OR ceftriaxone 50 mg/kg/day IV, IM q24h (BIII). Total therapy (IV plus PO) usually 4–6 wk for MSSA (with end-of-therapy normal ESR, radiograph to document healing) but may be as short as 3 wk for mild infection. May need longer than 4–6 wk for CA-MRSA (BII). Follow closely for clinical response to empiric therapy.	In children with open fractures secondary to trauma, add ceftazidime or cefepime for extended aerobic gram-negative bacilli activity. *Kingella* is often resistant to clindamycin and vancomycin. The proportion of MRSA in pediatric osteomyelitis is decreasing in some regions.[65] For MSSA (BI) and *Kingella* (BIII), step-down oral therapy with cephalexin 100 mg/kg/day PO div tid. *Kingella* is usually susceptible to amoxicillin. Oral step-down therapy options for CA-MRSA include clindamycin and linezolid,[66] with insufficient data to recommend TMP/SMX.[61] For prosthetic devices, biofilms may impair microbial eradication, requiring the addition of rifampin or other agents.[63]
– Acute, other organisms	See Chapter 7 for preferred antibiotics.	
– Chronic (staphylococcal)	For MSSA: cephalexin 100 mg/kg/day PO div tid OR dicloxacillin caps 75–100 mg/kg/day PO div qid for 3–6 mo or longer (CIII) For CA-MRSA: clindamycin or linezolid (CIII)	Surgery to debride sequestrum is usually required for cure. For prosthetic joint infection caused by staphylococci, add rifampin (CIII).[63] Watch for beta-lactam–associated neutropenia with high-dose, long-term therapy and linezolid-associated neutropenia/thrombocytopenia with long-term (>2 wk) therapy.[66]

Osteomyelitis of the foot[67,68] (osteochondritis after a puncture wound) *Pseudomonas aeruginosa* (occasionally *S aureus,* including CA-MRSA)	Cefepime 150 mg/kg/day IV div q8h (BIII); OR meropenem 60 mg/kg/day IV div q8h (BIII); OR ceftazidime 150 mg/kg/day IV, IM div q8h AND tobramycin 6–7.5 mg/kg/day IM, IV div q8h (BIII); if MRSA is suspected, ADD vancomycin OR ceftaroline OR clindamycin, pending culture results.	Cefepime and meropenem will provide coverage for MSSA in addition to *Pseudomonas.* Thorough surgical debridement required for *Pseudomonas* (second drainage procedure needed in at least 20% of children); oral convalescent therapy with ciprofloxacin is appropriate (BIII).[69] Treatment course 7–10 days after surgery.

C. EYE INFECTIONS

Clinical Diagnosis	Therapy (evidence grade)	Comments
Cellulitis, orbital[70–72] (cellulitis of the contents of the orbit; may be associated with orbital abscess; usually secondary to sinus infection; caused by respiratory tract flora and *Staphylococcus aureus,* including CA-MRSA)	Ceftriaxone 50 mg/kg/day q24h AND clindamycin 30 mg/kg/day IV div q8h (for *S aureus,* including CA-MRSA) or ceftaroline: 2 mo–<2 y, 24 mg/kg/day IV div q8h; ≥2 y, 36 mg/kg/day IV div q8h (max single dose 400 mg); >33 kg, either 400 mg/dose IV q8h or 600 mg/dose IV q12h (BIII) or vancomycin 40 mg/kg/day IV q8h (AIII). If MSSA isolated, use oxacillin/nafcillin IV OR cefazolin IV.	Surgical drainage of significant orbital or subperiosteal abscess if present by CT scan or MRI. Try medical therapy alone for small abscess (BIII).[73] Treatment course for 10–14 days after surgical drainage, up to 21 days. CT scan or MRI can confirm cure (BIII).
Cellulitis, periorbital[74] (preseptal cellulitis)	Periorbital tissues are TENDER with cellulitis. Periorbital edema with sinusitis can look identical but is NOT tender.	
– Associated with entry site lesion on skin (*S aureus,* including CA-MRSA, group A streptococcus) in the fully immunized child	Standard: oxacillin/nafcillin 150 mg/kg/day IV div q6h OR cefazolin 100 mg/kg/day IV div q8h (BII) CA-MRSA: clindamycin 30 mg/kg/day IV div q8h or ceftaroline: 2 mo–<2 y, 24 mg/kg/day IV div q8h; ≥2 y, 36 mg/kg/day IV div q8h (max single dose 400 mg); >33 kg, either 400 mg/dose IV q8h or 600 mg/dose IV q12h (BII)	Oral antistaphylococcal antibiotic (eg, clindamycin) for empiric therapy of less severe infection; treatment course for 7–10 days

C. EYE INFECTIONS (continued)

Clinical Diagnosis	Therapy (evidence grade)	Comments
– No associated entry site (in febrile, unimmunized infants): pneumococcal or *Haemophilus influenzae* type b	Ceftriaxone 50 mg/kg/day q24h OR cefuroxime 150 mg/kg/day IV div q8h (AII)	Treatment course for 7–10 days; rule out meningitis if bacteremic with *H influenzae*. Alternative agents for beta-lactamase–positive strains of *H influenzae:* other 2nd-, 3rd-, or 4th-generation cephalosporins or amoxicillin/clavulanate.
– Periorbital edema (not true cellulitis; usually associated with sinusitis); non-tender erythematous swelling Sinus pathogens *rarely* may erode anteriorly, causing cellulitis.	Ceftriaxone 50 mg/kg/day q24h OR cefuroxime 150 mg/kg/day IV div q8h (BIII). For suspect *S aureus* including CA-MRSA, can use ceftaroline instead of ceftriaxone. For chronic sinusitis ADD clindamycin (covers anaerobes) to either ceftriaxone or ceftaroline (AIII).	For oral convalescent antibiotic therapy, see Sinusitis, acute; total treatment course of 14–21 days or 7 days after resolution of symptoms.
Conjunctivitis, acute (*Haemophilus* and pneumococcus predominantly)[75–77]	Polymyxin/trimethoprim ophth soln OR polymyxin/bacitracin ophth ointment OR ciprofloxacin ophth soln (BII), for 7–10 days. For neonatal infection, see Chapter 5. Steroid-containing therapy only if HSV ruled out.	Other topical antibiotics (gentamicin, tobramycin, erythromycin, besifloxacin, moxifloxacin, norfloxacin, ofloxacin, levofloxacin) may offer advantages for particular pathogens (CII). High rates of resistance to sulfacetamide.
Conjunctivitis, herpetic[78–81]	1% trifluridine or 0.15% ganciclovir ophth gel (AII) AND acyclovir PO (80 mg/kg/day div qid; max daily dose: 3,200 mg/day) has been effective in limited studies (BIII). Oral valacyclovir (60 mg/kg/day div tid) has superior pharmacokinetics to oral acyclovir and can be considered for systemic treatment, as can parenteral (IV) acyclovir if extent of disease is severe (CIII).	Consultation with ophthalmologist required for assessment and management (eg, concomitant use of topical steroids in certain situations). Recurrences common; corneal scars may form. Long-term prophylaxis (≥1 y) for suppression of recurrent infection with oral acyclovir 300 mg/m^2/dose PO tid (max 400 mg/dose). Potential risks must balance potential benefits to vision (BIII).
Dacryocystitis	No antibiotic usually needed; oral therapy for more symptomatic infection, based on Gram stain and culture of pus; topical therapy as for conjunctivitis may be helpful.	Warm compresses; may require surgical probing of nasolacrimal duct.

Endophthalmitis[82,83]		
NOTE: Subconjunctival/sub-tenon antibiotics are likely to be required (vancomycin/ceftazidime or clindamycin/gentamicin); steroids commonly used (except for fungal infection); requires anterior chamber or vitreous tap for microbiological diagnosis. Listed systemic antibiotics to be used in addition to ocular injections.		Refer to ophthalmologist; vitrectomy may be necessary for advanced endophthalmitis. No prospective, controlled studies.
– Empiric therapy following open globe injury	Vancomycin 40 mg/kg/day IV div q8h AND cefepime 150 mg/kg/day IV div q8h (AIII)	
– Staphylococcal	Vancomycin 40 mg/kg/day IV div q8h pending susceptibility testing; oxacillin/nafcillin 150 mg/kg/day IV div q6h if susceptible (AIII)	Consider ceftaroline for MRSA treatment, as it may penetrate the vitreous better than vancomycin.
– Pneumococcal, meningococcal, *Haemophilus*	Ceftriaxone 100 mg/kg/day IV q24h; penicillin G 250,000 U/kg/day IV div q4h if susceptible (AIII)	Rule out meningitis; treatment course for 10–14 days.
– Gonococcal	Ceftriaxone 50 mg/kg q24h IV, IM AND azithromycin (AIII)	Treatment course 7 days or longer.
– *Pseudomonas*	Cefepime 150 mg/kg/day IV div q8h for 10–14 days (AIII)	Cefepime is preferred over ceftazidime for *Pseudomonas* based on decreased risk of development of resistance on therapy; meropenem IV or imipenem IV are alternatives (no clinical data). Very poor outcomes.
– *Candida*[84]	Fluconazole (25 mg/kg loading, then 12 mg/kg/day IV), OR voriconazole (9 mg/kg loading, then 8 mg/kg/day IV); for resistant strains, L-AmB (5 mg/kg/day IV). For chorioretinitis, systemic antifungals PLUS intravitreal amphotericin 5–10 mcg/0.1-mL sterile water OR voriconazole 100 mcg/0.1-mL sterile water or physiologic (normal) saline soln (AIII). Duration of therapy is at least 4–6 wk (AIII).	Echinocandins given IV may not be able to achieve adequate antifungal activity in the eye.
Hordeolum (sty) or chalazion	None (topical antibiotic not necessary)	Warm compresses; I&D when necessary

C. EYE INFECTIONS (continued)

Clinical Diagnosis	Therapy (evidence grade)	Comments
Retinitis		
– CMV[85–87] For neonatal, see Chapter 5. For HIV-infected children, see https://aidsinfo.nih.gov/guidelines/html/5/pediatric-opportunistic-infection/401/cytomegalovirus (accessed October 10, 2019).	Ganciclovir 10 mg/kg/day IV div q12h for 2 wk (BIII); if needed, continue at 5 mg/kg/day q24h to complete 6 wk total (BIII).	Neutropenia risk increases with duration of therapy. Foscarnet IV and cidofovir IV are alternatives but demonstrate significant toxicities. Letermovir approved for prophylaxis of CMV in stem cell transplant patients but has not been studied as treatment for CMV retinitis. Oral valganciclovir has not been evaluated in HIV-infected children with CMV retinitis but is an option primarily for older children who weigh enough to receive the adult dose of valganciclovir (CIII). Intravitreal ganciclovir and combination therapy for non-responding, immunocompromised hosts; however, intravitreal injections may not be practical for most children.

D. EAR AND SINUS INFECTIONS

Clinical Diagnosis	Therapy (evidence grade)	Comments
Bullous myringitis (See Otitis media, acute.)	Believed to be a clinical presentation of acute bacterial otitis media	
Mastoiditis, acute (pneumococcus [less since introduction of PCV13], *Staphylococcus aureus,* including CA-MRSA; group A streptococcus; increasing *Pseudomonas* in adolescents, *Haemophilus* rare)[88–90]	Ceftriaxone 50 mg/kg/day q24h AND clindamycin 40 mg/kg/day IV div q8h (BIII) For adolescents: cefepime 150 mg/kg/day IV div q8h AND clindamycin 40 mg/kg/day IV div q8h (BIII)	Rule out meningitis; surgery as needed for mastoid and middle ear drainage. Step down to appropriate oral therapy after clinical improvement, guided by culture results. Duration of therapy not well defined; look for evidence of mastoid osteomyelitis.
Mastoiditis, chronic (See also Otitis, chronic suppurative.) (anaerobes, *Pseudomonas, S aureus* [including CA-MRSA])[89]	Antibiotics only for acute superinfections (according to culture of drainage); for *Pseudomonas:* cefepime 150 mg/kg/day IV div q8h. Alternatives to enhance anaerobic coverage: meropenem 60 mg/kg/day IV div q8h, OR pip/tazo 240 mg/kg/day IV div q4–6h (BIII).	Daily cleansing of ear important; if no response to antibiotics, surgery. Be alert for CA-MRSA.
Otitis externa		
Bacterial, swimmer's ear (*Pseudomonas aeruginosa, S aureus,* including CA-MRSA)[91,92]	Topical antibiotics: fluoroquinolone (ciprofloxacin or ofloxacin) with steroid, OR neomycin/polymyxin B/hydrocortisone (BII) Irrigation and cleaning canal of detritus important	Wick moistened with Burow (aluminum acetate topical) soln, used for marked swelling of canal; to prevent swimmer's ear, 2% acetic acid to canal after water exposure will restore acid pH.
– Bacterial, malignant otitis externa (*P aeruginosa*)[93]	Cefepime 150 mg/kg/day IV div q8h (AIII)	Other antipseudomonal antibiotics should also be effective: ceftazidime IV AND tobramycin IV, OR meropenem IV or imipenem IV or pip/tazo IV. For more mild infection, ciprofloxacin PO.

D. EAR AND SINUS INFECTIONS (continued)

Clinical Diagnosis	Therapy (evidence grade)	Comments
– Bacterial furuncle of canal (*S aureus*, including CA-MRSA)	Standard: oxacillin/nafcillin 150 mg/kg/day IV div q6h OR cefazolin 100 mg/kg/day IV div q8h (BIII) CA-MRSA: clindamycin, ceftaroline, or vancomycin (BIII)	I&D; antibiotics for cellulitis. Oral therapy for mild disease, convalescent therapy. For MSSA: cephalexin. For CA-MRSA: clindamycin, TMP/SMX, OR linezolid (BIII).
– *Candida*	Fluconazole 6–12 mg/kg/day PO qd for 5–7 days (CIII)	May occur following antibiotic therapy of bacterial external otitis; debride canal.
Otitis media, acute		
NOTE: The natural history of AOM in different age groups by specific pathogens has not been well defined; therefore, the actual contribution of antibiotic therapy on resolution of disease had also been poorly defined until 2 blinded, prospective studies using amox/clav vs placebo were published in 2011,[94,95] although neither study used tympanocentesis to define a pathogen. The benefits and risks (including development of antibiotic resistance) of antibiotic therapy for AOM need to be further evaluated before the most accurate advice on the "best" antibiotic can be provided. However, based on available data, for most children, amoxicillin or amox/clav can be used initially. Considerations for the need for extended antimicrobial activity of amox/clav include severity of disease, young age of the child, previous antibiotic therapy within 6 months, and child care attendance, which address the issues of types of pathogens and antibiotic resistance patterns to expect. However, with universal PCV13 immunization, data suggest that the risk of antibiotic-resistant pneumococcal otitis has decreased but the percent of *Haemophilus* responsible for AOM have increased; therefore, some experts recommend use of amox/clav as first-line therapy for well-documented AOM. The most current AAP guidelines[96] and meta-analyses[97,98] suggest the greatest benefit with therapy occurs in children with bilateral AOM who are younger than 2 years; for other children, close observation is also an option. AAP guidelines provide an option to treatment in non-severe cases, particularly disease in older children, to provide a prescription to parents but have them only fill the prescription if the child deteriorates.[96] Although prophylaxis is only rarely indicated, amoxicillin or other antibiotics can be given at same mg/kg dose as for treatment but less frequently, once or twice daily to prevent infections (if the benefits outweigh the risks of development of resistant organisms for that child).[96]		
– Newborns	See Chapter 5.	
– Infants and children (pneumococcus, *Haemophilus influenzae* non–type b, *Moraxella* most common)[99–101]	Amox/clav (90 mg amox component/kg/day PO div bid). Amoxicillin is still a reasonable choice for empiric therapy, but failures will most likely be caused by beta-lactamase–producing *Haemophilus* (or *Moraxella*).	See Chapter 11 for dosages. Current data suggest that post-PCV13, *H influenzae* is now the most common pathogen, shifting the recommendation for empiric therapy from amoxicillin to amox/clav.[99–101] Published data document new emergence of penicillin

	a) For *Haemophilus* strains that are beta-lactamase positive, the following oral antibiotics offer better in vitro activity than amoxicillin: amox/clav, cefdinir, cefpodoxime, cefuroxime, ceftriaxone IM, levofloxacin. b) For pen-R pneumococci: high-dosage amoxicillin achieves greater middle ear activity than oral cephalosporins. Options include ceftriaxone IM 50 mg/kg/day q24h for 1–3 doses; OR levofloxacin 20 mg/kg/day PO div bid for children ≤5 y and 10 mg/kg PO qd for children >5 y; OR a macrolide-class antibiotic*: azithromycin PO at 1 of 3 dosages: (1) 10 mg/kg on day 1, followed by 5 mg/kg qd on days 2–5; (2) 10 mg/kg qd for 3 days; or (3) 30 mg/kg once. ***Caution:** Up to 40% of pneumococci are macrolide resistant.	resistance in pneumococci isolated in the post-PCV13 era,[102,103] suggesting that high-dosage amoxicillin (90 mg/kg/day) is still preferred for empiric therapy, although overall susceptibility in *Pneumococcus* is still far greater than in the pre-PCV7 era. The high serum and middle ear fluid concentrations achieved with 45 mg/kg/dose of amoxicillin, combined with a long half-life in middle ear fluid, allow for a therapeutic antibiotic exposure in the middle ear with only twice-daily dosing; high-dose amoxicillin (90 mg/kg/day) with clavulanate (Augmentin ES) is also available. If published data subsequently document low resistance to amoxicillin, standard dosage (45 mg/kg/day) can again be recommended. Tympanocentesis should be performed in children who fail second-line therapy.
Otitis, chronic suppurative (*P aeruginosa, S aureus,* including CA-MRSA, and other respiratory tract/skin flora)[92,103,104]	Topical antibiotics: fluoroquinolone (ciprofloxacin, ofloxacin, besifloxacin) with or without steroid (BIII) Cleaning of canal, view of tympanic membrane, for patency; cultures important	Presumed middle ear drainage through open tympanic membrane. Avoid aminoglycoside-containing therapy given risk of ototoxicity.[105] Other topical fluoroquinolones with/without steroids available.
Sinusitis, acute (*H influenzae* non–type b, pneumococcus, group A streptococcus, *Moraxella*)[99,106–110]	Same antibiotic therapy as for AOM as pathogens similar: amox/clav (90 mg amox component/kg/day PO div bid).[99] Therapy of 14 days may be necessary while mucosal swelling resolves and ventilation is restored.	IDSA sinusitis guidelines recommend amox/clav as first-line therapy,[109] while AAP guidelines recommend amoxicillin.[107] However, accumulating evidence for current isolates in the PCV13 era suggests that amox/clav is now the empiric therapy of choice for both sinusitis and otitis. There is no controlled evidence to determine whether the use of antihistamines, decongestants, or nasal irrigation is efficacious in children with acute sinusitis.[108]

E. OROPHARYNGEAL INFECTIONS

Clinical Diagnosis	Therapy (evidence grade)	Comments
Dental abscess (mixed aerobic/anaerobic oral flora)[111,112]	Clindamycin 30 mg/kg/day PO, IV, IM div q6–8h OR penicillin G 100–200,000 U/kg/day IV div q6h (AIII)	Amox/clav PO; amoxicillin PO is another option. Metronidazole has excellent anaerobic activity but no aerobic activity. Tooth extraction usually necessary. Erosion of abscess may occur into facial, sinusitis, deep head, and neck compartments.
Diphtheria pharyngitis[113]	Erythromycin 40–50 mg/kg/day PO div qid for 14 days OR penicillin G 150,000 U/kg/day IV div q6h; PLUS DAT (AIII)	DAT, a horse antisera, is investigational and only available from CDC Emergency Operations Center at 770/488-7100; www.cdc.gov/diphtheria/dat.html (accessed October 10, 2019).
Epiglottitis (supraglottitis; *Haemophilus influenzae* type b in an unimmunized child; rarely pneumococcus, *Staphylococcus aureus*)[114,115]	Ceftriaxone 50 mg/kg/day IV, IM q24h for 7–10 days	Emergency: provide airway. For suspected *S aureus* infection (causes only 5% of epiglottitis), consider substituting ceftaroline for ceftriaxone or adding clindamycin to ceftriaxone.
Gingivostomatitis, herpetic[116–118]	Acyclovir 80 mg/kg/day PO div qid (max dose: 800 mg) for 7 days (for severe disease, use IV therapy at 30 mg/kg/day div q8h) (BIII); OR for infants ≥3 mo, valacyclovir 20 mg/kg/dose PO bid (max dose: 1,000 mg; instructions for preparing liquid formulation with 28-day shelf life included in package insert) (CIII).[118]	Early treatment is likely to be the most effective. Start treatment as soon as oral intake is compromised. Valacyclovir is the prodrug of acyclovir that provides improved oral bioavailability compared with oral acyclovir. Extended duration of therapy may be needed for immunocompromised children. The oral acyclovir dose (80 mg/kg/day) provided is safe and effective for varicella, but 75 mg/kg/day div into 5 equal doses has been studied for HSV.[117] Maximum daily acyclovir dose should not exceed 3,200 mg.

Lemierre syndrome (*Fusobacterium necrophorum* primarily, new reports with MRSA)[119–123] (pharyngitis with internal jugular vein septic thrombosis, postanginal sepsis, necrobacillosis)	Empiric: meropenem 60 mg/kg/day div q8h (or 120 mg/kg/day div q8h for CNS metastatic foci) (AIII) OR ceftriaxone 100 mg/kg/day q24h AND metronidazole 40 mg/kg/day div q8h or clindamycin 40 mg/kg/day div q6h (BIII). ADD empiric vancomycin if MRSA suspected if clindamycin is not in the treatment regimen.	Anecdotal reports suggest metronidazole may be effective for apparent failures with other agents. Often requires anticoagulation. Metastatic and recurrent abscesses often develop while on active, appropriate therapy, requiring multiple debridements and prolonged antibiotic therapy. Treat until CRP and ESR are normal (AIII).
Peritonsillar cellulitis or abscess (group A streptococcus with mixed oral flora, including anaerobes, CA-MRSA)[124]	Clindamycin 30 mg/kg/day PO, IV, IM div q8h; for preschool infants with consideration of enteric bacilli, ADD ceftriaxone 50 mg/kg/day IV q24h (BIII).	Consider I&D for abscess. Alternatives: meropenem or imipenem or pip/tazo. Amox/clav for convalescent oral therapy (BIII). No controlled prospective data on benefits/risks of steroids.[125]
Pharyngitis (group A streptococcus primarily)[9,126–128]	Amoxicillin 50–75 mg/kg/day PO, either qd, bid, or tid for 10 days OR penicillin V 50–75 mg/kg/day PO, either qid, bid, or tid, OR benzathine penicillin 600,000 units IM for children <27 kg, 1.2 million units IM if >27 kg, as a single dose (AII) For penicillin-allergic children: erythromycin (estolate) at 20–40 mg/kg/day PO div bid to qid; OR 40 mg/kg/day PO div bid to qid) for 10 days; OR azithromycin 12 mg/kg qd for 5 days* (AII); OR clindamycin 30 mg/kg/day PO div tid *This is the dose investigated and FDA approved for children since 1994.	Although penicillin V is the most narrow spectrum treatment, amoxicillin displays better GI absorption than oral penicillin V; the suspension is better tolerated. These advantages should be balanced by the unnecessary increased spectrum of activity. Once-daily amoxicillin dosage: for children 50 mg/kg (max 1,000–1,200 mg).[9] Meta-analysis suggests that oral cephalosporins are more effective than penicillin for treatment of strep.[129] A 5-day treatment course is FDA approved for azithromycin at 12 mg/kg/day for 5 days, and some oral cephalosporins have been approved (cefdinir, cefpodoxime), with rapid clinical response to treatment that can also be seen with other antibiotics; a 10-day course is preferred for the prevention of ARF, particularly areas where ARF is prevalent, as no data exist on efficacy of 5 days of therapy for prevention of ARF.[128,130]

E. OROPHARYNGEAL INFECTIONS (continued)

Clinical Diagnosis	Therapy (evidence grade)	Comments
Retropharyngeal, parapharyngeal, or lateral pharyngeal cellulitis or abscess (mixed aerobic/anaerobic flora, now including CA-MRSA)[124,131–133]	Clindamycin 40 mg/kg/day IV div q8h AND ceftriaxone 50 mg/kg/day IV q24h	Consider I&D; possible airway compromise, mediastinitis. Alternatives: meropenem or imipenem (BIII); pip/tazo. Can step-down to less broad-spectrum coverage based on cultures. Amox/clav for convalescent oral therapy (but no activity for MRSA) (BIII).
Tracheitis, bacterial (*S aureus,* including CA-MRSA; group A streptococcus; pneumococcus; *H influenzae* type b, rarely *Pseudomonas*)[134,135]	Vancomycin 40 mg/kg/day IV div q8h or clindamycin 40 mg/kg/day IV div q8h AND ceftriaxone 50 mg/kg/day q24h OR ceftaroline single drug therapy: 2 mo–<2 y, 24 mg/kg/day IV div q8h; ≥2 y, 36 mg/kg/day IV div q8h (max single dose 400 mg); >33 kg, either 400 mg/dose IV q8h or 600 mg/dose IV q12h (BIII)	For susceptible *S aureus,* oxacillin/nafcillin or cefazolin. May represent bacterial superinfection of viral laryngotracheobronchitis, including influenza.

F. LOWER RESPIRATORY TRACT INFECTIONS

Clinical Diagnosis	Therapy (evidence grade)	Comments
Abscess, lung		
– Primary (severe, necrotizing community-acquired pneumonia caused by pneumococcus, *Staphylococcus aureus,* including CA-MRSA, group A streptococcus)[136–138]	Empiric therapy with ceftriaxone 50–75 mg/kg/day q24h AND clindamycin 40 mg/kg/day div q8h or vancomycin 45 mg/kg/day IV div q8h for 14–21 days or longer (AIII) OR (for MRSA) ceftaroline: 2–<6 mo, 30 mg/kg/day IV div q8h (each dose given over 2 h); ≥6 mo, 45 mg/kg/day IV div q8h (each dose given over 2 h) (max single dose 600 mg) (BII)	For severe CA-MRSA infections, see Chapter 4. Bronchoscopy may be necessary if abscess fails to drain; surgical excision rarely necessary for pneumococcus but may be important for CA-MRSA and MSSA. Focus antibiotic coverage based on culture results. For MSSA: oxacillin/nafcillin or cefazolin.
– Secondary to aspiration (ie, foul smelling; polymicrobial infection with oral aerobes and anaerobes)[139]	Clindamycin 40 mg/kg/day IV div q8h or meropenem 60 mg/kg/day IV div q8h for 10 days or longer (AIII)	Alternatives: imipenem IV or pip/tazo IV (BIII) Oral step-down therapy with clindamycin or amox/clav (BIII)
Allergic bronchopulmonary aspergillosis[140]	Prednisone 0.5 mg/kg qd for 1–2 wk and then taper (BII) for mild, acute stage illness AND (for more severe disease) voriconazole[141] 18 mg/kg/day PO div q12h load followed by 16 mg/kg/day div q12h (AIII) OR itraconazole[142] 10 mg/kg/day PO div q12h (BII). Voriconazole and itraconazole require trough concentration monitoring.	Not all allergic pulmonary disease is associated with true fungal infection. Larger steroid dosages to control inflammation may lead to tissue invasion by *Aspergillus.* Corticosteroids are the cornerstone of therapy for exacerbations, and itraconazole and voriconazole have a demonstrable corticosteroid-sparing effect.
Aspiration pneumonia (polymicrobial infection with oral aerobes and anaerobes)[139]	Clindamycin 40 mg/kg/day IV div q8h; ADD ceftriaxone 50–75 mg/kg/day q24h for additional *Haemophilus* activity OR, as a single agent, meropenem 60 mg/kg/day IV div q8h; for 10 days or longer (BIII).	Alternatives: imipenem IV or pip/tazo IV (BIII) Oral step-down therapy with clindamycin or amox/clav (BIII)

F. LOWER RESPIRATORY TRACT INFECTIONS (continued)

Clinical Diagnosis	Therapy (evidence grade)	Comments
Atypical pneumonia (See *Mycoplasma pneumoniae*, Legionnaires disease.)		
Bronchitis (bronchiolitis), acute[143]	For bronchitis/bronchiolitis in children, no antibiotic needed for most cases, as disease is usually viral	With PCR multiplex diagnosis now widely available, a nonbacterial diagnosis will allow clinician to avoid use of antibiotics, but viral/bacterial coinfection can still occur.
Community-acquired pneumonia (See Pneumonia: Community-acquired, bronchopneumonia; Pneumonia: Community-acquired, lobar consolidation.)		
Cystic fibrosis: Seek advice from experts in acute and chronic management. Larger than standard dosages of beta-lactam antibiotics are required in most patients with cystic fibrosis.[144] Dosages of beta-lactams should achieve their pharmacokinetic/pharmacodynamic goals to increase chances of response.[145] The Cystic Fibrosis Foundation posts guidelines (https://www.cff.org/Care/Clinical-Care-Guidelines/Respiratory-Clinical-Care-Guidelines/Pulmonary-Exacerbations-Clinical-Care-Guidelines; accessed October 10, 2019).		
– Acute exacerbation (*Pseudomonas aeruginosa* primarily; also *Burkholderia cepacia, Stenotrophomonas maltophilia, S aureus,* including CA-MRSA, nontuberculous mycobacteria)[146–151]	Cefepime 150–200 mg/kg/day div q8h or meropenem 120 mg/kg/day div q6h AND tobramycin 6–10 mg/kg/day IM, IV div q6–8h for treatment of acute exacerbation (AII); alternatives: imipenem, ceftazidime, or ciprofloxacin 30 mg/kg/day PO, IV div tid. May require vancomycin 60–80 mg/kg/day IV div q8h for MRSA, OR ceftaroline 45 mg/kg/day IV div q8h (each dose given over 2 h) (max single dose 600 mg) (BIII). Duration of therapy not well defined: 10–14 days (BIII).[147]	Monitor concentrations of aminoglycosides, vancomycin. Insufficient evidence to recommend routine use of inhaled antibiotics for acute exacerbations.[152] Cultures with susceptibility and synergy testing will help select antibiotics, as multidrug resistance is common, but synergy testing is not well standardized.[153,154] Combination therapy may provide synergistic killing and delay the emergence of resistance (BIII). Attempt at early eradication of new onset *Pseudomonas* may decrease progression of disease.[149,155] Failure to respond to antibacterials should prompt evaluation for appropriate drug doses and for invasive/allergic fungal disease as well as maximizing pulmonary hygiene.

– Chronic inflammation (Minimize long-term damage to lung.)	Inhaled tobramycin 300 mg bid, cycling 28 days on therapy, 28 days off therapy, is effective adjunctive therapy between exacerbation, with new data suggesting a benefit of alternating inhaled tobramycin with inhaled aztreonam (AI).[153,156,157] Azithromycin adjunctive chronic therapy, greatest benefit for those colonized with *Pseudomonas* (AII).[158,159]	Alternative inhaled antibiotics: colistin[152,160] (BIII). Two newer powder preparations of inhaled tobramycin are available.
Pertussis[161–163]	Azithromycin: those ≥6 mo, 10 mg/kg/day for day 1, then 5 mg/kg/day for days 2–5; for those <6 mo, 10 mg/kg/day for 5 days; OR clarithromycin 15 mg/kg/day div bid for 7 days; or erythromycin (estolate preferable) 40 mg/kg/day PO div qid for 7–10 days (AII) Alternative: TMP/SMX 8 mg/kg/day TMP div bid for 14 days (BIII)	Azithromycin and clarithromycin are better tolerated than erythromycin; azithromycin is preferred in young infants to reduce pyloric stenosis risk (see Chapter 5). Provide prophylaxis to family members. Unfortunately, no adjunctive therapy has been shown beneficial in decreasing the cough.[164]
Pneumonia: Community-acquired, bronchopneumonia		
– Mild to moderate illness (overwhelmingly viral, especially in preschool children)[165]	No antibiotic therapy unless epidemiologic, clinical, or laboratory reasons to suspect bacteria or *Mycoplasma*.	Broad-spectrum antibiotics may increase risk of subsequent infection with antibiotic-resistant pathogens.

F. LOWER RESPIRATORY TRACT INFECTIONS (continued)

Clinical Diagnosis	Therapy (evidence grade)	Comments
– Moderate to severe illness (pneumococcus; group A streptococcus; *S aureus,* including CA-MRSA; *Mycoplasma pneumoniae*[136,137,166–168]; for those with aspiration and underlying comorbidities, *H influenzae,* non-typable); and for unimmunized children, *H influenzae* type b	Empiric therapy For regions with high PCV13 vaccine use or low pneumococcal resistance to penicillin: ampicillin 150–200 mg/kg/day div q6h. For regions with low rates of PCV13 use or high pneumococcal resistance to penicillin: ceftriaxone 50–75 mg/kg/day q24h(AI). For suspected CA-MRSA: ceftaroline: 2–<6 mo, 30 mg/kg/day IV div q8h (each dose given over 2 h); ≥6 mo, 45 mg/kg/day IV div q8h (each dose given over 2 h) (max single dose 600 mg) (BII),[167] OR vancomycin 40–60 mg/kg/day (AIII).[3] For suspect *Mycoplasma*/atypical pneumonia agents, particularly in school-aged children, ADD azithromycin 10 mg/kg IV, PO on day 1, then 5 mg/kg qd for days 2–5 of treatment (AII).	Tracheal aspirate or bronchoalveolar lavage for Gram stain/culture for severe infection in intubated children. Check vancomycin serum concentrations and renal function, particularly at the higher dosage needed to achieve an AUC:MIC of 400 for CA-MRSA pneumonia. Alternatives to azithromycin for atypical pneumonia include erythromycin IV, PO, or clarithromycin PO, or doxycycline IV, PO for children >7 y, or levofloxacin. New data suggest that combination empiric therapy with a beta-lactam and a macrolide confers no benefit over beta-lactam monotherapy.[169,170] Empiric oral outpatient therapy for less severe illness: high-dosage amoxicillin 80–100 mg/kg/day PO div tid (NOT bid, which is used for otitis) (BIII).
Pneumonia: Community-acquired, lobar consolidation		
Pneumococcus (May occur with non-PCV13[136,137,166–168]	Empiric therapy For regions with high PCV13 vaccine use or low pneumococcal resistance to penicillin: ampicillin 150–200 mg/kg/day div q6h. For regions with low rates of PCV13 use or high pneumococcal resistance to penicillin: ceftriaxone 50–75 mg/kg/day q24h (AI) Empiric oral outpatient therapy for less severe illness: high-dosage amoxicillin 80–100 mg/kg/day PO div tid (NOT bid, which is used for otitis).	Change to PO after improvement (decreased fever, no oxygen needed); treat until clinically asymptomatic and chest radiography significantly improved (7–21 days) (BIII). No reported failures of ceftriaxone for pen-R pneumococcus; no need to add empiric vancomycin for this reason (CIII). Oral therapy for pneumococcus may also be successful with amox/clav, cefdinir, cefixime, cefpodoxime, or cefuroxime. Levofloxacin is an alternative, particularly for those with severe allergy to beta-lactam antibiotics (BI),[171] but due to theoretical cartilage toxicity concerns for humans, should not be first-line therapy.

– Pneumococcal, pen-S	Penicillin G 250,000–400,000 U/kg/day IV div q4–6h for 10 days (BII) OR ampicillin 150–200 mg/kg/day IV div q6h	After improvement, change to PO amoxicillin 50–75 mg/kg/day PO div tid OR penicillin V 50–75 mg/kg/day div qid.
– Pneumococcal, pen-R	Ceftriaxone 75 mg/kg/day q24h for 10–14 days (BIII)	Addition of vancomycin has not been required for eradication of pen-R strains. Ceftaroline is more active against pneumococcus than ceftriaxone, but with no current ceftriaxone resistance, ceftaroline is not required. For oral convalescent therapy, high-dosage amoxicillin (100–150 mg/kg/day PO div tid), clindamycin (30 mg/kg/day PO div tid), linezolid (30 mg/kg/day PO div tid), or levofloxacin PO.
Staphylococcus aureus (including CA-MRSA)[4,8,136,166,172,173]	For MSSA: oxacillin/nafcillin 150 mg/kg/day IV div q6h or cefazolin 100 mg/kg/day IV div q8h (AII). For suspected CA-MRSA: ceftaroline: 2–<6 mo, 30 mg/kg/day IV div q8h (each dose given over 2 h); ≥6 mo, 45 mg/kg/day IV div q8h (each dose given over 2 h) (max single dose 600 mg) (BII),[167] OR vancomycin 40–60 mg/kg/day (AIII)[3]; may need addition of rifampin, clindamycin, or gentamicin (AIII) (see Chapter 4).	Check vancomycin serum concentrations and renal function, particularly at the higher dosage designed to attain an AUC:MIC of 400, or serum trough concentrations of 15 mcg/mL for invasive CA-MRSA disease. For life-threatening disease, optimal therapy of CA-MRSA is not defined: add gentamicin and/or rifampin for combination therapy (CIII). Linezolid 30 mg/kg/day IV, PO div q8h is another option, more effective in adults than vancomycin for MRSA nosocomial pneumonia[174] (follow platelets and WBC count weekly).

F. LOWER RESPIRATORY TRACT INFECTIONS (continued)

Clinical Diagnosis	Therapy (evidence grade)	Comments
Pneumonia: Immunosuppressed, neutropenic host[175] (*P aeruginosa*, other community-associated or nosocomial gram-negative bacilli, *S aureus*, fungi, AFB, *Pneumocystis*, viral [adenovirus, CMV, EBV, influenza, RSV, others])	Cefepime 150 mg/kg/day IV div q8h (AII), OR meropenem 60 mg/kg/day div q8h (AII) (BIII); AND if *S aureus* (including MRSA) is suspected clinically, ADD vancomycin 40–60 mg/kg/day IV div q8h (AIII) OR ceftaroline: 2–<6 mo, 30 mg/kg/day IV div q8h; ≥6 mo, 45 mg/kg/day IV div q8h (max single dose 600 mg) (BIII).	Biopsy or bronchoalveolar lavage, or cell-free serum for next-generation sequencing testing, usually needed to determine need for antifungal, antiviral, antimycobacterial treatment. Antifungal therapy usually started if no response to antibiotics in 48–72 h (AmB, voriconazole, or caspofungin/micafungin — see Chapter 8). For septic patients, the addition of tobramycin will increase coverage for gram-negative pathogens. For those with mucositis, anaerobic coverage may be needed. Consider use of 2 active agents for definitive therapy for *Pseudomonas* for neutropenic hosts to assist clearing the pathogen and potentially decrease risk of resistance (BIII).
– **Pneumonia: Interstitial pneumonia syndrome of early infancy**	If *Chlamydia trachomatis* suspected, azithromycin 10 mg/kg on day 1, followed by 5 mg/kg/day qd days 2–5 OR erythromycin 40 mg/kg/day PO div qid for 14 days (BII)	Most often respiratory viral pathogens, CMV, or chlamydial; role of *Ureaplasma* uncertain
– **Pneumonia, nosocomial (health care–associated/ ventilator-associated)** (*P aeruginosa*, gram-negative enteric bacilli [*Enterobacter, Klebsiella, Serratia, Escherichia coli*], *Acinetobacter, Stenotrophomonas*, and gram-positive organisms including CA-MRSA and *Enterococcus*)[176–178]	Commonly used regimens Meropenem 60 mg/kg/day div q8h, OR pip/tazo 240–300 mg/kg/day div q6–8h, OR cefepime 150 mg/kg/day div q8h; ± gentamicin 6.0–7.5 mg/kg/day div q8h (AIII); ADD vancomycin or ceftaroline for suspect CA-MRSA (AIII).	Empiric therapy should be institution specific, based on your hospital's nosocomial pathogens and susceptibilities. Pathogens that cause nosocomial pneumonia often have multidrug resistance. Cultures are critical. Empiric therapy also based on child's prior colonization/infection. Do not treat colonization, though. For MDR gram-negative bacilli, available IV therapy options include ceftazidime/avibactam (now FDA approved for children), ceftolozane/tazobactam, meropenem/vaborbactam, plazomicin, or colistin. Aerosol delivery of antibiotics may be required for MDR pathogens, but little high-quality controlled data are available for children.[179]

– **Pneumonia: With pleural fluid/empyema** (same pathogens as for community-associated bronchopneumonia) (Based on extent of fluid and symptoms, may benefit from chest tube drainage with fibrinolysis or video-assisted thoracoscopic surgery.)[166,180–183]	Empiric therapy: ceftriaxone 50–75 mg/kg/day q24h AND vancomycin 40–60 mg/kg/day IV div q8h (BIII) OR ceftaroline as single drug therapy: 2–<6 mo, 30 mg/kg/day IV div q8h; ≥6 mo, 45 mg/kg/day IV div q8h (each dose given over 2 h) (max single dose 600 mg) (BII)	Initial therapy based on Gram stain of empyema fluid; typically, clinical improvement is slow, with persisting but decreasing "spiking" fever for 2–3 wk. Concerns about the effectiveness of vancomycin monotherapy in influenza-associated MRSA pneumonia.[183]
– Group A streptococcal	Penicillin G 250,000 U/kg/day IV div q4–6h for 10 days (BII)	Change to PO amoxicillin 75 mg/kg/day div tid or penicillin V 50–75 mg/kg/day div qid to tid after clinical improvement (BIII).
– Pneumococcal	(See Pneumonia: Community-acquired, lobar consolidation.)	
S aureus (including CA-MRSA)[4,8,136,172]	For MSSA: oxacillin/nafcillin or cefazolin (AII). For CA-MRSA: ceftaroline: 2–<6 mo, 30 mg/kg/day IV div q8h (each dose given over 2 h); ≥6 mo, 45 mg/kg/day IV div q8h (each dose given over 2 h) (max single dose 600 mg) (BII),[167] OR vancomycin 60 mg/kg/day (AIII) (designed to attain an AUC:MIC of 400, or serum trough concentrations of 15 mcg/mL); follow serum concentrations and renal function; (see Chapter 4).	For life-threatening disease, optimal therapy of CA-MRSA is not defined; add gentamicin and/or rifampin. For influenza-associated MRSA pneumonia, vancomycin monotherapy was inferior to combination therapies.[183] Alternatives include clindamycin and linezolid. Do NOT use daptomycin for pneumonia. For MRSA nosocomial pneumonia in adults, linezolid was superior to vancomycin.[174] Oral convalescent therapy for MSSA: cephalexin PO; for CA-MRSA: clindamycin or linezolid PO. Total course for 21 days or longer (AIII).
Pneumonias of other established etiologies (See Chapter 7 for treatment by pathogen.)		
– *Chlamydia*[184] *pneumoniae, Chlamydophila psittaci,* or *Chlamydia trachomatis*	Azithromycin 10 mg/kg on day 1, followed by 5 mg/kg/day qd days 2–5 or erythromycin 40 mg/kg/day PO div qid; for 14 days	Doxycycline (patients >7 y). Levofloxacin should also be effective.

F. LOWER RESPIRATORY TRACT INFECTIONS (continued)

Clinical Diagnosis	Therapy (evidence grade)	Comments
– CMV (immunocompromised host)[185,186] (See chapters 5 and 9 for CMV infection in newborns and older children, respectively.)	Ganciclovir IV 10 mg/kg/day IV div q12h for 2 wk (BIII); if needed, continue at 5 mg/kg/day q24h to complete 4–6 wk total (BIII).	Bone marrow transplant recipients with CMV pneumonia who fail to respond to ganciclovir therapy alone may benefit from therapy with IV CMV hyperimmunoglobulin and ganciclovir given together (BII).[187–189] Oral valganciclovir may be used for convalescent therapy (BIII). Foscarnet for ganciclovir-resistant strains.
– *E coli*	Ceftriaxone 50–75 mg/kg/day q24h (AII)	For cephalosporin-resistant strains (ESBL producers), use meropenem, imipenem, or ertapenem (AIII). Use high-dose ampicillin if susceptible.
– *Enterobacter* spp	Cefepime 100 mg/kg/day div q12h or meropenem 60 mg/kg/day div q8h; OR ceftriaxone 50–75 mg/kg/day q24h AND gentamicin 6.0–7.5 mg/kg/day IM, IV div q8h (AIII)	Addition of aminoglycoside to 3rd-generation cephalosporins may retard the emergence of ampC-mediated constitutive high-level resistance, but concern exists for inadequate aminoglycoside concentration in airways; not an issue with beta-lactams (cefepime, meropenem, or imipenem).
– *Francisella tularensis*[190]	Gentamicin 6.0–7.5 mg/kg/day IM, IV div q8h for 10 days or longer for more severe disease (AIII); for less severe disease, doxycycline PO for 14–21 days (AIII)	Alternatives for oral therapy of mild disease: ciprofloxacin or levofloxacin (BIII)

– Fungi (See Chapter 8.) Community-associated pathogens, vary by region (eg, *Coccidioides*,[191,192] *Histoplasma*)[193,194] *Aspergillus*, mucormycosis, other mold infections in immunocompromised hosts (See Chapter 8.)	For detailed pathogen-specific recommendations, see Chapter 8. For suspected endemic fungi or mucormycosis in immunocompromised host, treat empirically with a lipid AmB and not voriconazole; biopsy needed to guide therapy. Posaconazole has in vitro activity against some *Rhizopus* spp. For suspected invasive aspergillosis, treat with voriconazole (AI) (load 18 mg/kg/day div q12h on day 1, then continue 16 mg/kg/day div q12h).	For normal hosts, triazoles (fluconazole, itraconazole, voriconazole, posaconazole, isavuconazole) are better tolerated than AmB and equally effective for many community-associated pathogens (see Chapter 2). For dosage, see Chapter 8. Check voriconazole trough concentrations; need to be at least >2 mcg/mL. For refractory *Coccidioides* infection, posaconazole or combination therapy with voriconazole and caspofungin may be effective[191] (AIII).
– Influenza virus[195,196] – Recent seasonal influenza A and B strains continue to be resistant to adamantanes.	Empiric therapy, or documented influenza A or B Oseltamivir[196,197] (AII): <12 mo: Term infants 0–8 mo: 3 mg/kg/dose bid 9–11 mo: 3.5 mg/kg/dose bid ≥12 mo: ≤15 kg: 30 mg PO bid >15–23 kg: 45 mg PO bid >23–40 kg: 60 mg PO bid >40 kg: 75 mg PO bid Zanamivir inhaled (AII): for those ≥7 y 10 mg (two 5-mg inhalations) bid Peramivir (BII): 2–12 y: single IV dose of 12 mg/kg, up to 600 mg max 13–17 y: Single IV dose of 600 mg Baloxavir (BI): ≥12 y: 40–79 kg: single PO dose of 40 mg ≥80 kg: single PO dose of 80 mg	Check for antiviral susceptibility each season at www.cdc.gov/flu/professionals/antivirals/index.htm (reviewed July 10, 2019; accessed October 10, 2019). For children 12–23 mo, the unit dose of 30 mg/dose may provide inadequate drug exposure. 3.5 mg/kg/dose PO bid has been studied,[197] but sample sizes have been inadequate to recommend weight-based dosing at this time. Limited data for oseltamivir in preterm neonates[196]: <38 wk PMA (gestational plus chronologic age): 1.0 mg/kg/dose PO bid 38–40 wk PMA: 1.5 mg/kg/dose PO bid Baloxavir under study in children <12 y. The adamantanes (amantadine and rimantadine) had activity against influenza A prior to the late 1990s, but all circulating A strains of influenza have been resistant for many years. Influenza B is intrinsically resistant to adamantanes.

F. LOWER RESPIRATORY TRACT INFECTIONS (continued)

Clinical Diagnosis	Therapy (evidence grade)	Comments
– *Klebsiella pneumoniae*[198,199]	Ceftriaxone 50–75 mg/kg/day IV, IM q24h (AIII); for ceftriaxone-resistant strains (ESBL strains), use meropenem 60 mg/kg/day IV div q8h (AIII) or other carbapenem.	For *K pneumoniae* that contain ESBLs, pip/tazo and fluoroquinolones are other options. New data presented in 2018 in adults suggest that outcomes with pip/tazo are inferior to carbapenems.[199] For KPC-producing strains that are resistant to meropenem: alternatives include ceftazidime/avibactam (FDA-approved for adults and now pediatrics in 2019), fluoroquinolones, or colistin (BIII).
– Legionnaires disease (*Legionella pneumophila*)	Azithromycin 10 mg/kg IV, PO q24h for 5 days (AIII)	Alternatives: clarithromycin, erythromycin, ciprofloxacin, levofloxacin, doxycycline
– Mycobacteria, nontuberculous (*Mycobacterium avium* complex most common)[200]	In a normal host: azithromycin PO or clarithromycin PO for 6–12 wk if susceptible For more extensive disease: a macrolide AND rifampin AND ethambutol; ± amikacin or streptomycin (AIII)	Highly variable susceptibilities of different nontuberculous mycobacterial species. Culture and susceptibility data are important for success. Check if immunocompromised: HIV or gamma-interferon receptor deficiency
– *Mycobacterium tuberculosis* (See Tuberculosis.)		
– *Mycoplasma pneumoniae*[166,201]	Azithromycin 10 mg/kg on day 1, followed by 5 mg/kg/day qd days 2–5, or clarithromycin 15 mg/kg/day div bid for 7–14 days, or erythromycin 40 mg/kg/day PO div qid for 14 days	*Mycoplasma* often causes self-limited infection and does not routinely require treatment (AIII). Little prospective, well-controlled data exist for treatment of documented mycoplasma pneumonia specifically in children.[201] Doxycycline (patients $>$7 y) or levofloxacin. Macrolide-resistant strains have recently appeared worldwide.[202]
– *Paragonimus westermani*	See Chapter 10.	

– *Pneumocystis jiroveci* (formerly *Pneumocystis carinii*)[203]; disease in immunosuppressed children and those with HIV	Severe disease: preferred regimen is TMP/SMX, 15–20 mg TMP component/kg/day IV div q8h for 3 wk (AI). Mild to moderate disease: may start with IV therapy, then after acute pneumonitis is resolving, TMP/SMX 20 mg of TMP/kg/day PO div qid for 21 days (AII). Use steroid adjunctive treatment for more severe disease (AII).	Alternatives for TMP/SMX intolerant, or clinical failure: pentamidine 3–4 mg IV qd, infused over 60–90 min (AII); TMP AND dapsone; OR primaquine AND clindamycin; OR atovaquone. Prophylaxis: TMP/SMX as 5 mg TMP/kg/day PO, divided in 2 doses, q12h, daily or 3 times/wk on consecutive days (AI); OR TMP/SMX 5 mg TMP/kg/day PO as a single dose, once daily, given 3 times/wk on consecutive days (AI); once-weekly regimens have also been successful[204]; OR dapsone 2 mg/kg (max 100 mg) PO qd, or 4 mg/kg (max 200 mg) once weekly; OR atovaquone: 30 mg/kg/day for infants 1–3 mo, 45 mg/kg/day for infants 4–24 mo, and 30 mg/kg/day for children >24 mo.
– *P aeruginosa*[179,205–207]	Cefepime 150 mg/kg/day IV div q8h ± tobramycin 6.0–7.5 mg/kg/day IM, IV div q8h (AII). Alternatives: meropenem 60 mg/kg/day div q8h, OR pip/tazo 240–300 mg/kg/day div q6–8h (AII) ± tobramycin (BIII).	Ciprofloxacin IV, or colistin IV for MDR strains of *Enterobacteriaceae* or *Pseudomonas* (See Chapter 4.)[207]
RSV infection (bronchiolitis, pneumonia)[208]	For immunocompromised hosts, the only FDA-approved treatment is ribavirin aerosol: 6-g vial (20 mg/mL in sterile water), by SPAG-2 generator, over 18–20 h daily for 3–5 days, although questions remain regarding efficacy.	Treat only for severe disease, immunocompromised, severe underlying cardiopulmonary disease, as aerosol ribavirin only provides a small benefit. Airway reactivity with inhalation precludes routine use. Palivizumab (Synagis) is not effective for treatment of an active RSV infection, only cost-effective for prevention of hospitalization in high-risk patients. One RSV antiviral, JNJ-53718678, is currently under investigation in children.

F. LOWER RESPIRATORY TRACT INFECTIONS (continued)

Clinical Diagnosis	Therapy (evidence grade)	Comments
— Tuberculosis		
– Primary pulmonary disease[15,16]	INH 10–15 mg/kg/day (max 300 mg) PO qd for 6 mo AND rifampin 10–20 mg/kg/day (max 600 mg) PO qd for 6 mo AND PZA 30–40 mg/kg/day (max 2 g) PO qd for first 2 mo therapy only (AII). Twice weekly treatment, particularly with DOT, is acceptable.[15] If risk factors present for multidrug resistance, ADD ethambutol 20 mg/kg/day PO qd OR streptomycin 30 mg/kg/day IV, IM div q12h initially.	Obtain baseline LFTs. Consider monthly LFTs for at least 3 mo or as needed for symptoms. It is common to have mildly elevated liver transaminase concentrations (2–3 times normal) that do not further increase during the entire treatment interval. Obese children may have mild elevation when started on therapy. Contact TB specialist for therapy of drug-resistant TB. Fluoroquinolones may play a role in treating MDR strains. Bedaquiline, in a new drug class for TB therapy, is approved for adults with MDR TB when used in combination therapy. Toxicities and lack of pediatric data preclude routine use in children. Directly observed therapy preferred; after 2 wk of daily therapy, can change to twice-weekly dosing double dosage of INH (max 900 mg), PZA (max 2 g), and ethambutol (max 2.5 g); rifampin remains same dosage (10–20 mg/kg/day, max 600 mg) (AII). LP ± CT of head for children ≤2 y to rule out occult, concurrent CNS infection; consider testing for HIV infection (AIII). *Mycobacterium bovis* infection from unpasteurized dairy products is also called "tuberculosis" but rarely causes pulmonary disease; all strains of *M bovis* are PZA resistant. Treat 9–12 mo with INH and rifampin.

– Latent TB infection[16,209] (skin test conversion)	Many options now: For children ≥2 y, once-weekly DOT for 12 wk: INH (15 mg/kg/dose, max 900 mg), AND rifapentine: 10.0–14.0 kg: 300 mg 14.1–25.0 kg: 450 mg 25.1–32.0 kg: 600 mg 32.1–49.9 kg: 750 mg ≥50.0 kg: 900 mg (max) Rifampin (15–20 mg/kg/dose daily (max 600 mg), for 4 mo. INH 10–15 mg/kg/day (max 300 mg) PO daily for 9 mo (12 mo for immunocompromised patients) (AIII); treatment with INH at 20–30 mg/kg twice weekly for 9 mo is also effective (AIII).	Obtain baseline LFTs. Consider monthly LFTs or as needed for symptoms. Stop INH-rifapentine if AST or ALT ≥5 times the ULN even in the absence of symptoms or ≥3 times the ULN in the presence of symptoms. For children <2 y: INH and rifapentine may be used, but less data on safety and efficacy. For exposure to known INH-R but rifampin-S strains, use rifampin 6 mo (AIII).
– Exposed child <4 y, or immunocompromised patient (high risk of dissemination)	Prophylaxis for possible infection with INH 10–15 mg/kg PO daily for 2–3 mo after last exposure with repeated skin test or interferon-gamma release assay test negative at that time (AIII). Also called "window prophylaxis."	If PPD remains negative at 2–3 mo and child well, consider stopping empiric therapy. PPD may not be reliable in immunocompromised patients. Not much data to assess reliability of interferon-gamma release assays in very young infants or immunocompromised hosts, but not likely to be much better than the PPD skin test.

G. CARDIOVASCULAR INFECTIONS

Clinical Diagnosis	Therapy (evidence grade)	Comments
Bacteremia		
– Occult bacteremia/serious bacterial infection (late-onset neonatal sepsis; fever without focus), infants <1–2 mo (group B streptococcus, *Escherichia coli, Listeria,* pneumococcus, meningococcus)[210–215]	In general, hospitalization for late-onset neonatal sepsis, with cultures of blood, urine, and CSF; start ampicillin for group B streptococcus and *Listeria* 200 mg/kg/day IV div q6h AND cefepime or ceftazidime for *E coli*/enterics (cefotaxime is no longer available in the United States); higher dosages if meningitis is documented. In areas with low (<20%) ampicillin resistance in *E coli,* consider ampicillin and gentamicin (gentamicin will not cover CNS infection caused by ampicillin-resistant *E coli*).	Current data document the importance of ampicillin-resistant *E coli* in bacteremia and UTI in infants <90 days.[213–215] For a nontoxic, febrile infant with good access to medical care: cultures may be obtained of blood and urine, and we are getting much closer to eliminating CSF cultures in low-risk infants. Risk scores incorporate various combinations of clinical status, urinalysis, WBC count, and procalcitonin. Ceftriaxone 50 mg/kg IM (lacks *Listeria* activity) may be given with outpatient follow-up the next day (Boston criteria) (BII) to minimize the very small risk of untreated meningitis; alternative is home without antibiotics if evaluation is negative (Rochester; modified Philadelphia criteria)[211–215] (BI).
– Occult bacteremia/serious bacterial infection (fever without focus) in age 2–3 mo to 36 mo (*Haemophilus influenzae* type b, pneumococcus, meningococcus; increasingly *Staphylococcus aureus*)[213]	Empiric therapy: if unimmunized, febrile, mild to moderate toxic: after blood culture: ceftriaxone 50 mg/kg IM (BII). If fully immunized (*Haemophilus* and *Pneumococcus*) and nontoxic, routine *empiric* therapy of fever with antibiotics is no longer recommended, but follow closely in case of vaccine failure or meningococcal bacteremia (BIII).	Oral convalescent therapy is selected by susceptibility of blood isolate, following response to IM/IV treatment, with CNS and other foci ruled out by examination ± laboratory tests ± imaging. LP is not recommended for routine evaluation of fever.[210]
– *H influenzae* type b, non-CNS infections	Ceftriaxone IM/IV OR, if beta-lactamase negative, ampicillin IV, followed by oral convalescent therapy (AII)	If beta-lactamase negative: amoxicillin 75–100 mg/kg/day PO div tid (AII) If positive: high-dosage cefixime, ceftibuten, cefdinir PO, or levofloxacin PO (CIII)

– Meningococcus	Ceftriaxone IM/IV or penicillin G IV, followed by oral convalescent therapy (AII)	Amoxicillin 75–100 mg/kg/day PO div tid (AIII)
– Pneumococcus, non-CNS infections	Ceftriaxone IM/IV or penicillin G/ampicillin IV (if pen-S), followed by oral convalescent therapy (AII)	If pen-S: amoxicillin 75–100 mg/kg/day PO div tid (AII). If pen-R: continue ceftriaxone IM or switch to clindamycin if susceptible (CIII); linezolid or levofloxacin may also be options (CIII).
– *S aureus*[4,8,216–219] usually associated with focal infection	MSSA: nafcillin or oxacillin/nafcillin IV 150–200 mg/kg/day div q6h ± gentamicin 6 mg/kg/day div q8h (AII). MRSA: vancomycin[217] 40–60 mg/kg/day IV div q8h OR ceftaroline: 2 mo–<2 y, 24 mg/kg/day IV div q8h; ≥2 y, 36 mg/kg/day IV div q8h (max single dose 400 mg) (BIII) ± gentamicin 6 mg/kg/day div q8h ± rifampin[218] 20 mg/kg/day div q12h (AIII). Treat for 2 wk (IV plus PO) from negative blood cultures unless endocarditis/endovascular thrombus present, which may require up to 6 wk of therapy (BIII).	For persisting bacteremia caused by MRSA, consider adding gentamicin, or changing from vancomycin (particularly for MRSA with vancomycin MIC of >2 mcg/mL) to ceftaroline or daptomycin (but daptomycin will not treat pneumonia). For toxic shock syndrome, clindamycin should be added for the initial 48–72 h of therapy to decrease toxin production (linezolid may also act in this way); IVIG may be added to bind circulating toxin (linezolid may also act in this way); no controlled data exist for these measures. Watch for the development of metastatic foci of infection, including endocarditis. If catheter-related, remove catheter.

Endocarditis: Surgical indications: intractable heart failure; persistent infection; large mobile vegetations; peripheral embolism; and valve dehiscence, perforation, rupture or fistula, or a large perivalvular abscess.[220–224] Consider community versus nosocomial pathogens based on recent surgeries, prior antibiotic therapy, and possible entry sites for bacteremia (skin, oropharynx and respiratory tract, gastrointestinal tract). Children with congenital heart disease are more likely to have more turbulent cardiovascular blood flow, which increases risk of endovascular infection. Catheter-placed bovine jugular valves appear to have an increased risk of infection.[223,224] Immunocompromised hosts may become bacteremic with a wide range of bacteria, fungi, and mycobacteria.

Prospective, controlled data on therapy for endocarditis in neonates, infants, and children is quite limited, and many recommendations provided are extrapolations from adults, where some level of evidence exists, or from other invasive bacteremia infections.

G. CARDIOVASCULAR INFECTIONS (continued)

Clinical Diagnosis	Therapy (evidence grade)	Comments
– **Native valve**[220–222]		
– Empiric therapy for presumed endocarditis (viridans streptococci, *S aureus*, HACEK group)	Ceftriaxone IV 100 mg/kg q24h AND gentamicin IV, IM 6 mg/kg/day div q8h (AII). For more acute, severe infection, ADD vancomycin 40–60 mg/kg/day IV div q8h to cover *S aureus* (AIII) (insufficient data to recommend ceftaroline for endocarditis).	Combination (ceftriaxone + gentamicin) provides bactericidal activity against most strains of viridans streptococci, the most common pathogens in infective endocarditis. Cefepime is recommended for adults,[220] but resistance data in enteric bacilli in children suggest that ceftriaxone remains a reasonable choice. May administer gentamicin with a qd regimen (CIII). For beta-lactam allergy, use vancomycin 45 mg/kg/day IV div q8h AND gentamicin 6 mg/kg/day IV div q8h.
Culture-negative native valve endocarditis: treat 4–6 wk (please obtain advice from an infectious diseases specialist for an appropriate regimen that is based on likely pathogens).[220]		
– Viridans streptococci: Follow echocardiogram for resolution of vegetation (BIII); for beta-lactam allergy: vancomycin.		
Fully susceptible to penicillin	Ceftriaxone 50 mg/kg IV, IM q24h for 4 wk OR penicillin G 200,000 U/kg/day IV div q4–6h for 4 wk (BII); OR penicillin G or ceftriaxone AND gentamicin 6 mg/kg/day IM, IV div q8h (AII) for 14 days for adults (4 wk for children per AHA guidelines due to lack of data in children)	AHA recommends higher dosage of ceftriaxone similar to that for penicillin non-susceptible strains.
Relatively resistant to penicillin	Penicillin G 300,000 U/kg/day IV div q4–6h for 4 wk, or ceftriaxone 100 mg/kg IV q24h for 4 wk; AND gentamicin 6 mg/kg/day IM, IV div q8h for the first 2 wk (AIII)	Gentamicin is used for the first 2 wk of a total of 4 wk of therapy for relatively resistant strains. Vancomycin-containing regimens should use at least a 4-wk treatment course, with gentamicin used for the entire course.
– Enterococcus (dosages for native or prosthetic valve infections)		

Ampicillin-susceptible (gentamicin-S)	Ampicillin 300 mg/kg/day IV, IM div q6h or penicillin G 300,000 U/kg/day IV div q4–6h; AND gentamicin 6.0 mg/kg/day IV div q8h; for 4–6 wk (AII)	Combined treatment with cell-wall active antibiotic plus aminoglycoside used to achieve bactericidal activity. For beta-lactam allergy: vancomycin. Little data exist in children for daptomycin or linezolid. For gentamicin-R strains, use streptomycin or other aminoglycoside if susceptible.
Ampicillin-resistant (gentamicin-S)	Vancomycin 40 mg/kg/day IV div q8h AND gentamicin 6.0 mg/kg/day IV div q8h; for 6 wk (AIII)	
Vancomycin-resistant (gentamicin-S)	Daptomycin IV if also ampicillin-resistant (dose is age-dependent; see Chapter 11) AND gentamicin 6.0 mg/kg/day IV div q8h; for 4–6 wk (AIII)	
– Staphylococci: *S aureus*, including CA-MRSA; *S epidermidis*[8,217] Consider continuing therapy at end of 6 wk if vegetations persist on echocardiogram. The risk of persisting organisms in deep venous thromboses subsequent to bacteremia is not defined.	MSSA or MSSE: nafcillin or oxacillin/nafcillin 150–200 mg/kg/day IV div q6h for 4–6 wk AND gentamicin 6 mg/kg/day div q8h for first 14 days. CA-MRSA or MRSE: vancomycin 40–60 mg/kg/day IV div q8h AND gentamicin for 6 wk; consider for slow response, ADD rifampin 20 mg/kg/day IV div q8–12h. Insufficient data to recommend ceftaroline routinely for MRSA endocarditis.	Surgery may be necessary in acute phase; avoid 1st-generation cephalosporins (conflicting data on efficacy). AHA suggests gentamicin for only the first 3–5 days for MSSA or MSSE and optional gentamicin for MRSA. For failures on therapy, or vancomycin-resistant MRSA, consider daptomycin (dose is age-dependent; see Chapter 11) AND gentamicin 6 mg/kg/day div q8h.
– Pneumococcus, gonococcus, group A streptococcus	Penicillin G 200,000 U/kg/day IV div q4–6h for 4 wk (BII); alternatives: ceftriaxone or vancomycin	Ceftriaxone plus azithromycin for suspected gonococcus until susceptibilities known. For penicillin non-susceptible strains of pneumococcus, use high-dosage penicillin G 300,000 U/kg/day IV div q4–6h or high-dosage ceftriaxone 100 mg/kg IV q12h or q24h for 4 wk.
HACEK (*Haemophilus*, *Aggregatibacter* [formerly *Actinobacillus*], *Cardiobacterium*, *Eikenella*, *Kingella* spp)	Usually susceptible to ceftriaxone 100 mg/kg IV q24h for 4 wk (BIII)	Some organisms will be ampicillin-susceptible. Usually do not require the addition of gentamicin.

G. CARDIOVASCULAR INFECTIONS (continued)

Clinical Diagnosis	Therapy (evidence grade)	Comments
– Enteric gram-negative bacilli	Antibiotics specific to pathogen (usually ceftriaxone plus gentamicin); duration at least 6 wk (AIII)	For ESBL organisms, carbapenems or beta-lactam/beta-lactamase inhibitor combinations PLUS gentamicin, should be effective.
– *Pseudomonas aeruginosa*	Antibiotic specific to susceptibility: cefepime or meropenem PLUS tobramycin	Cefepime and meropenem are both more active against *Pseudomonas* and less likely to allow beta-lactamase–resistant pathogens to emerge than ceftazidime.
– **Prosthetic valve/ material**[220,224]	Follow echocardiogram for resolution of vegetation. For beta-lactam allergy: vancomycin.	
– Viridans streptococci		
Fully susceptible to penicillin	Ceftriaxone 100 mg/kg IV, IM q24h for 6 wk OR penicillin G 300,000 U/kg/day IV div q4–6h for 6 wk (AII); OR penicillin G or ceftriaxone AND gentamicin 6.0 mg/kg/day IM, IV div q8h for first 2 wk of 6 wk course (AII)	Gentamicin is optional for the first 2 wk of a total of 6 wk of therapy for prosthetic valve/material endocarditis.
Relatively resistant to penicillin	Penicillin G 300,000 U/kg/day IV div q4–6h for 6 wk, or ceftriaxone 100 mg/kg IV q24h for 6 wk; AND gentamicin 6 mg/kg/day IM, IV div q8h for 6 wk (AIII)	Gentamicin is used for all 6 wk of therapy for prosthetic valve/material endocarditis caused by relatively resistant strains.
– Enterococcus (See dosages under native valve.) Treatment course is at least 6 wk, particularly if vancomycin is used.[220,224]		
– Staphylococci: *S aureus*, including CA-MRSA; *S epidermidis*[8,220] Consider continuing therapy at end of 6 wk if vegetations persist on echocardiogram.	MSSA or MSSE: nafcillin or oxacillin/nafcillin 150–200 mg/kg/day IV div q6h for ≥6 wk AND gentamicin 6 mg/kg/day div q8h for first 14 days. CA-MRSA or MRSE: vancomycin 40–60 mg/kg/day IV div q8h AND gentamicin for ≥6 wk; ADD rifampin 20 mg/kg/day IV div q8–12h.	For failures on therapy, consider daptomycin (dose is age-dependent; see Chapter 11) AND gentamicin 6 mg/kg/day div q8h.

– *Candida*[84,220,221,225]	AmB preparations have more experience (no comparative trials against echinocandins), OR caspofungin 70 mg/m^2 load on day 1, then 50 mg/m^2/day or micafungin 2–4 mg/kg/day (BIII). Do not use fluconazole as initial therapy because of inferior fungistatic effect.	Poor prognosis; please obtain advice from an infectious diseases specialist. Surgery may be required to resect infected valve. Long-term suppressive therapy with fluconazole. Suspect *Candida* vegetations when lesions are large on echocardiography.
– Culture-negative prosthetic valve endocarditis: treat at least 6 wk.		
Endocarditis prophylaxis[218,221,222,226]: Given that (1) endocarditis is rarely caused by dental/GI procedures and (2) prophylaxis for procedures prevents an exceedingly small number of cases, the risks of antibiotics outweigh the benefits. Highest risk conditions currently recommended for prophylaxis: (1) prosthetic heart valve (or prosthetic material used to repair a valve); (2) previous endocarditis; (3) cyanotic congenital heart disease that is unrepaired (or palliatively repaired with shunts and conduits); (4) congenital heart disease that is repaired but with defects at the site of repair adjacent to prosthetic material; (5) completely repaired congenital heart disease using prosthetic material, for the first 6 mo after repair; or (6) cardiac transplant patients with valvulopathy. Routine prophylaxis no longer is required for children with native valve abnormalities. Assessment of new prophylaxis guidelines documents a possible increase in viridans streptococcal endocarditis in children 10–17 y old but not 0–9 y old.[227] However, no changes in prophylaxis recommendations are being made at this time.		
– In highest risk patients: dental procedures that involve manipulation of the gingival or periodontal region of teeth	Amoxicillin 50 mg/kg PO 60 min before procedure OR ampicillin or ceftriaxone or cefazolin, all at 50 mg/kg IM/IV 30–60 min before procedure	If penicillin allergy: clindamycin 20 mg/kg PO (60 min before) or IV (30 min before); OR azithromycin 15 mg/kg or clarithromycin 15 mg/kg, 60 min before (little data to support alternative regimens).
– Genitourinary and GI procedures	None	No longer recommended
Lemierre syndrome (*Fusobacterium necrophorum* primarily, new reports with MRSA)[119–123] (pharyngitis with internal jugular vein septic thrombosis, postanginal sepsis, necrobacillosis)	Empiric: meropenem 60 mg/kg/day div q8h (or 120 mg/kg/day div q8h for CNS metastatic foci) (AIII) OR ceftriaxone 100 mg/kg/day q24h AND metronidazole 40 mg/kg/day div q8h or clindamycin 40 mg/kg/day div q6h (BIII). ADD empiric vancomycin if MRSA suspected if clindamycin is not in the treatment regimen.	Anecdotal reports suggest metronidazole may be effective for apparent failures with other agents. Often requires anticoagulation. Metastatic and recurrent abscesses often develop while on active, appropriate therapy, requiring multiple debridements and prolonged antibiotic therapy. Treat until CRP and ESR are normal (AIII).

G. CARDIOVASCULAR INFECTIONS (continued)

Clinical Diagnosis	Therapy (evidence grade)	Comments
Purulent pericarditis		
– Empiric (acute, bacterial: *S aureus* [including MRSA], group A streptococcus, pneumococcus, meningococcus, *H influenzae* type b)[228,229]	Vancomycin 40 mg/kg/day IV div q8h AND ceftriaxone 50–75 mg/kg/day q24h (AIII), OR ceftaroline: 2–<6 mo, 30 mg/kg/day IV div q8h; ≥6 mo, 45 mg/kg/day IV div q8h (max single dose 600 mg) (BIII)	For presumed staphylococcal infection, ADD gentamicin (AIII). Increasingly uncommon with immunization against pneumococcus and *H influenzae* type b.[229] Pericardiocentesis is essential to establish diagnosis. Surgical drainage of pus with pericardial window or pericardiectomy is important to prevent tamponade.
– *S aureus*	For MSSA: oxacillin/nafcillin 150–200 mg/kg/day IV div q6h OR cefazolin 100 mg/kg/day IV div q8h. Treat for 2–3 wk after drainage (BIII). For CA-MRSA: continue vancomycin or ceftaroline. Treat for 3–4 wk after drainage (BIII).	Continue therapy with gentamicin; consider use of rifampin in severe cases due to tissue penetration characteristics.
– *H influenzae* type b in unimmunized children	Ceftriaxone 50 mg/kg/day q24h for 10–14 days (AIII)	Ampicillin for beta-lactamase–negative strains
– Pneumococcus, meningococcus, group A streptococcus	Penicillin G 200,000 U/kg/day IV, IM div q6h for 10–14 days OR ceftriaxone 50 mg/kg qd for 10–14 days (AIII)	Ceftriaxone for penicillin non-susceptible pneumococci
– Coliform bacilli	Ceftriaxone 50–75 mg/kg/day q24h for 3 wk or longer (AIII)	Alternative drugs depending on susceptibilities; for *Enterobacter, Serratia,* or *Citrobacter,* use cefepime or meropenem. For ESBL *E coli* or *Klebsiella,* use a carbapenem.
– Tuberculous[15,16]	INH 10–15 mg/kg/day (max 300 mg) PO, IV qd, for 6 mo AND rifampin 10–20 mg/kg/day (max 600 mg) PO qd, IV for 6 mo. ADD PZA 20–40 mg/kg/day PO qd for first 2 mo therapy; if suspected multidrug resistance, also add ethambutol 20 mg/kg/day PO qd (AIII).	Current guidelines do not suggest a benefit from routine use of corticosteroids. However, for those at highest risk of restrictive pericarditis, steroid continues to be recommended.[15] For children: prednisone 2 mg/kg/day for 4 wk, then 0.5 mg/kg/day for 4 wk, then 0.25 mg/kg/day for 2 wk, then 0.1 mg/kg/day for 1 wk.

H. GASTROINTESTINAL INFECTIONS (See Chapter 10 for parasitic infections.)

Clinical Diagnosis	Therapy (evidence grade)	Comments
Diarrhea/Gastroenteritis		
Note on *Escherichia coli* and diarrheal disease: Antibiotic susceptibility of *E coli* varies considerably from region to region. For mild to moderate disease, TMP/SMX may be started as initial therapy, but for more severe disease and for locations with rates of TMP/SMX resistance greater than 10% to 20%, azithromycin, an oral 3rd-generation cephalosporin (eg, cefixime, cefdinir, ceftibuten), or ciprofloxacin should be used (AIII). Diagnostic testing (molecular and traditions cultures) and antibiotic susceptibility testing are recommended for significant disease (AIII). Updated IDSA guidelines were recently published.[230]		
– Empiric therapy of community-associated diarrhea in the United States (*E coli* [STEC, including O157:H7 strains, and ETEC], *Salmonella*, *Campylobacter*, and *Shigella* predominate; *Yersinia* and parasites causing <5%; however, viral pathogens are far more common, especially for children <3 y.)[230,231]	Azithromycin 10 mg/kg qd for 3 days (BII); OR ciprofloxacin 30 mg/kg/day PO div bid for 3 days; OR cefixime 8 mg/kg/day PO qd (BII). Current recommendations are to avoid treatment of STEC O157:H7 strains.[230]	Alternatives: 3rd-generation cephalosporins (eg, ceftriaxone); have been shown effective in uncomplicated *Salmonella typhi* infections. Rifaximin 600 mg/day div tid for 3 days (for nonfebrile, non-bloody diarrhea for children >11 y). Retrospective data exist for treatment of O157:H7 strains to support either withholding treatment or treatment (including retrospective data on treatment with azithromycin).[232–236]

H. GASTROINTESTINAL INFECTIONS (continued) (See Chapter 10 for parasitic infections.)

Clinical Diagnosis	Therapy (evidence grade)	Comments
– Traveler's diarrhea: empiric therapy (*E coli, Campylobacter, Salmonella, Shigella,* plus many other pathogens, including protozoa)[237–244]	For mild diarrhea, treatment is not recommended.[240] Azithromycin 10 mg/kg qd for 1–3 days (AII); OR rifaximin 200 mg PO tid for 3 days (age ≥12 y) (BIII); OR ciprofloxacin (BII); OR rifaximin 200 mg tid for 3 days for age ≥12 y (BII)	Susceptibility patterns of *E coli, Campylobacter, Salmonella,* and *Shigella* vary widely by country; check country-specific data for departing or returning travelers. Azithromycin preferable to ciprofloxacin for travelers to Southeast Asia given high prevalence of quinolone-resistant *Campylobacter.* Rifaximin is less effective than ciprofloxacin for invasive bloody bacterial enteritis; rifaximin may also not be as effective for *Shigella, Salmonella,* and *Campylobacter* as other agents. Another, nonabsorbable rifamycin, in a delayed release formulation, was recently approved for adults ≥18 y.[243] Interestingly, for adults who travel and take antibiotics (mostly fluoroquinolones), colonization with ESBL-positive *E coli* is more frequent on return home.[245] Adjunctive therapy with loperamide (antimotility) is not recommended for children $<$2 y and should be used only in nonfebrile, non-bloody diarrhea.[238,244,246,247] May shorten symptomatic illness by about 24 h.
– Traveler's diarrhea: prophylaxis[237,238,240]	– Prophylaxis: Early self-treatment with agents listed previously is preferred over long-term prophylaxis, but may use prophylaxis for a short-term ($<$14 days) visit to very high-risk region: rifaximin (for older children), azithromycin, or bismuth subsalicylate (BIII). Fluoroquinolones should not be used.[240]	
– *Aeromonas hydrophila*[248]	Ciprofloxacin 30 mg/kg/day PO div bid for 5 days OR azithromycin 10 mg/kg qd for 3 days OR cefixime 8 mg/kg/day PO qd (BIII)	Not all strains produce enterotoxins and diarrhea; role in diarrhea questioned.[248] Resistance to TMP/SMX about 10%–15%. Choose narrowest spectrum agent based on in vitro susceptibilities.

– *Campylobacter jejuni*[249–251]	Azithromycin 10 mg/kg/day for 3 days (BII) or erythromycin 40 mg/kg/day PO div qid for 5 days (BII)	Alternatives: doxycycline or ciprofloxacin (high rate of fluoroquinolone resistance in Thailand, India, and now the United States). Single-dose azithromycin (1 g, once) is effective in adults.
– Cholera[242,252]	Azithromycin 20 mg/kg once; OR erythromycin 50 mg/kg/day PO div qid for 3 days; OR doxycycline 4.4 mg/kg/day (max 200 mg/day) PO div bid, for all ages	Ciprofloxacin or TMP/SMX (if susceptible)
– *Clostridioides* (formerly *Clostridium) difficile* (antibiotic-associated colitis)[253–258]	Now stratified by severity and recurrence. First episode: Mild to moderate illness: metronidazole 30 mg/kg/day PO div qid. Moderate to severe illness: vancomycin 40 mg/kg/day PO div qid for 7 days. Severe and complicated/systemic: vancomycin PO AND metronidazole IV; consider vancomycin enema (500 mg/100 mL physiologic [normal] saline) q8h until improvement).[254,255] For relapsing *C difficile* enteritis, consider pulse therapy (1 wk on/1 wk off for 3–4 cycles) or prolonged tapering therapy.[253] Stool transplantation for failure of medical therapy in recurrent enteritis.	Attempt to stop antibiotics that may have represented the cause of *C difficile* infection. Vancomycin is more effective for severe infection.[254,255] Fidaxomicin approved for adults; pediatric studies successfully completed with similar results to those in adults.[257] Many infants and children may have asymptomatic colonization with *C difficile*.[255] Higher risk of relapse in children with multiple comorbidities.
– *E coli*		
Enterotoxigenic (etiology of most traveler's diarrhea)[238–241]	Azithromycin 10 mg/kg qd for 3 days; OR ciprofloxacin 30 mg/kg/day PO div bid for 3 days; OR cefixime 8 mg/kg/day PO qd for 3 days	Most illnesses brief and self-limited and may not require treatment. Alternatives: rifaximin 600 mg/day div tid for 3 days (for nonfebrile, non-bloody diarrhea for children >11 y, as rifaximin is not absorbed systemically); OR TMP/SMX. Resistance increasing worldwide; check country-specific rates, if possible.

H. GASTROINTESTINAL INFECTIONS (continued) (See Chapter 10 for parasitic infections.)

Clinical Diagnosis	Therapy (evidence grade)	Comments
Enterohemorrhagic (O157:H7; STEC, etiology of HUS)[230,232–236]	Current recommendations are to avoid treatment of STEC O157:H7 strains.[230] Retrospective data exist for treatment of O157:H7 strains to support either withholding treatment or treatment (including retrospective data on treatment with azithromycin).[232–236]	Injury to colonic mucosa may lead to invasive bacterial colitis that does require antimicrobial therapy.
Enteropathogenic	Neomycin 100 mg/kg/day PO div q6–8h for 5 days	Most traditional "enteropathogenic" strains are not toxigenic or invasive. Postinfection diarrhea may be problematic.
– Gastritis, peptic ulcer disease (*Helicobacter pylori*)[259–262]	Either triple agent therapy in areas of low clarithromycin resistance: clarithromycin 7.5 mg/kg/dose 2–3 times each day, AND amoxicillin 40 mg/kg/dose (max 1 g) PO bid AND omeprazole 0.5 mg/kg/dose PO bid 14 days (BII), OR quadruple therapy that includes metronidazole (15 mg/kg/day div bid) added to the regimen previously described.[263]	New pediatric guidelines recommend some restriction of testing for those at high risk of complications. Resistance to clarithromycin is as high as 20% in some regions.[259,261,264] Current approach for empiric therapy if clarithromycin resistance may be present: high-dose triple therapy is recommended with proton pump inhibitor, amoxicillin, and metronidazole for 14 days ± bismuth to create quadruple therapy.[259]
– Giardiasis (See Chapter 10.) (*Giardia intestinalis*, formerly *lamblia*)[265]	Metronidazole 30–40 mg/kg/day PO div tid for 7–10 days (BII); OR tinidazole (for age ≥3 y) 50 mg/kg/day (max 2 g) for 1 day (BII); OR nitazoxanide PO (take with food), age 12–47 mo, 100 mg/dose bid for 7 days; age 4–11 y, 200 mg/dose bid for 7 days; age ≥12 y, 1 tab (500 mg)/dose bid for 7 days (BII)	If therapy is unsuccessful, another course of the same agent is usually curative. Alternatives: paromomycin OR albendazole (CII). Prolonged or combination drug courses may be needed for immunocompromised conditions (eg, hypogammaglobulinemia). Treatment of asymptomatic carriers not usually recommended.
– Salmonellosis[266–268] (See Chapter 10 for discussion of traveler's diarrhea for typhoid infection outside of North America.)		

Non-typhoid strains[266–268]	Usually none for self-limited diarrhea in immunocompetent child (eg, diarrhea is often much improved by the time culture results are available). Treat those with persisting symptomatic infection and all infants <3 months: azithromycin 10 mg/kg PO qd for 3 days (AII); OR ceftriaxone 75 mg/kg/day IV, IM q24h for 5 days (AII); OR cefixime 20–30 mg/kg/day PO for 5–7 days (BII); OR for susceptible strains: TMP/SMX 8 mg/kg/day of TMP PO div bid for 14 days (AI).	Alternatives: ciprofloxacin 30 mg/kg/day PO div bid for 5 days (AI). Carriage of strains may be prolonged in treated children. For bacteremic infection, ceftriaxone IM/IV may be initially used until secondary sites of infection (bone/joint, liver/spleen, CNS) are ruled out.
Typhoid fever[268–272]	Azithromycin 10 mg/kg qd for 5 days (AII); OR ceftriaxone 75 mg/kg/day IV, IM q24h for 5 days (AII); OR cefixime 20–30 mg/kg/day PO, div q12h for 14 days (BII); OR for susceptible strains: amoxicillin OR TMP/SMX 8 mg/kg/day of TMP PO div bid for 14 days (AI)	Increasing cephalosporin resistance. For newly emergent MDR strains, may require prolonged IV therapy. Amoxicillin does not achieve high colonic intraluminal concentrations or high intracellular concentrations. Longer treatment courses for focal invasive disease (eg, osteomyelitis). Alternative: ciprofloxacin 30 mg/kg/day PO div bid for 5–7 days (AI).
– Shigellosis[273–275]	Mild episodes do not require treatment. Cefixime 8 mg/kg/day PO qd for 5 days (AII); OR azithromycin 10 mg/kg/day PO for 3 days (AII); OR ciprofloxacin 30 mg/kg/day PO div bid for 3–5 days (BII)	Alternatives for susceptible strains: TMP/SMX 8 mg/kg/day of TMP PO div bid for 5 days; OR ampicillin (*not* amoxicillin). Ceftriaxone 50 mg/kg/day IM, IV if parenteral therapy necessary, for 2–5 days. Avoid antiperistaltic drugs. Treatment for the improving child is not usually necessary to hasten recovery, but some experts would treat to decrease communicability.

H. GASTROINTESTINAL INFECTIONS (continued) (See Chapter 10 for parasitic infections.)

Clinical Diagnosis	Therapy (evidence grade)	Comments
– *Yersinia enterocolitica*[276–278]	Antimicrobial therapy probably not of value for mild disease in normal hosts. TMP/SMX PO, IV; OR ciprofloxacin PO, IV (BIII).	Alternatives: ceftriaxone or gentamicin. High rates of resistance to ampicillin. May mimic appendicitis in older children. Limited clinical data exist on oral therapy.
Intra-abdominal infection (abscess, peritonitis secondary to bowel/appendix contents)		
– Appendicitis; bowel-associated (enteric gram-negative bacilli, *Bacteroides* spp, *Enterococcus* spp, increasingly *Pseudomonas*)[279–284]	Source control is critical to curing this infection. Newer data suggest that stratification of cases is important to assess the effect of surgical and medical therapy on outcomes.[279,280] Meropenem 60 mg/kg/day IV div q8h or imipenem 60 mg/kg/day IV div q6h; OR pip/tazo 240 mg pip/kg/day div q6h; for 4–5 days for patients with adequate source control,[283] 7–10 days or longer if suspicion of persisting intra-abdominal abscess (AII). *Pseudomonas* is found consistently in up to 30% of children)[280,281,285] providing evidence to document the need for empiric use of an antipseudomonal drug (preferably one with anaerobic activity), such as a carbapenem or pip/tazo, *unless the surgery was highly effective at drainage/source control* (gentamicin is not active in an abscess), which may explain successful outcomes in retrospective studies that did not include antipseudomonal coverage.[286–288]	Many other regimens may be effective, including ampicillin 150 mg/kg/day div q8h AND gentamicin 6–7.5 mg/kg/day IV, IM div q8h AND metronidazole 40 mg/kg/day IV div q8h; OR ceftriaxone 50 mg/kg q24h AND metronidazole 40 mg/kg/day IV div q8h. Data support IV outpatient therapy or oral step-down therapy[284,285] when clinically improved, particularly when oral therapy can be focused on the most prominent, invasive cultured pathogens. Publications on outcomes of antibiotic therapy regimens (IV or PO) without culture data cannot be accurately interpreted.

– Tuberculosis, abdominal (*Mycobacterium bovis,* from unpasteurized dairy products)[15,16,289,290]	INH 10–15 mg/kg/day (max 300 mg) PO qd for 6–9 mo AND rifampin 10–20 mg/kg/day (max 600 mg) PO qd for 6–9 mo (AII). Some experts recommend routine use of ethambutol in the empiric regimen. *M bovis* is resistant to PZA. If risk factors are present for multidrug resistance (eg, poor adherence to previous therapy), ADD ethambutol 20 mg/kg/day PO qd OR a fluoroquinolone (moxifloxacin or levofloxacin).	Corticosteroids have been routinely used as adjunctive therapy to decrease morbidity from inflammation.[291] Directly observed therapy preferred; after 2+ wk of daily therapy, can change to twice-weekly dosing double dosage of INH (max 900 mg); rifampin remains same dosage (10–20 mg/kg/day, max 600 mg) (AII). LP ± CT of head for children ≤2 y with active disease to rule out occult, concurrent CNS infection (AIII). No published prospective comparative data on a 6 mo vs 9 mo treatment course in children.
Perirectal abscess (*Bacteroides* spp, other anaerobes, enteric bacilli, and *S aureus* predominate)[292]	Clindamycin 30–40 mg/kg/day IV div q8h AND ceftriaxone or gentamicin (BIII)	Surgical drainage alone may be curative. Obtaining cultures and susceptibilities is increasingly important with rising resistance to cephalosporins in community *E coli* isolates. May represent inflammatory bowel disease.
Peritonitis		
– Peritoneal dialysis indwelling catheter infection (staphylococcal; enteric gram-negatives; yeast)[293,294]	Antibiotic added to dialysate in concentrations approximating those attained in serum for systemic disease (eg, 4 mcg/mL for gentamicin, 25 mcg/mL for vancomycin, 125 mcg/mL for cefazolin, 25 mcg/mL for ciprofloxacin) after a larger loading dose (AII)[294]	Selection of antibiotic based on organism isolated from peritoneal fluid; systemic antibiotics if there is accompanying bacteremia/fungemia
– Primary (pneumococcus or group A streptococcus)[295]	Ceftriaxone 50 mg/kg/day q24h; if pen-S, then penicillin G 150,000 U/kg/day IV div q6h; for 7–10 days (AII)	Other antibiotics according to culture and susceptibility tests. Spontaneous pneumococcal peritonitis now infrequent in PCV13 immunized children.

I. GENITAL AND SEXUALLY TRANSMITTED INFECTIONS

Clinical Diagnosis	Therapy (evidence grade)	Comments
Consider testing for HIV and other STIs in a child with one documented STI; consider sexual abuse in prepubertal children. The most recent CDC STI treatment guidelines (2015)[57] are posted online with STI surveillance (2017) at www.cdc.gov/std (accessed October 10, 2019).		
Chancroid (*Haemophilus ducreyi*)[57]	Azithromycin 1 g PO as single dose OR ceftriaxone 250 mg IM as single dose	Alternative: erythromycin 1.5 g/day PO div tid for 7 days OR ciprofloxacin 1,000 mg PO qd, div bid for 3 days
Chlamydia trachomatis (cervicitis, urethritis)[57,296]	Azithromycin 20 mg/kg (max 1 g) PO for 1 dose; OR doxycycline (patients >7 y) 4.4 mg/kg/day (max 200 mg/day) PO div bid for 7 days	Alternatives: erythromycin 2 g/day PO div qid for 7 days; OR levofloxacin 500 mg PO q24h for 7 days
Epididymitis (associated with positive urine cultures and STIs)[57,297,298]	Ceftriaxone 50 mg/kg/day q24h for 7–10 days AND (for older children) doxycycline 200 mg/day div bid for 10 days	Microbiology not well studied in children; in infants, also associated with urogenital tract anomalies. Treat infants for *Staphylococcus aureus* and *Escherichia coli;* may resolve spontaneously; in STI, treat for *Chlamydia* and gonococcus.
Gonorrhea[57,296,299–301]	Antibiotic resistance is an ongoing problem, with new data to suggest the emergence of global azithromycin resistance being tracked closely by the CDC.[301]	
– Newborns	See Chapter 5.	
– Genital infections (uncomplicated vulvovaginitis, cervicitis, urethritis, or proctitis)[57,296,299,300]	Ceftriaxone 250 mg IM for 1 dose (regardless of weight) AND azithromycin 1 g PO for 1 dose or doxycycline 200 mg/day div q12h for 7 days	Cefixime no longer recommended due to increasing cephalosporin resistance.[57] Fluoroquinolones are no longer recommended at all due to resistance. Dual therapy has not been evaluated yet in children but should be effective.
– Pharyngitis[57,301]	Ceftriaxone 250 mg IM for 1 dose (regardless of weight) AND azithromycin 1 g PO for 1 dose or doxycycline 200 mg/day div q12h for 7 days	
– Conjunctivitis[57]	Ceftriaxone 1g IM for 1 dose AND azithromycin 1 g PO for 1 dose	Lavage the eye with saline.

– Disseminated gonococcal infection[57,301]	Ceftriaxone 50 mg/kg/day IM, IV q24h (max: 1 g) AND azithromycin 1 g PO for 1 dose; total course for 7 days	No studies in children: increase dosage for meningitis.
Granuloma inguinale (donovanosis, *Klebsiella granulomatis,* formerly *Calymmatobacterium*)[57]	Azithromycin 1 g orally once per week or 500 mg daily for at least 3 weeks and until all lesions have completely healed	Primarily in tropical regions of India, Pacific, and Africa. Options: Doxycycline 4.4 mg/kg/day div bid (max 200 mg/day) PO for at least 3 wk OR ciprofloxacin 750 mg PO bid for at least 3 wk, OR erythromycin base 500 mg PO qid for at least 3 wk OR TMP/SMX 1 double-strength (160 mg/800 mg) tab PO bid for at least 3 wk; all regimens continue until all lesions have completely healed.
Herpes simplex virus, genital infection[57,302–305]	Acyclovir 20 mg/kg/dose (max 400 mg) PO tid for 7–10 days (first episode) (AI); OR valacyclovir 20 mg/kg/dose of extemporaneous suspension (directions on package label), max 1 g PO bid for 7–10 days (first episode) (AI); OR famciclovir 250 mg PO tid for 7–10 days (AI); for more severe infection: acyclovir 15 mg/kg/day IV div q8h as 1-h infusion for 7–10 days (AII)	For recurrent episodes: treat with acyclovir PO, valacyclovir PO, or famciclovir PO, immediately when symptoms begin, for 5 days. For suppression[305]: acyclovir 20 mg/kg/dose (max 400 mg) PO bid; OR valacyclovir 20 mg/kg/dose PO qd (little long-term safety data in children; no efficacy data in children). Prophylaxis is recommended by ACOG in pregnant women.[304,305]
Lymphogranuloma venereum (*C trachomatis*)[57]	Doxycycline 4.4 mg/kg/day (max 200 mg/day) PO (patients >7 y) div bid for 21 days	Alternatives: erythromycin 2 g/day PO div qid for 21 days; OR azithromycin 1 g PO once weekly for 3 wk
Pelvic inflammatory disease (*Chlamydia,* gonococcus, plus anaerobes)[57,306]	Cefoxitin 2 g IV q6h; AND doxycycline 200 mg/day PO or IV div bid; OR cefotetan 2 g IV q12h AND doxycycline 100 mg orally or IV q12h, OR clindamycin 900 mg IV q8h AND gentamicin 1.5 mg/kg IV, IM q8h until clinical improvement for 24 h, followed by doxycycline 200 mg/day PO div bid (AND clindamycin 1,800 mg/day PO div qid for tubo-ovarian abscess) to complete 14 days of therapy	Optional regimen: ceftriaxone 250 mg IM for 1 dose AND doxycycline 200 mg/day PO div bid; WITH/WITHOUT metronidazole 1 g/day PO div bid; for 14 days

I. GENITAL AND SEXUALLY TRANSMITTED INFECTIONS (continued)

Clinical Diagnosis	Therapy (evidence grade)	Comments
Syphilis[57,307] **(Test for HIV.)**		
– Congenital	See Chapter 5.	
– Neurosyphilis (positive CSF VDRL or CSF pleocytosis with serologic diagnosis of syphilis)	Crystalline penicillin G 200–300,000 U/kg/day (max 24,000,000 U/day) div q6h for 10–14 days (AIII)	
– Primary, secondary	Benzathine penicillin G 50,000 U/kg (max 2,400,000 U) IM as a single dose (AIII); do not use benzathine-procaine penicillin mixtures.	Follow-up serologic tests at 6, 12, and 24 mo; 15% may remain seropositive despite adequate treatment. If allergy to penicillin: doxycycline (patients >7 y) 4.4 mg/kg/day (max 200 mg) PO div bid for 14 days. CSF examination should be obtained for children being treated for primary or secondary syphilis to rule out asymptomatic neurosyphilis. Test for HIV.
– Syphilis of <1 y duration, without clinical symptoms (early latent syphilis)	Benzathine penicillin G 50,000 U/kg (max 2,400,000 U) IM as a single dose (AIII)	Alternative if allergy to penicillin: doxycycline (patients >7 y) 4.4 mg/kg/day (max 200 mg/day) PO div bid for 14 days
– Syphilis of >1 y duration, without clinical symptoms (late latent syphilis) or syphilis of unknown duration	Benzathine penicillin G 50,000 U/kg (max 2,400,000 U) IM weekly for 3 doses (AIII)	Alternative if allergy to penicillin: doxycycline (patients >7 y) 4.4 mg/kg/day (max 200 mg/day) PO div bid for 28 days. Look for neurologic, eye, and aortic complications of tertiary syphilis.
Trichomoniasis[57]	Tinidazole 50 mg/kg (max 2 g) PO for 1 dose (BII) OR metronidazole 2 g PO for 1 dose OR metronidazole 500 mg PO bid for 7 days (BII)	
Urethritis, nongonococcal (See Gonorrhea for gonorrhea therapy.)[57,308]	Azithromycin 20 mg/kg (max 1 g) PO for 1 dose, OR doxycycline (patients >7 y) 4.4 mg/kg/day (max 200 mg/day) PO div bid for 7 days (AII)	Erythromycin, levofloxacin, or ofloxacin Increasing resistance noted in *Mycoplasma genitalium*[308]

Vaginitis[57]		
– Bacterial vaginosis[57,309]	Metronidazole 500 mg PO twice daily for 7 days OR metronidazole vaginal gel (0.75%) qd for 5 days, OR clindamycin vaginal cream for 7 days	Alternative: tinidazole 1 g PO qd for 5 days, OR clindamycin 300 mg PO bid for 7 days Relapse common Caused by synergy of *Gardnerella* with anaerobes
– Candidiasis, vulvovaginal[57,310]	Topical vaginal cream/tabs/suppositories (alphabetic order): butoconazole, clotrimazole, econazole, fenticonazole, miconazole, sertaconazole, terconazole, or tioconazole for 3–7 days (AI); OR fluconazole 10 mg/kg (max 150 mg) as a single dose (AII)	For uncomplicated vulvovaginal candidiasis, no topical agent is clearly superior. Avoid azoles during pregnancy. For recurring disease, consider 10–14 days of induction with topical agent or fluconazole, followed by fluconazole once weekly for 6 mo (AI).
– Prepubertal vaginitis[311]	No prospective studies	Cultures from symptomatic prepubertal girls are statistically more likely to yield *E coli*, enterococcus, coagulase-negative staphylococci, and streptococci (viridans strep and group A strep), but these organisms may also be present in asymptomatic girls.
– *Shigella*[312]	Cefixime 8 mg/kg/day PO qd for 5 days OR ciprofloxacin 30 mg/kg/day PO div bid for 5 days	50% have bloody discharge; usually not associated with diarrhea.
– *Streptococcus,* group A[313]	Penicillin V 50–75 mg/kg/day PO div tid for 10 days	Amoxicillin 50–75 mg/kg/day PO div tid

J. CENTRAL NERVOUS SYSTEM INFECTIONS

Clinical Diagnosis	Therapy (evidence grade)	Comments
Abscess, brain (respiratory tract flora, skin flora, or bowel flora, depending on the pathogenesis of infection based on underlying comorbid disease and origin of bacteremia)[314,315]	Until etiology established, use empiric therapy for presumed mixed-flora infection with origins from the respiratory tract, skin, and/or bowel, based on individual patient evaluation and risk for brain abscess (see Comments for MRSA considerations): meropenem 120 mg/kg/day div q8h (AIII); OR nafcillin 150–200 mg/kg/day IV div q6h AND ceftriaxone 100 mg/kg/day IV q24h AND metronidazole 30 mg/kg/day IV div q8h (BIII); for 2–3 wk after successful drainage (depending on pathogen, size of abscess, and response to therapy); longer course if no surgery (3–6 wk) (BIII). Follow resolution by imaging. For single pathogen abscess, use a single agent in doses that will achieve effective CNS exposure. The blood-brain barrier is not intact in brain abscesses.	Surgery for abscesses ≥2 cm diameter. If CA-MRSA suspected, ADD vancomycin 60 mg/kg/day IV div q8h ± rifampin 20 mg/kg/day IV div q12h, pending culture results. We have successfully treated MRSA intracranial infections with ceftaroline, but no prospective data exist. If secondary to chronic otitis, include meropenem or cefepime in regimen for anti-*Pseudomonas* activity. For enteric gram-negative bacilli, consider ESBL-producing *Escherichia coli* and *Klebsiella* that require meropenem and are resistant to ceftriaxone.
Encephalitis[316] (May be infectious or immune-complex mediated)[317]		
– Amebic (*Naegleria fowleri, Balamuthia mandrillaris,* and *Acanthamoeba*)	See Chapter 10, Amebiasis.	
– CMV	See Chapter 9, CMV. Not well studied in children. Consider ganciclovir 10 mg/kg/day IV div q12h; for severe immunocompromised, ADD foscarnet 180 mg/kg/day IV div q8h for 3 wk.	Follow quantitative PCR for CMV. Reduce dose for renal insufficiency. Watch for neutropenia.
– Enterovirus	Supportive therapy; no antivirals currently FDA approved.	Pocapavir PO is currently under investigation for enterovirus (poliovirus). As of October 2019, it is not available for compassionate use.

		Pleconaril PO is currently under consideration for submission to FDA for approval for treatment of neonatal enteroviral sepsis syndrome.[318] As of October 2019, it is not available for compassionate use.
– EBV[319]	Not studied in a controlled comparative trial. Consider ganciclovir 10 mg/kg/day IV div q12h or acyclovir 60 mg/kg/day IV div q8h for 3 wk.	Follow quantitative PCR in CSF for EBV. Efficacy of antiviral therapy not well defined.
– Herpes simplex virus[320] (See Chapter 5 for neonatal infection).	Acyclovir 60 mg/kg/day IV as 1–2 h infusion div q8h for 21 days for ≤4 mo; for those ≥5 mo, 45 mg/kg/day IV for 21 days (AIII)	Perform CSF HSV PCR near end of 21 days of therapy and continue acyclovir until PCR negative. Safety of high-dose acyclovir (60 mg/kg/day) not well defined beyond the neonatal period; can be used, but monitor for neurotoxicity and nephrotoxicity; FDA has approved acyclovir at this dosage for encephalitis for children up to 12 y.
– *Toxoplasma* (See Chapter 5 for neonatal congenital infection.)	See Chapter 10.	
– Arbovirus (flavivirus—Zika, West Nile, St. Louis encephalitis, tick-borne encephalitis; togavirus—western equine encephalitis, eastern equine encephalitis; bunyavirus—La Crosse encephalitis, California encephalitis)[316]	Supportive therapy	Investigational only (antiviral, interferon, immune globulins). No specific antiviral agents are yet commercially available for any of the arboviruses, including Zika or West Nile.

J. CENTRAL NERVOUS SYSTEM INFECTIONS (continued)

Clinical Diagnosis	Therapy (evidence grade)	Comments
Meningitis, bacterial, community-associated		
NOTES – In areas where pen-R pneumococci exist (>5% of invasive strains, which is quite uncommon in the era of conjugate pneumococcal vaccines), initial empiric therapy for suspect pneumococcal meningitis should be with vancomycin AND ceftriaxone until susceptibility test results are available. Although ceftaroline is more active than ceftriaxone against pneumococci and, as a beta-lactam, should be expected to achieve therapeutic CSF concentrations, no substantial pediatric data yet exist on treatment of CNS infections. – Dexamethasone 0.6 mg/kg/day IV div q6h for 2 days as an adjunct to antibiotic therapy decreases hearing deficits and other neurologic sequelae in adults and children (for *Haemophilus* and pneumococcus; not prospectively studied in children for meningococcus or *E coli*). The first dose of dexamethasone is given before or concurrent with the first dose of antibiotic; probably little benefit if given ≥1 h after the antibiotic.[321,322]		
– Empiric therapy[323]	Ceftriaxone 100 mg/kg/day IV q24h (AII)	If Gram stain or cultures demonstrate a pathogen other than pneumococcus, vancomycin is not needed; vancomycin used empirically for possible pen-R pneumococcus in unimmunized children, or for possible MRSA; high-dose ceftaroline (MRSA dosing) should also prove effective for both pathogens, but no data exist currently for CNS infections.
– *Haemophilus influenzae* type b[323] in unimmunized children	Ceftriaxone 100 mg/kg/day IV q24h; for 10 days (AI)	Alternative: ampicillin 200–400 mg/kg/day IV div q6h (for beta-lactamase–negative strains)
– Meningococcus (*Neisseria meningitidis*)[323]	Penicillin G 250,000 U/kg/day IV div q4h; or ceftriaxone 100 mg/kg/day IV q24h, or cefotaxime 200 mg/kg/day IV div q6h; treatment course for 7 days (AI)	Meningococcal prophylaxis: rifampin 10 mg/kg PO q12h for 4 doses OR ceftriaxone 125–250 mg IM once OR ciprofloxacin 500 mg PO once (adolescents and adults)
– Neonatal	See Chapter 5.	
– Pneumococcus (*Streptococcus pneumoniae*)[323]	For pen-S and cephalosporin-susceptible strains: penicillin G 250,000 U/kg/day IV div q4–6h, OR ceftriaxone 100 mg/kg/day IV q24h; for 10 days (AI).	Some pneumococci may be resistant to penicillin but susceptible to ceftriaxone and may be treated with the cephalosporin alone. For the rare ceftriaxone-resistant strain, add vancomycin to ceftriaxone (once resistance is suspected or documented) to complete a 14-day course.

	For pen-R pneumococci (assuming ceftriaxone susceptibility): continue ceftriaxone IV for total course (AIII).	With the efficacy of current pneumococcal conjugate vaccines, primary bacterial meningitis is uncommon, and penicillin resistance has decreased substantially. Test-of-cure LP may be helpful in those with pen-R pneumococci.
Meningitis, TB (*Mycobacterium tuberculosis; Mycobacterium bovis*)[15,16]	For non-immunocompromised children: INH 15 mg/kg/day PO, IV div q12–24h AND rifampin 15 mg/kg/day PO, IV div q12–24h for 12 mo AND PZA 30 mg/kg/day PO div q12–24h for first 2 mo of therapy, AND streptomycin 30 mg/kg/day IV, IM div q12h or ethionamide for first 4–8 wk of therapy; followed by INH and rifampin combination therapy to complete at least 12 mo for the total course.	Hyponatremia from inappropriate ADH secretion is common; ventricular drainage may be necessary for obstructive hydrocephalus. Corticosteroids (can use the same dexamethasone dose as for bacterial meningitis, 0.6 mg/kg/day IV div q6h) for 4 wk until neurologically stable, then taper dose for 1–3 mo to decrease neurologic complications and improve prognosis by decreasing the incidence of infarction.[324] Watch for rebound inflammation during taper; increase dose to previously effective level, then taper more slowly. For recommendations for drug-resistant strains and treatment of TB in HIV-infected patients, visit the CDC website for TB: www.cdc.gov/tb (accessed October 10, 2019).
Shunt infections: The use of antibiotic-impregnated shunts has decreased the frequency of this infection.[325] Shunt removal is usually necessary for cure, with placement of a new external ventricular drain; intraventricular injection of antibiotics should be considered in children who are responding poorly to systemic antibiotic therapy. Duration of therapy varies by pathogen and response to treatment.[326]		
– Empiric therapy pending Gram stain and culture[323,326]	Vancomycin 60 mg/kg/day IV div q8h, AND ceftriaxone 100 mg/kg/day IV q24h (AII)	If Gram stain shows only gram-positive cocci, can use vancomycin alone. Cefepime, meropenem, or ceftazidime should be used instead of ceftriaxone if *Pseudomonas* is suspected. For ESBL-containing gram-negative bacilli, meropenem should be used as the preferred carbapenem for CNS infection.

J. CENTRAL NERVOUS SYSTEM INFECTIONS (continued)

Clinical Diagnosis	Therapy (evidence grade)	Comments
– *Staphylococcus epidermidis* or *Staphylococcus aureus*[323,326]	Vancomycin (for *S epidermidis* and CA-MRSA) 60 mg/kg/day IV div q8h; OR nafcillin (if organisms susceptible) 150–200 mg/kg/day AND rifampin; for 10–14 days (AIII)	For children who cannot tolerate vancomycin, ceftaroline has anecdotally been successful: ceftaroline: 2–<6 mo, 30 mg/kg/day IV div q8h (each dose given over 2 h); ≥6 mo, 45 mg/kg/day IV div q8h (each dose given over 2 h) (max single dose 600 mg) (BIII). Linezolid, daptomycin, and TMP/SMX are other untested options.
– Gram-negative bacilli[323,326]	Empiric therapy with meropenem 120 mg/kg/day IV div q8h OR cefepime 150 mg/kg/day IV div q8h (AIII). For *E coli* (without ESBLs): ceftriaxone 100 mg/kg/day IV q12h for at least 10–14 days, preferably 21 days.	Remove shunt. Select appropriate therapy based on in vitro susceptibilities. Meropenem, ceftriaxone, cefotaxime, and cefepime have all been studied in pediatric meningitis. Systemic gentamicin as combination therapy is not routinely recommended. Intrathecal therapy with aminoglycosides not routinely necessary with highly active beta-lactam therapy and shunt removal.

K. URINARY TRACT INFECTIONS

Clinical Diagnosis	Therapy (evidence grade)	Comments
NOTE: Antibiotic susceptibility profiles of *Escherichia coli,* the most common cause of UTI, vary considerably. For mild disease, TMP/SMX may be started as initial empiric therapy if local susceptibility ≥80% and a 20% failure rate is acceptable. For moderate to severe disease (possible pyelonephritis), obtain cultures and begin an oral 2nd- or 3rd-generation cephalosporin (cefuroxime, cefaclor, cefprozil, cefixime, ceftibuten, cefdinir, cefpodoxime), ciprofloxacin PO, or ceftriaxone IM. Antibiotic susceptibility testing will help direct your therapy to the narrowest spectrum agent.		
Cystitis, acute (*E coli*)[327,328]	For mild disease: TMP/SMX, 8 mg/kg/day of TMP PO div bid for 3 days (See NOTE about resistance to TMP/SMX.) For moderate to severe disease: cefixime 8 mg/kg/day PO qd; OR ceftriaxone 50 mg/kg IM q24h for 3–5 days (with normal anatomy) (BII); follow-up culture after 36–48 h treatment ONLY if still symptomatic	Alternative: amoxicillin 30 mg/kg/day PO div tid OR amoxicillin/clavulanate PO if susceptible (BII); ciprofloxacin 20–30 mg/kg/day PO div bid for suspected or documented resistant organisms[329]
Nephronia, lobar *E coli* and other enteric rods (also called focal bacterial nephritis)[329–331]	Ceftriaxone 50 mg/kg/day IV, IM q24h. Duration depends on resolution of renal cellulitis vs development of abscess (10–21 days) (AIII). For ESBL-positive *E coli,* carbapenems and fluoroquinolones are often active agents.	Invasive, consolidative parenchymal infection; complication of pyelonephritis, can evolve into renal abscess. Step-down therapy with oral cephalosporins once cellulitis/abscess has initially responded to therapy.

K. URINARY TRACT INFECTIONS (continued)

Clinical Diagnosis	Therapy (evidence grade)	Comments
Pyelonephritis, acute (*E coli*)[199,327-329,332-336]	Ceftriaxone 50 mg/kg/day IV, IM q24h OR gentamicin 5–6 mg/kg/day IV, IM q24h (yes, once daily). For documented or suspected ceftriaxone-resistant ESBL-positive strains, use meropenem IV, imipenem IV, or ertapenem IV[199,333,334]; OR gentamicin IV, IM, OR pip/tazo. Switch to oral therapy following clinical response (BII). If organism resistant to amoxicillin and TMP/SMX, use an oral 1st-, 2nd-, or 3rd-generation cephalosporin (BII); if cephalosporin-R, can use ciprofloxacin PO 30 mg/kg/day div q12h (up to 40 mg/kg/day for *Pseudomonas*)[329] (BIII); for 7–14 days total (depending on response to therapy).	For mild to moderate infection, oral therapy is likely to be as effective as IV/IM therapy for susceptible strains, down to 3 mo of age.[332,335] If bacteremia documented and infant is <2–3 mo, rule out meningitis and treat 14 days IV + PO (AIII). Aminoglycosides at any dose are more nephrotoxic than beta-lactams but represent effective therapy (AI). Once-daily dosing of gentamicin is preferred to tid.[332]
Recurrent urinary tract infection, prophylaxis[327,337-340]	Only for those with grade III–V reflux or with recurrent febrile UTI: TMP/SMX 2 mg/kg/dose of TMP PO qd OR nitrofurantoin 1–2 mg/kg PO qd at bedtime; more rapid resistance may develop using beta-lactams (BII).	Prophylaxis not recommended for patients with grade I–II reflux and no evidence of renal damage (although the RIVUR study[339] included these children, and they may also benefit, but early treatment of new infections is recommended for these children). *Resistance eventually develops to every antibiotic;* follow resistance patterns for each patient. The use of periodic urine cultures is controversial, as there are no comparative data to guide management of asymptomatic bacteriuria in a child at high risk of recurrent UTI.

L. MISCELLANEOUS SYSTEMIC INFECTIONS

Clinical Diagnosis	Therapy (evidence grade)	Comments
Actinomycosis[341–343]	Penicillin G 250,000 U/kg/day IV div q6h, OR ampicillin 150 mg/kg/day IV div q8h until improved (often up to 6 wk for extensive infection); then long-term convalescent therapy with penicillin V 100 mg/kg/day (up to 4 g/day) PO for 6–12 mo (AII)	Surgery with debridement as indicated Alternatives: amoxicillin, clindamycin, erythromycin; ceftriaxone IM/IV, doxycycline for children >7 y, or meropenem IV.
Anaplasmosis[344,345] (human granulocytotropic anaplasmosis, *Anaplasma phagocytophilum*)	Doxycycline 4.4 mg/kg/day IV, PO (max 200 mg/day) div bid for 7–10 days (regardless of age) (AIII)	For mild disease, consider rifampin 20 mg/kg/day PO div bid for 7–10 days (BIII).
Anthrax, sepsis/pneumonia, community vs bioterror exposure (inhalation, cutaneous, gastrointestinal, meningoencephalitis)[17]	For community-associated anthrax infection, amoxicillin 75 mg/kg/day div q8h OR doxycycline for children >7 y. For bioterror-associated exposure (regardless of age): ciprofloxacin 20–30 mg/kg/day IV div q12h, OR levofloxacin 16 mg/kg/day IV div q12h not to exceed 250 mg/dose (AIII); OR doxycycline 4.4 mg/kg/day PO (max 200 mg/day) div bid (regardless of age).	For invasive infection after bioterror exposure, 2 or 3 antibiotics may be required.[17] For oral step-down therapy, can use oral ciprofloxacin or doxycycline; if susceptible, can use penicillin, amoxicillin, or clindamycin. May require long-term postexposure prophylaxis after bioterror event.
Appendicitis (See Table 6H, Gastrointestinal Infections, Intra-abdominal infection, Appendicitis.)		
Brucellosis[346–349]	Doxycycline 4.4 mg/kg/day PO (max 200 mg/day) div bid (for children >7 y) AND rifampin (15–20 mg/kg/day div q12h) (BIII); OR for children <8 y: TMP/SMX 10 mg/kg/day TMP IV, PO div q12h AND rifampin 15–20 mg/kg/day div q12h (BIII); for at least 6 wk	Combination therapy with rifampin will decrease the risk of relapse. For more serious infections, ADD gentamicin 6–7.5 mg/kg/day IV, IM div q8h for the first 1–2 wk of therapy to further decrease risk of relapse[349] (BIII), particularly for endocarditis, osteomyelitis, or meningitis. Prolonged treatment for 4–6 mo and surgical debridement may be necessary for deep infections (AIII).

L. MISCELLANEOUS SYSTEMIC INFECTIONS (continued)

Clinical Diagnosis	Therapy (evidence grade)	Comments
Cat-scratch disease (*Bartonella henselae*)[350–352]	Supportive care for adenopathy (I&D of infected lymph node); azithromycin 12 mg/kg/day PO qd for 5 days shortens the duration of adenopathy (AIII). No prospective data exist for invasive CSD: gentamicin (for 14 days) AND TMP/SMX AND rifampin for hepatosplenic disease and osteomyelitis (AIII). For CNS infection, use ceftriaxone AND gentamicin ± TMP/SMX (AIII). Alternatives: ciprofloxacin, doxycycline.	This dosage of azithromycin has been documented to be safe and effective for streptococcal pharyngitis and may offer greater deep tissue exposure than the dosage studied by Bass et al[10] and used for otitis media.
Chickenpox/shingles (varicella-zoster virus)	See Chapter 9, Varicella virus.	
Ehrlichiosis (human monocytic ehrlichiosis, caused by *Ehrlichia chaffeensis*, and *Ehrlichia ewingii*)[344,353–355]	Doxycycline 4.4 mg/kg/day IV, PO div bid (max 100 mg/dose) for 7–10 days (regardless of age) (AIII)	For mild disease, consider rifampin 20 mg/kg/day PO div bid (max 300 mg/dose) for 7–10 days (BIII).
Febrile neutropenic patient (empiric therapy of invasive infection: *Pseudomonas*, enteric gram-negative bacilli, staphylococci, streptococci, yeast, fungi)[356,357]	Cefepime 150 mg/kg/day div q8h (AI); or meropenem 60 mg/kg/day div q8h (AII); OR pip/tazo (300-mg pip component/kg/day div q8h for 9 mo; 240 mg/kg/day div q8h for 2–9 mo), OR ceftazidime 150 mg/kg/day IV div q8h AND tobramycin 6 mg/kg/day IV q8h (AII). ADD vancomycin 40 mg/kg/day IV div q8h if MRSA or coagulation-negative staph suspected (eg, central catheter infection) (AIII). ADD metronidazole to ceftazidime or cefepime if colitis or other deep anaerobic infection suspected (AIII).	Alternatives: other anti-*Pseudomonas* beta-lactams (imipenem) AND antistaphylococcal antibiotics. If no response in 3–4 days and no alternative etiology demonstrated, begin additional empiric therapy with antifungals (BII)[348]; dosages and formulations outlined in Chapter 8. Increasingly resistant pathogens (ESBL *E coli* and KPC *Klebsiella*) will require alternative empiric therapy if MDR organisms are colonizing or present on the child's hospital unit.

		For low-risk patients with negative cultures and close follow-up, alternative management strategies are being explored: oral therapy with amox/clav and ciprofloxacin may be used, cautious discontinuation of antibiotics (even in those without marrow recovery).[356,358]
Human immunodeficiency virus infection	See Chapter 9.	
Infant botulism[359]	Botulism immune globulin for infants (BabyBIG) 50 mg/kg IV for 1 dose (AI); BabyBIG can be obtained from the California Department of Public Health at www.infantbotulism.org, through your state health department.	www.infantbotulism.org provides information for physicians and parents. Website organized by the California Department of Public Health (accessed October 10, 2019. Aminoglycosides should be avoided because they potentiate the neuromuscular effect of botulinum toxin.
Kawasaki syndrome[360–363]	No antibiotics; IVIG 2 g/kg as single dose (AI); may need to repeat dose in up to 15% of children for persisting fever that lasts 24 h after completion of the IVIG infusion (AII). For subsequent relapse, many children will respond to a second IVIG infusion, otherwise consult an infectious diseases physician or pediatric cardiologist. Adjunctive therapy with corticosteroids for those at high risk for the development of aneurysms.[361]	Aspirin 80–100 mg/kg/day div qid in acute, febrile phase; once afebrile for 24–48 h, initiate low-dosage (3–5 mg/kg/day) aspirin therapy for 6–8 wk (assuming echocardiogram is normal). Role of corticosteroids, infliximab, calcineurin inhibitors, and anti-thrombotic therapy, as well as methotrexate and cyclosporin, for IVIG-resistant Kawasaki syndrome under investigation and may improve outcome in severe cases.[362,363]
Leprosy (Hansen disease)[364]	Dapsone 1 mg/kg/day PO qd AND rifampin 10 mg/kg/day PO qd; ADD (for multibacillary disease) clofazimine 1 mg/kg/day PO qd; for 12 mo for paucibacillary disease; for 24 mo for multibacillary disease (AII).	Consult Health Resources and Services Administration National Hansen's Disease (Leprosy) Program, reviewed June 2019, at www.hrsa.gov/hansens-disease (accessed October 10, 2019) for advice about treatment and free antibiotics: 800/642-2477.

L. MISCELLANEOUS SYSTEMIC INFECTIONS (continued)

Clinical Diagnosis	Therapy (evidence grade)	Comments
Leptospirosis[365,366]	Penicillin G 250,000 U/kg/day IV div q6h, or ceftriaxone 50 mg/kg/day IV, IM q24h; for 7 days (BII) For mild disease in all age groups, doxycycline (>7 y) 4.4 mg/kg/day (max 200 mg/day) PO div bid for 7–10 days (BII)	Alternative: for those with mild disease, intolerant of doxycycline, azithromycin 20 mg/kg on day 1, 10 mg/kg on days 2 and 3, or amoxicillin
Lyme disease (*Borrelia burgdorferi*)[355,367–369]	Neurologic evaluation, including LP, if there is clinical suspicion of CNS involvement	
– Early localized disease (Erythema migrans, single or multiple) (any age)	Doxycycline 4.4 mg/kg/day (max 200 mg/day) PO div bid for 14 days for all ages (AII) OR amoxicillin 50 mg/kg/day (max 1.5 g/day) PO div tid for 14 days (AII)	Alternative: cefuroxime, 30 mg/kg/day (max 1,000 mg/day) PO, in 2 div doses for 14 days OR azithromycin 10 mg/kg/day PO qd for 7 days
– Arthritis (no CNS disease)	Oral therapy as outlined in early localized disease, but for 28 days (AIII).	Persistent or recurrent joint swelling after treatment: repeat a 4-wk course of oral antibiotics or give ceftriaxone 50–75 mg/kg IV q24h for 14–28 days. For persisting arthritis after 2 defined antibiotic treatment courses, use symptomatic therapy.
– Isolated facial (Bell) palsy	Doxycycline as outlined previously, for 14 days (AIII); efficacy of amoxicillin unknown.	LP is not routinely required unless CNS symptoms present. Treatment to prevent late sequelae; will not provide a quick response for palsy.
– Carditis	Oral therapy as outlined in early localized disease, for 14 days (range: 14–21 days) OR ceftriaxone 50–75 mg/kg IV q24h for 14 days (range: 14–21 days) (AIII)	
– Neuroborreliosis	Doxycycline 4.4 mg/kg/day (max 200 mg/day) PO div bid for 14 days (AII) OR ceftriaxone 50–75 mg/kg IV q24h OR penicillin G 300,000 U/kg/day IV div q4h; for 14 days (AIII)	

Melioidosis (*Burkholderia pseudomallei*)[370,371]	Acute sepsis: meropenem 75 mg/kg/day div q8h; OR ceftazidime 150 mg/kg/day IV div q8h; followed by TMP/SMX (10 mg/kg/day of TMP) PO div bid for 3–6 mo	Alternative convalescent therapy: amox/clav (90 mg/kg/day amox div tid, not bid) for children ≤7 y, or doxycycline for children >7 y; for 20 wk (AII)
Mycobacteria, nontuberculous[11,13,14,372]		
– Adenitis in normal host (See Adenitis entries in this table and Table 6A.)	Excision usually curative (BII); azithromycin PO OR clarithromycin PO for 6–12 wk (with or without rifampin) if susceptible (BII)	Antibiotic susceptibility patterns are quite variable; cultures should guide therapy; medical therapy 60%–70% effective. Newer data suggest toxicity of antimicrobials may not be worth the small clinical benefit.
– Pneumonia or disseminated infection in compromised hosts (HIV, gamma-interferon receptor deficiency, cystic fibrosis)[13,372–375]	Usually treated with 3 or 4 active drugs (eg, clarithromycin OR azithromycin, AND amikacin, cefoxitin, meropenem). Also test for ciprofloxacin, TMP/SMX, ethambutol, rifampin, linezolid, clofazimine, and doxycycline (BII).	Outcomes particularly poor for *Mycobacterium abscessus*.[376] See Chapter 11 for dosages; cultures are essential, as the susceptibility patterns of nontuberculous mycobacteria are varied.
Nocardiosis (*Nocardia asteroides* and *Nocardia brasiliensis*)[377,378]	TMP/SMX 8 mg/kg/day TMP div bid or sulfisoxazole 120–150 mg/kg/day PO div qid for 6–12 wk or longer. For severe infection, particularly in immunocompromised hosts, use ceftriaxone or imipenem or meropenem AND amikacin 15–20 mg/kg/day IM, IV div q8h (AIII).	Wide spectrum of disease from skin lesions to brain abscess. Surgery when indicated. Alternatives: doxycycline (for children >7 y), amox/clav, or linezolid. Immunocompromised children may require months of therapy.
Plague (*Yersinia pestis*)[379–381]	Gentamicin 7.5 mg/kg/day IV div q8h (AII) OR doxycycline 4.4 mg/kg/day (max 200 mg/day) PO div bid OR ciprofloxacin 30 mg/kg/day PO div bid. Gentamicin is poorly active in abscesses; consider alternatives for bubonic plague.	A complete listing of options for children is provided on the CDC website: https://www.cdc.gov/plague/healthcare/clinicians.html (accessed October 10, 2019).

L. MISCELLANEOUS SYSTEMIC INFECTIONS (continued)

Clinical Diagnosis	Therapy (evidence grade)	Comments
Q fever (*Coxiella burnetii*)[382,383]	Acute stage: doxycycline 4.4 mg/kg/day (max 200 mg/day) PO div bid for 14 days (AII) for children of any age. Endocarditis and chronic disease (ongoing symptoms for 6–12 mo): doxycycline for children >7 y AND hydroxychloroquine for 18–36 mo (AIII). Seek advice from pediatric infectious diseases specialist for children ≤7 y: may require TMP/SMX, 8–10 mg TMP/kg/day div q12h with doxycycline; OR levofloxacin with rifampin for 18 mo.	Follow doxycycline and hydroxychloroquine serum concentrations during endocarditis/chronic disease therapy. CNS: Use fluoroquinolone (no prospective data) (BIII). Clarithromycin may be an alternative based on limited data (CIII).
Rocky Mountain spotted fever (fever, petechial rash with centripetal spread; *Rickettsia rickettsii*)[384,385]	Doxycycline 4.4 mg/kg/day (max 200 mg/day) PO div bid for 7–10 days (AI) for children of any age	Start empiric therapy early.
Tetanus (*Clostridium tetani*)[386,387]	Metronidazole 30 mg/kg/day IV, PO div q8h OR penicillin G 100,000 U/kg/day IV div q6h for 10–14 days; AND TIG 3,000–6,000 U IM (AII)	Wound debridement essential; may infiltrate wound with a portion of TIG dose, but not well-studied; IVIG may provide antibody to toxin if TIG not available. Immunize with Td or Tdap. See Chapter 14 for prophylaxis recommendations.
Toxic shock syndrome (toxin-producing strains of *S aureus* [including MRSA] or group A streptococcus)[3,8,9,388,389]	Empiric: vancomycin 45 mg/kg/day IV div q8h AND oxacillin/nafcillin 150 mg/kg/day IV div q6h, AND clindamycin 30–40 mg/kg/day div q8h ± gentamicin for 7–10 days (AIII)	Clindamycin added for the initial 48–72 h of therapy to decrease toxin production. Ceftaroline is an option for MRSA treatment, particularly with renal injury from shock and vancomycin (BIII). IVIG may provide additional benefit by binding circulating toxin (CIII). For MSSA: oxacillin/nafcillin AND clindamycin ± gentamicin.

		For CA-MRSA: vancomycin AND clindamycin ± gentamicin. For group A streptococcus: penicillin G AND clindamycin.
Tularemia (*Francisella tularensis*)[190,390]	Gentamicin 6–7.5 mg/kg/day IM, IV div q8h; for 10–14 days (AII) Alternative for mild disease: ciprofloxacin (for 10 days) Additional information from CDC: https://www.cdc.gov/tularemia/clinicians/index.html (reviewed December 13, 2018; accessed October 10, 2019)	CDC also recommends doxycycline as an alternative, although relapse rates may be higher than with other antibiotics.

7. Preferred Therapy for Specific Bacterial and Mycobacterial Pathogens

NOTES

- For fungal, viral, and parasitic infections, see chapters 8, 9, and 10, respectively.
- Limitations of space do not permit listing of all possible alternative antimicrobials.
- Cefotaxime, a third-generation cephalosporin approved by the US Food and Drug Administration (FDA) for children more than 3 decades ago, is no longer available in the United States. Ceftriaxone has a virtually identical antibacterial spectrum of activity to cefotaxime; cefepime is very similar in gram-positive activity but adds *Pseudomonas aeruginosa* (and some enhanced activity for *Enterobacter, Serratia*, and *Citrobacter*) to the gram-negative activity of cefotaxime; ceftazidime adds *Pseudomonas* activity but loses gram-positive activity, compared with cefotaxime. Cefepime[1] and ceftazidime[2] have been documented to be effective in pediatric meningitis clinical trials.
- **Abbreviations:** amox/clav, amoxicillin/clavulanate (Augmentin); amp/sul, ampicillin/sulbactam; CA-MRSA, community-associated methicillin-resistant *Staphylococcus aureus;* CAZ/AVI, ceftazidime/avibactam; CDC, Centers for Disease Control and Prevention; CNS, central nervous system; ESBL, extended spectrum beta-lactamase; FDA, US Food and Drug Administration; HACEK, *Haemophilus aphrophilus, Actinobacillus actinomycetemcomitans, Cardiobacterium hominis, Eikenella corrodens,* and *Kingella* spp; HRSA, Health Resources and Services Administration; IM, intramuscular; IMI/REL, imipenem/relebactam; INH, isoniazid; IV, intravenous; IVIG, intravenous immunoglobulin; KPC, *Klebsiella pneumoniae* carbapenemase; MDR, multidrug resistant; mero/vabor, meropenem/vaborbactam; MIC, minimal inhibitory concentration; MRSA, methicillin-resistant *S aureus;* MSSA, methicillin-susceptible *S aureus;* NARMS, National Antimicrobial Resistance Monitoring System for Enteric Bacteria; NDM, New Delhi metallo-beta-lactamase; PCV13, pneumococcal 13-valent conjugate vaccine; pen-S, penicillin-susceptible; pip/tazo, piperacillin/tazobactam; PO, oral; PZA, pyrazinamide; spp, species; tid, 3 times daily; TIG, tetanus immune globulin; TMP/SMX, trimethoprim/sulfamethoxazole; UTI, urinary tract infection.

A. COMMON BACTERIAL PATHOGENS AND USUAL PATTERN OF SUSCEPTIBILITY TO ANTIBIOTICS (GRAM POSITIVE)

	Commonly Used Antibiotics (One Agent per Class Listed) (scale — to ++ defined in footnote)			
	Penicillin	Ampicillin/ Amoxicillin	Amoxicillin/ Clavulanate	Methicillin/ Oxacillin
Enterococcus faecalis[a]	++	++	+	—
Enterococcus faecium[a]	++	++	+	—
Staphylococcus, coagulase negative	—	—	—	±
Staphylococcus aureus, methicillin-resistant	—	—	—	—
Staphylococcus aureus, methicillin-susceptible	—	—	—	++
Streptococcus pneumoniae	++	++	++	+
Streptococcus pyogenes	++	++	++	++

NOTE: ++ = preferred; + = acceptable; ± = possibly effective (see text for further discussion); — = unlikely to be effective; [blank cell] = untested.

[a] Need to add gentamicin or other aminoglycoside to ampicillin/penicillin or vancomycin for in vitro bactericidal activity.

Commonly Used Antibiotics (One Agent per Class Listed) (scale — to ++ defined in footnote)					
Cefazolin/ Cephalexin	Vancomycin	Clindamycin	Linezolid	Daptomycin	Ceftaroline
–	+	–	+	+	–
–	+	–	+	+	–
±	++	+	++	++	++
–	++	++	++	++	++
++	++	+	++	++	++
++	+	+	++	+	++
++	+	++	+	+	+

B. COMMON BACTERIAL PATHOGENS AND USUAL PATTERN OF SUSCEPTIBILITY TO ANTIBIOTICS (GRAM NEGATIVE)[a]

	Commonly Used Antibiotics (One Agent per Class Listed) (scale — to ++ defined in footnote)					
	Ampicillin/ Amoxicillin	**Amoxicillin/ Clavulanate**	**Cefazolin/ Cephalexin**	**Cefuroxime**	**Ceftriaxone**	**Ceftazidime/ Avibactam**
Acinetobacter spp	—	—	—	—	+	+
Citrobacter spp	—	—	—	+	+	++
Enterobacter spp[b]	—	—	—	±	+	++
Escherichia coli[c]	+	+	+	++[d]	++[d]	++
Haemophilus influenzae[f]	+	++	+	++	++	++
Klebsiella spp[c]	—	—	+	++	++	++
Neisseria meningitidis	++	++		+	++	
Pseudomonas aeruginosa	—	—	—	—	—	++
Salmonella, non-typhoid spp	+	++			++	++
Serratia spp[b]	—	—	—	±	+	++
Shigella spp	+	++	+	+	++	++
Stenotrophomonas maltophilia	—	—	—	—	—	+

NOTE: ++ = preferred; + = acceptable; ± = possibly effective (see text for further discussion); — = unlikely to be effective; [blank cell] = untested.

[a] CDC (NARMS) statistics for each state, by year, are found for many enteric pathogens on the CDC website at https://wwwn.cdc.gov/narmsnow and are also provided by the SENTRY surveillance system (JMI Laboratories); we also use current pediatric hospital antibiograms from the editors' hospitals to assess pediatric trends. When sufficient data are available, pediatric community isolate susceptibility data are used. Nosocomial resistance patterns may be quite different, usually with increased resistance, particularly in adults; please check your local/regional hospital antibiogram for your local susceptibility patterns.

[b] AmpC will be constitutively produced in low frequency in every population of organisms and will be selected out during therapy with third-generation cephalosporins if used as single agent therapy.

[c] Rare carbapenem-resistant isolates in pediatrics (KPC, NDM strains).

[d] Will be resistant to virtually all current cephalosporins if ESBL producing.

[e] Follow the MIC, and not the report for susceptible (S), intermediate (I), or resistant (R), as some ESBL producers will have low MICs and can be effectively treated with higher dosages.

[f] Will be resistant to ampicillin/amoxicillin if beta-lactamase producing.

Commonly Used Antibiotics (One Agent per Class Listed) (scale – to ++ defined in footnote)						
Ceftazidime	Cefepime	Meropenem/ Imipenem	Piperacillin/ Tazobactam	TMP/SMX	Ciprofloxacin	Gentamicin
+	+	+	+	+	+	+
+	++	++	+	++	++	+
+	++	++	+	++	++	+
++[d]	++[e]	++	++	+	++	+
++	++	++	++	++	++	±
++	++[e]	++	++	++	++	++
+	++	++	++		++	
+	++	++	++	–	++	+
++	++	++	++	++	++	
+	++	++	+	++	++	++
++	++	++	++	±	++	
+	±	–	+	++	++	±

C. COMMON BACTERIAL PATHOGENS AND USUAL PATTERN OF SUSCEPTIBILITY TO ANTIBIOTICS (ANAEROBES)

	Commonly Used Antibiotics (One Agent per Class Listed) (scale — to ++ defined in footnote)				
	Penicillin	**Ampicillin/ Amoxicillin**	**Amoxicillin/ Clavulanate**	**Cefazolin**	**Cefoxitin**
Anaerobic streptococci	++	++	++	++	++
Bacteroides fragilis	±	±	++	—	+
Clostridia (eg, *tetani, perfringens*)	++	++	++		+
Clostridium difficile	—	—	—		—

NOTE: ++ = preferred; + = acceptable; ± = possibly effective (see text for further discussion); — = unlikely to be effective; [blank cell] = untested.

Commonly Used Antibiotics (One Agent per Class Listed) (scale – to ++ defined in footnote)					
Ceftriaxone/ Cefotaxime	Meropenem/ Imipenem	Piperacillin/ Tazobactam	Metronidazole	Clindamycin	Vancomycin
++	++	++	++	++	++
–	++	++	++	+	
±	++	++	++	+	++
–	++		++	–	++

D. PREFERRED THERAPY FOR SPECIFIC BACTERIAL AND MYCOBACTERIAL PATHOGENS

Organism	Clinical Illness	Drug of Choice (evidence grade)	Alternatives
Acinetobacter baumannii[3–6]	Sepsis, meningitis, nosocomial pneumonia, wound infection	Meropenem (BIII) or other carbapenem	Use culture results to guide therapy: ceftazidime, amp/sul, pip/tazo, TMP/SMX, ciprofloxacin, tigecycline, colistin/polymyxin B. Watch for emergence of resistance *during* therapy, including to colistin. Consider combination therapy for life-threatening infection.[5,6] Inhaled colistin for pneumonia caused by MDR strains (BIII).
Actinomyces israelii[7]	Actinomycosis (cervicofacial, thoracic, abdominal)	Penicillin G; ampicillin (CIII)	Amoxicillin, doxycycline, clindamycin, ceftriaxone, meropenem, pip/tazo, linezolid
Aeromonas hydrophila[8]	Diarrhea	Ciprofloxacin (CIII)	Azithromycin, cefepime, TMP/SMX
	Sepsis, cellulitis, necrotizing fasciitis	Cefepime (BIII)	Meropenem, ciprofloxacin, TMP/SMX
Aggregatibacter (formerly *Actinobacillus*) *actinomycetemcomitans*[9]	Periodontitis, abscesses (including brain), endocarditis	Ceftriaxone (CIII)	Ampicillin/amoxicillin for beta-lactamase–negative strains, or amox/clav, doxycycline, TMP/SMX, ciprofloxacin
Anaplasma (formerly *Ehrlichia*) *phagocytophilum*[10,11]	Human granulocytic anaplasmosis	Doxycycline (all ages) (AII)	Rifampin, levofloxacin
Arcanobacterium haemolyticum[12]	Pharyngitis, cellulitis, Lemierre syndrome	Azithromycin; penicillin (BIII)	Erythromycin, amoxicillin, ceftriaxone, clindamycin, doxycycline, vancomycin
Bacillus anthracis[13]	Anthrax (cutaneous, gastrointestinal, inhalational, meningoencephalitis)	Ciprofloxacin (regardless of age) (AIII). For invasive, systemic infection, use combination therapy.	Doxycycline, amoxicillin, levofloxacin, clindamycin, penicillin G, vancomycin, meropenem. Bioterror strains may be antibiotic resistant.

Bacillus cereus or *subtilis*[14,15]	Sepsis; toxin-mediated gastroenteritis	Vancomycin (BIII)	Clindamycin, ciprofloxacin, linezolid, daptomycin
Bacteroides fragilis[16,17]	Peritonitis, sepsis, abscesses	Metronidazole (AI)	Meropenem or imipenem (AI); pip/tazo (AI); amox/clav (BII). Recent surveillance suggests resistance of up to 25% for clindamycin.
Bacteroides, other spp[16,17]	Pneumonia, sepsis, abscesses	Metronidazole (BII)	Meropenem or imipenem; penicillin G or ampicillin if beta-lactamase negative
Bartonella henselae[18,19]	Cat-scratch disease	Azithromycin for lymph node disease (BII); gentamicin in combination with TMP/SMX AND rifampin for invasive disease (BIII)	Cefotaxime, ciprofloxacin, doxycycline
Bartonella quintana[19,20]	Bacillary angiomatosis, peliosis hepatis, endocarditis	Gentamicin plus doxycycline (BIII); erythromycin; ciprofloxacin (BIII)	Azithromycin, doxycycline
Bordetella pertussis, parapertussis[21,22]	Pertussis	Azithromycin (AIII); erythromycin (BII)	Clarithromycin, TMP/SMX, ciprofloxacin (in vitro data)
Borrelia burgdorferi, Lyme disease[23–25]	Treatment based on stage of infection (See Lyme disease in Chapter 6.)	Doxycycline for all ages (AII); amoxicillin or cefuroxime can be used in children $\leq$7 y (AIII); ceftriaxone IV for CNS/meningitis (AII)	
Borrelia hermsii, turicatae, parkeri, tick-borne relapsing fever[26,27]	Relapsing fever	Doxycycline for all ages (AIII)	Penicillin or erythromycin in children intolerant of doxycycline (BIII)
Borrelia recurrentis, louse-borne relapsing fever[26,27]	Relapsing fever	Single-dose doxycycline for all ages (AIII)	Penicillin or erythromycin in children intolerant of doxycycline (BIII). Amoxicillin; ceftriaxone.

D. PREFERRED THERAPY FOR SPECIFIC BACTERIAL AND MYCOBACTERIAL PATHOGENS (continued)

Organism	Clinical Illness	Drug of Choice (evidence grade)	Alternatives
Brucella spp[28–30]	Brucellosis (See Chapter 6.)	Doxycycline AND rifampin (BIII); OR, for children ≤7 y: TMP/SMX AND rifampin (BIII)	For serious infection: doxycycline AND gentamicin AND rifampin; or TMP/SMX AND gentamicin AND rifampin (AIII). May require extended therapy (months).
Burkholderia cepacia complex[31–33]	Pneumonia, sepsis in immunocompromised children; pneumonia in children with cystic fibrosis[34]	Meropenem (BIII); for severe disease consider combination therapy with TMP/SMX (AIII).	Ceftolozane/tazobactam, doxycycline, ceftazidime, pip/tazo, ciprofloxacin, TMP-SMX. Aerosolized antibiotics may provide higher concentrations in lung.
Burkholderia pseudomallei[35–37]	Melioidosis	Meropenem (AIII) or ceftazidime (BIII), followed by prolonged TMP/SMX for 12 wk (AII)	TMP/SMX, doxycycline, or amox/clav for chronic disease
Campylobacter fetus[38,39]	Sepsis, meningitis in the neonate	Meropenem (BIII)	Ampicillin, gentamicin, erythromycin, ciprofloxacin
Campylobacter jejuni[40,41]	Diarrhea	Azithromycin (BII); erythromycin (BII)	Amox/clav, doxycycline, ciprofloxacin (very high rates of ciprofloxacin-resistant strains in Thailand, Hong Kong, and Spain)
Capnocytophaga canimorsus[42,43]	Sepsis after dog bite (increased risk with asplenia)	Pip/tazo OR meropenem OR amp/sul; amox/clav (BIII)	Clindamycin, linezolid, penicillin G, ciprofloxacin
Capnocytophaga ochracea[44]	Sepsis, abscesses	Ampicillin, clindamycin (BIII); amox/clav (BIII)	Meropenem, pip/tazo, ciprofloxacin
Cellulosimicrobium (formerly *Oerskovia*) *cellulans*[45]	Wound infection; catheter infection	Vancomycin ± rifampin (AIII)	Linezolid; resistant to beta-lactams, macrolides, clindamycin, aminoglycosides

Chlamydia trachomatis[46–48]	Lymphogranuloma venereum	Doxycycline (AII)	Azithromycin, erythromycin
	Urethritis, cervicitis	Doxycycline (AII)	Azithromycin, erythromycin, ofloxacin
	Inclusion conjunctivitis of newborn	Azithromycin (AIII)	Erythromycin
	Pneumonia of infancy	Azithromycin (AIII)	Erythromycin, ampicillin
	Trachoma	Azithromycin (AI)	Doxycycline, erythromycin
Chlamydophila (formerly *Chlamydia*) *pneumoniae*[46,47,49,50]	Pneumonia	Azithromycin (AII); erythromycin (AII)	Doxycycline, ciprofloxacin
Chlamydophila (formerly *Chlamydia*) *psittaci*[51]	Psittacosis	Doxycycline (AII) for >7 y; azithromycin (AIII) OR erythromycin (AIII) for ≤ 7 y	Doxycycline, levofloxacin
Chromobacterium violaceum[52,53]	Sepsis, pneumonia, abscesses	Meropenem AND ciprofloxacin (AIII)	TMP/SMX AND ciprofloxacin. Susceptibility is variable.
Citrobacter koseri (formerly *diversus*) and *freundii*[54,55]	Meningitis, sepsis	Meropenem (AIII) for ampC beta-lactamase resistance	Cefepime, ciprofloxacin, pip/tazo, ceftriaxone AND gentamicin, TMP/SMX Carbapenem-resistant strains now reported

D. PREFERRED THERAPY FOR SPECIFIC BACTERIAL AND MYCOBACTERIAL PATHOGENS (continued)

Organism	Clinical Illness	Drug of Choice (evidence grade)	Alternatives
Clostridium botulinum[56–58]	Botulism: foodborne; wound; potentially bioterror related	Botulism antitoxin heptavalent (equine) types A–G FDA approved in 2013 (https://www.fda.gov/vaccines-blood-biologics/approved-blood-products/bat-botulism-antitoxin-heptavalent-b-c-d-e-f-g-equine; accessed October 2, 2019) No antibiotic treatment except for wound botulism when treatment for vegetative organisms can be provided after antitoxin administered (no controlled data)	For more information, call your state health department or the CDC clinical emergency botulism service, 770/488-7100 (https://www.cdc.gov/botulism/health-professional.html; accessed October 2, 2019). For bioterror exposure, treatment recommendations per www.cdc.gov.
	Infant botulism	Human botulism immune globulin for infants (BabyBIG) (AII) No antibiotic treatment	BabyBIG available nationally from the California Department of Public Health at 510/231-7600 (www.infantbotulism.org; accessed October 2, 2019)
Clostridium difficile[59–61]	Antibiotic-associated colitis (See Chapter 6, Table 6H, Gastrointestinal Infections, *Clostridium difficile*.)	Metronidazole PO for mild to moderate infection (AI)	Vancomycin PO ± metronidazole PO for severe infection. Vancomycin PO for metronidazole failures. Stop the predisposing antimicrobial therapy, if possible. New pediatric data on fidaxomicin PO.[62] No pediatric data on fecal transplantation for recurrent disease.

Clostridium perfringens[63,64]	Gas gangrene/necrotizing fasciitis/sepsis (also caused by *Clostridium sordellii, Clostridium septicum, Clostridium novyi*) Food poisoning	Penicillin G AND clindamycin for invasive infection (BII); no antimicrobials indicated for foodborne illness	Meropenem, metronidazole, clindamycin monotherapy No defined benefit of hyperbaric oxygen over aggressive surgery/antibiotic therapy
Clostridium tetani[65,66]	Tetanus	Tetanus immune globulin 3,000–6,000 U IM, with part injected directly into the wound (IVIG at 200–400 mg/kg if TIG not available) Metronidazole (AIII) OR penicillin G (BIII)	Prophylaxis for contaminated wounds: 250 U IM for those with <3 tetanus immunizations. Start/continue immunization for tetanus. Alternative antibiotics: meropenem; doxycycline, clindamycin.
Corynebacterium diphtheriae[67]	Diphtheria	Diphtheria equine antitoxin (available through CDC under an investigational protocol [www.cdc.gov/diphtheria/dat.html; accessed October 2, 2019]) AND erythromycin or penicillin G (AIII)	Antitoxin from the CDC Emergency Operations Center, 770/488-7100; protocol: www.cdc.gov/diphtheria/downloads/protocol.pdf (accessed October 2, 2019)
Corynebacterium jeikeium[68,69]	Sepsis, endocarditis	Vancomycin (AIII)	Penicillin G AND gentamicin, daptomycin, tigecycline, linezolid
Corynebacterium minutissimum[70,71]	Erythrasma; bacteremia in compromised hosts	Erythromycin PO for erythrasma (BIII); vancomycin IV for bacteremia (BIII)	Topical clindamycin for cutaneous infection; meropenem, penicillin/ampicillin, ciprofloxacin
Coxiella burnetii[72,73]	Q fever (See Chapter 6, Table 6L, Miscellaneous Systemic Infections, Q fever.)	Acute infection: doxycycline (all ages) (AII) Chronic infection: TMP/SMX AND doxycycline (BII); OR levofloxacin AND rifampin	Alternative for acute infection: TMP/SMX

D. PREFERRED THERAPY FOR SPECIFIC BACTERIAL AND MYCOBACTERIAL PATHOGENS (continued)

Organism	Clinical Illness	Drug of Choice (evidence grade)	Alternatives
Ehrlichia chaffeensis[11] *Ehrlichia muris*[74,75]	Human monocytic ehrlichiosis	Doxycycline (all ages) (AII)	Rifampin
Ehrlichia ewingii[11]	*E ewingii* ehrlichiosis	Doxycycline (all ages) (AII)	Rifampin
Eikenella corrodens[76,77]	Human bite wounds; abscesses, meningitis, endocarditis	Amox/clav; meropenem/imipenem; ceftriaxone For beta-lactamase–negative strains: ampicillin; penicillin G (BIII)	Pip/tazo, amp/sul, ciprofloxacin Resistant to clindamycin, cephalexin, erythromycin
Elizabethkingia (formerly *Chryseobacterium*) *meningoseptica*[78,79]	Sepsis, meningitis (particularly in neonates)	Levofloxacin; TMP/SMX (BIII)	Add rifampin to another active drug; pip/tazo.
Enterobacter spp[55,80,81]	Sepsis, pneumonia, wound infection, UTI	Cefepime; meropenem; pip/tazo (BII)	CAZ/AVI, ertapenem, imipenem, ceftriaxone AND gentamicin, TMP/SMX, ciprofloxacin Newly emerging carbapenem-resistant strains worldwide[82]
Enterococcus spp[83–85]	Endocarditis, UTI, intra-abdominal abscess	Ampicillin AND gentamicin (AI); bactericidal activity only present with combination	Vancomycin AND gentamicin. For strains that are resistant to gentamicin on synergy testing, use streptomycin or other active aminoglycoside for invasive infections. Ampicillin AND ceftriaxone in combination also effective.[86] For vancomycin-resistant strains that are also ampicillin resistant: daptomycin OR linezolid.[84,85]

Erysipelothrix rhusiopathiae[86]	Cellulitis (erysipeloid), sepsis, abscesses, endocarditis[87]	Invasive infection: ampicillin (BIII); penicillin G (BIII) Cutaneous infection: penicillin V; amoxicillin; clindamycin	Resistance to penicillin reported. Ceftriaxone, meropenem, ciprofloxacin, erythromycin. Resistant to vancomycin, daptomycin, TMP/SMX.
Escherichia coli See Chapter 6 for specific infection entities and references. *Increasing resistance to 3rd-generation cephalosporins due to ESBLs.*	UTI, community acquired, not hospital acquired	A 1st-, 2nd- or 3rd-generation cephalosporin PO, IM as empiric therapy (BI)	Amoxicillin; TMP/SMX if susceptible. Ciprofloxacin if resistant to other options. For hospital-acquired UTI, review hospital antibiogram for choices.
	Traveler's diarrhea	Azithromycin (AII)	Rifaximin (for nonfebrile, non-bloody diarrhea for children >11 y); cefixime
	Sepsis, pneumonia, hospital-acquired UTI	A 2nd- or 3rd-generation cephalosporin IV (BI)	For ESBL-producing strains: meropenem (AIII) or other carbapenem; pip/tazo and ciprofloxacin if resistant to other antibiotics For KPC-producing strains: CAZ/AVI
	Meningitis	Ceftriaxone; cefotaxime (AIII)	For ESBL-producing strains: meropenem (AIII)
Francisella tularensis[88,89]	Tularemia	Gentamicin (AII)	Doxycycline, ciprofloxacin. Resistant to beta-lactam antibiotics.
Fusobacterium spp[90,91]	Sepsis, soft tissue infection, Lemierre syndrome	Metronidazole (AIII); clindamycin (BIII)	Penicillin G, meropenem, pip/tazo. Combinations often used for Lemierre syndrome.
Gardnerella vaginalis[48,92]	Bacterial vaginosis	Metronidazole (BII)	Tinidazole, clindamycin, metronidazole gel, clindamycin cream
Haemophilus (now *Aggregatibacter*) *aphrophilus*[93]	Sepsis, endocarditis, abscesses (including brain abscess)	Ceftriaxone (AII); OR ampicillin (if beta-lactamase negative) AND gentamicin (BII)	Ciprofloxacin, amox/clav (for strains resistant to ampicillin) One of the HACEK organisms that cause endocarditis
Haemophilus ducreyi[48]	Chancroid	Azithromycin (AIII); ceftriaxone (BIII)	Erythromycin, ciprofloxacin

D. PREFERRED THERAPY FOR SPECIFIC BACTERIAL AND MYCOBACTERIAL PATHOGENS (continued)

Organism	Clinical Illness	Drug of Choice (evidence grade)	Alternatives
Haemophilus influenzae[94]	Nonencapsulated strains: upper respiratory tract infections	Beta-lactamase negative: ampicillin IV (AI); amoxicillin PO (AI) Beta-lactamase positive: ceftriaxone IV, IM (AI) or cefotaxime IV (AI); amox/clav (AI) OR 2nd- or 3rd-generation cephalosporins PO (AI)	Levofloxacin, azithromycin, TMP/SMX
	Type b strains: meningitis, arthritis, cellulitis, epiglottitis, pneumonia	Beta-lactamase negative: ampicillin IV (AI); amoxicillin PO (AI) Beta-lactamase positive: ceftriaxone IV, IM (AI); amox/clav (AI) OR 2nd- or 3rd-generation cephalosporins PO (AI)	Other regimens: meropenem IV, levofloxacin IV Full IV course (10 days) for meningitis, but oral step-down therapy well documented after response to treatment for non-CNS infections Levofloxacin PO for step-down therapy
Helicobacter pylori[95,96]	Gastritis, peptic ulcer	Triple agent therapy: clarithromycin (susceptible strains) AND amoxicillin AND omeprazole (AII); ADD metronidazole for suspected resistance to clarithromycin.	Other regimens include bismuth[96,97] in addition to other proton-pump inhibitors.
Kingella kingae[98,99]	Osteomyelitis, arthritis	Ampicillin; penicillin G (AII)	Ceftriaxone, TMP/SMX, cefuroxime, ciprofloxacin. Resistant to clindamycin.
Klebsiella spp (*K pneumoniae, K oxytoca*)[100–103] *Increasing resistance to 3rd-generation cephalosporins (ESBLs) and carbapenems (KPC), as well as to colistin*	UTI	A 2nd- or 3rd-generation cephalosporin (AII)	Use most narrow spectrum agent active against pathogen: TMP/SMX, ciprofloxacin, gentamicin. ESBL producers should be treated with a carbapenem (meropenem, ertapenem, imipenem), but KPC (carbapenemase)-containing bacteria may require ciprofloxacin, colistin, CAZ/AVI.[102]

	Sepsis, pneumonia, meningitis, hospital-acquired infection	Ceftriaxone; cefepime (AIII) CAZ/AVI or mero/vabor for carbapenem-R strains	Carbapenem or ciprofloxacin if resistant to other routine antibiotics. Meningitis caused by ESBL producer: meropenem if susceptible. KPC (carbapenemase) producers: ciprofloxacin, colistin, OR CAZ/AVI (approved by FDA for children in 2019 and is active against current strains of KPC[104]).
Klebsiella granulomatis[48]	Granuloma inguinale	Azithromycin (AII)	Doxycycline, TMP/SMX, ciprofloxacin
Legionella spp[105]	Legionnaires disease	Azithromycin (AI) OR levofloxacin (AII)	Erythromycin, clarithromycin, TMP/SMX, doxycycline
Leptospira spp[106]	Leptospirosis	Penicillin G IV (AII); ceftriaxone IV (AII)	Amoxicillin, doxycycline, azithromycin
Leuconostoc[107]	Bacteremia	Penicillin G (AIII); ampicillin (BIII)	Clindamycin, erythromycin, doxycycline (resistant to vancomycin)
Listeria monocytogenes[108]	Sepsis, meningitis in compromised host; neonatal sepsis	Ampicillin (ADD gentamicin for severe infection, compromised hosts.) (AII)	Ampicillin AND TMP/SMX; ampicillin AND linezolid; levofloxacin
Moraxella catarrhalis[109]	Otitis, sinusitis, bronchitis	Amox/clav (AI)	TMP/SMX; a 2nd- or 3rd-generation cephalosporin
Morganella morganii[55,81,110,111]	UTI, neonatal sepsis, wound infection	Cefepime (AIII); meropenem (AIII). Has intrinsic inducible ampC beta-lactamase; 3rd-generation cephalosporins may select for resistance.	Pip/tazo, ceftriaxone AND gentamicin, ciprofloxacin

D. PREFERRED THERAPY FOR SPECIFIC BACTERIAL AND MYCOBACTERIAL PATHOGENS (continued)

Organism	Clinical Illness	Drug of Choice (evidence grade)	Alternatives
Mycobacterium abscessus[112–115] *3 subspecies now identified*	Skin and soft tissue infections; pneumonia in cystic fibrosis	Clarithromycin or azithromycin (AIII); ADD cefoxitin or imipenem AND amikacin for invasive disease (AIII).	Also test for susceptibility to meropenem, tigecycline, linezolid. May need pulmonary resection. Initial intensive phase of therapy followed by months of "maintenance" therapy.
Mycobacterium avium complex[112,116,117]	Cervical adenitis	Clarithromycin (AII); azithromycin (AII)	Surgical excision is more likely to lead to cure than sole medical therapy. May increase cure rate with addition of rifampin or ethambutol.
	Pneumonia	Clarithromycin (AII) or azithromycin (AII) AND ethambutol ± rifampin	Depending on susceptibilities and the severity of illness, ADD amikacin ± ciprofloxacin.
	Disseminated disease in competent host, or disease in immuno-compromised host	Clarithromycin or azithromycin AND ethambutol AND rifampin (AIII)	Depending on susceptibilities and the severity of illness, ADD amikacin ± ciprofloxacin.
Mycobacterium bovis[118,119]	Tuberculosis (historically not differentiated from *M tuberculosis* infection; causes adenitis, abdominal tuberculosis, meningitis)	Isoniazid AND rifampin (AII); ADD ethambutol for suspected resistance (AIII).	ADD streptomycin for severe infection. *M bovis* is always resistant to PZA.
Mycobacterium chelonae[112,119,120]	Abscesses; catheter infection	Clarithromycin or azithromycin (AIII); ADD amikacin ± cefoxitin for invasive disease (AIII).	Also test for susceptibility to cefoxitin, TMP/SMX, doxycycline, tobramycin, imipenem, moxifloxacin, linezolid.
Mycobacterium fortuitum complex[111,116,120,121]	Skin and soft tissue infections; catheter infection	Amikacin AND cefoxitin or meropenem (AIII) ± levofloxacin (AIII)	Also test for susceptibility to clarithromycin, sulfonamides, doxycycline, linezolid.

Mycobacterium leprae[122]	Leprosy	Dapsone AND rifampin for paucibacillary (1–5 patches) (AII). ADD clofazimine for lepromatous, multibacillary (>5 patches) disease (AII).	Consult HRSA (National Hansen's Disease [Leprosy] Program) at www.hrsa.gov/hansens-disease for advice about treatment and free antibiotics: 800/642-2477 (accessed August 16, 2019).
Mycobacterium marinum/balnei[112,123]	Papules, pustules, abscesses (swimming pool granuloma)	Clarithromycin ± ethambutol (AIII)	TMP/SMX AND rifampin, ethambutol AND rifampin, doxycycline ± 1 or 2 additional antibiotics Surgical debridement
Mycobacterium tuberculosis[118,124] See Tuberculosis in Chapter 6, Table 6F, Lower Respiratory Tract Infections, for detailed recommendations for active infection, latent infection, and exposures in high-risk children.	Tuberculosis (pneumonia; meningitis; cervical adenitis; mesenteric adenitis; osteomyelitis)	For active infection: isoniazid AND rifampin AND PZA (AI); ADD ethambutol for suspect resistance. For latent infection: INH AND rifapentine once weekly for 12 wk (AII) OR rifampin daily for 4 mo, OR INH daily or biweekly (AII).	Add streptomycin for severe infection. For MDR tuberculosis, bedaquiline is FDA approved for adults and available for children. Corticosteroids should be added to regimens for meningitis, mesenteric adenitis, and endobronchial infection (AIII).
Mycoplasma hominis[125,126]	Neonatal infection including meningitis/ventriculitis; nongonococcal urethritis	Neonates: doxycycline; moxifloxacin Urethritis: clindamycin (AIII)	Usually erythromycin resistant
Mycoplasma pneumoniae[127,128]	Pneumonia	Azithromycin (AI); erythromycin (BI); macrolide resistance emerging worldwide[129]	Doxycycline and fluoroquinolones are active against macrolide-susceptible and macrolide-resistant strains.
Neisseria gonorrhoeae[48]	Gonorrhea; arthritis	Ceftriaxone AND azithromycin or doxycycline (AIII)	Oral cefixime as single drug therapy no longer recommended due to increasing resistance[130] Spectinomycin IM

D. PREFERRED THERAPY FOR SPECIFIC BACTERIAL AND MYCOBACTERIAL PATHOGENS (continued)

Organism	Clinical Illness	Drug of Choice (evidence grade)	Alternatives
Neisseria meningitidis[131,132]	Sepsis, meningitis	Ceftriaxone (AI)	Penicillin G or ampicillin if susceptible with amoxicillin step-down therapy for non-CNS infection.
			For prophylaxis following exposure: rifampin or ciprofloxacin (ciprofloxacin-resistant strains have now been reported). Azithromycin may be less effective.
Nocardia asteroides or *brasiliensis*[133–135]	Pneumonia with abscess, cutaneous cellulitis/abscess, brain abscess	TMP/SMX (AII); sulfisoxazole (BII); imipenem or meropenem AND amikacin for severe infection (AII)	Linezolid, ceftriaxone, clarithromycin, minocycline, levofloxacin, tigecycline, amox/clav
Pasteurella multocida[136,137]	Sepsis, abscesses, animal bite wound	Penicillin G (AIII); ampicillin (AIII); amoxicillin (AIII)	Amox/clav, pip/tazo, doxycycline, ceftriaxone, cefpodoxime, cefuroxime, TMP/SMX. Cephalexin may not demonstrate adequate activity. Not usually susceptible to clindamycin.
Peptostreptococcus[138]	Sepsis, deep head/neck space and intra-abdominal infection	Penicillin G (AII); ampicillin (AII)	Clindamycin, vancomycin, meropenem, imipenem, metronidazole
Plesiomonas shigelloides[139,140]	Diarrhea, neonatal sepsis, meningitis	Antibiotics may not be necessary to treat diarrhea: TMP/SMX (AIII); 2nd- and 3rd-generation cephalosporins (AIII); azithromycin (BIII); ciprofloxacin (CIII). For meningitis/sepsis: ceftriaxone.	Meropenem, amox/clav

Prevotella (formerly *Bacteroides*) spp,[141] *melaninogenica*	Deep head/neck space abscess; dental abscess	Metronidazole (AII); meropenem or imipenem (AII)	Pip/tazo, cefoxitin, clindamycin, tigecycline
Propionibacterium acnes[142,143]	In addition to acne, invasive infection: sepsis, post-op wound/shunt infection	Penicillin G (AIII); vancomycin (AIII)	Ceftriaxone, doxycycline, clindamycin, linezolid, daptomycin Resistant to metronidazole
Proteus mirabilis[144]	UTI, sepsis, meningitis	Ceftriaxone (AII); cefepime; ciprofloxacin; gentamicin Oral therapy: amox/clav; TMP/SMX, ciprofloxacin	Carbapenem; pip/tazo; increasing resistance to ampicillin, TMP/SMX, and fluoroquinolones, particularly in nosocomial isolates Colistin resistant
Proteus vulgaris, other spp (indole-positive strains)[55]	UTI, sepsis, meningitis	Cefepime; ciprofloxacin; gentamicin (BIII) AmpC producer (and some strains with ESBLs), so at risk of 3rd-generation cephalosporin resistance	Meropenem or other carbapenem; pip/tazo; TMP/SMX Colistin resistant
Providencia spp[55,145]	Sepsis	Cefepime; ciprofloxacin, gentamicin (BIII)	Meropenem or other carbapenem; pip/tazo; TMP/SMX Colistin and tigecycline resistant

D. PREFERRED THERAPY FOR SPECIFIC BACTERIAL AND MYCOBACTERIAL PATHOGENS (continued)

Organism	Clinical Illness	Drug of Choice (evidence grade)	Alternatives
Pseudomonas aeruginosa[146–151]	UTI	Cefepime (AII); other antipseudomonal beta-lactams; tobramycin	Amikacin, ciprofloxacin
	Nosocomial sepsis, pneumonia	Cefepime (AI) or meropenem (AI); OR pip/tazo AND tobramycin (BI); ceftazidime AND tobramycin (BII)	Ciprofloxacin AND tobramycin; colistin.[151] Controversy regarding additional clinical benefit in outcomes using newer, more potent beta-lactams over aminoglycoside combinations, but combinations may increase the likelihood of empiric active coverage and decrease emergence of resistance.[152,153] Prolonged infusion of beta-lactam antibiotics will allow greater therapeutic exposure to high-MIC pathogens.
	Pneumonia in cystic fibrosis[154–157] See Cystic Fibrosis in Chapter 6, Table 6F, Lower Respiratory Tract Infections.	Cefepime (AII) or meropenem (AI); OR ceftazidime AND tobramycin (BII); ADD aerosol tobramycin (AI). Azithromycin provides benefit in prolonging interval between exacerbations.	Inhalational antibiotics for prevention of acute exacerbations: tobramycin; aztreonam; colistin. Many organisms are MDR; consider ciprofloxacin or colistin parenterally; in vitro synergy testing may suggest effective combinations. For MDR organism treatment for acute deterioration, little prospective data on aerosolized antibiotics exist.
Pseudomonas cepacia, mallei, or *pseudomallei* (See *Burkholderia*.)			
Rhodococcus equi[158]	Necrotizing pneumonia	Imipenem AND vancomycin (AIII)	Combination therapy with ciprofloxacin or levofloxacin AND azithromycin or rifampin

Rickettsia[159,160]	Rocky Mountain spotted fever, Q fever, typhus, rickettsialpox	Doxycycline (all ages) (AII)	Chloramphenicol is less effective than doxycycline.
Salmonella, non-*typhi* strains[161–163]	Gastroenteritis (may not require therapy if clinically improving and not immunocompromised). Consider treatment for those at higher risk of invasion (<1 y [or, at highest risk, those <3 mo], immunocompromised, and with focal infections or bacteremia).	Azithromycin (AII) or ceftriaxone (AII); cefixime (AII)	For susceptible strains: ciprofloxacin; TMP/SMX; ampicillin
Salmonella typhi[161,164]	Typhoid fever	Azithromycin (AII); ceftriaxone (AII); TMP/SMX (AII); ciprofloxacin (AII)	Prefer antibiotics with high intracellular concentrations (eg, TMP/SMX, fluoroquinolones). Amoxicillin acceptable for susceptible strains.
Serratia marcescens[55,81]	Nosocomial sepsis, pneumonia	Cefepime; meropenem; pip/tazo (BII)	Ertapenem, imipenem, cefotaxime or ceftriaxone AND gentamicin, TMP/SMX, ciprofloxacin Resistant to colistin
Shewanella spp[165,166]	Wound infection, nosocomial pneumonia, peritoneal-dialysis peritonitis, ventricular shunt infection, neonatal sepsis	Ceftazidime (AIII); gentamicin (AIII)	Ampicillin, meropenem, pip/tazo, ciprofloxacin Resistant to TMP/SMX and colistin

D. PREFERRED THERAPY FOR SPECIFIC BACTERIAL AND MYCOBACTERIAL PATHOGENS (continued)

Organism	Clinical Illness	Drug of Choice (evidence grade)	Alternatives
Shigella spp[167,168]	Enteritis, UTI, prepubertal vaginitis	Ceftriaxone (AII); azithromycin[169] (AII); cefixime (AII); ciprofloxacin[170] (AII)	Resistance to azithromycin now reported. Use most narrow spectrum agent active against pathogen: PO ampicillin (not amoxicillin for enteritis); TMP/SMX.
Spirillum minus[171]	Rat-bite fever (sodoku)	Penicillin G IV (AII); for endocarditis, ADD gentamicin or streptomycin (AIII).	Ampicillin, doxycycline, cefotaxime, vancomycin, streptomycin
Staphylococcus aureus (See chapters 4 and 6 for specific infections.)[172,173]			
– Mild to moderate infections	Skin infections, mild to moderate	MSSA: a 1st-generation cephalosporin (cefazolin IV, cephalexin PO) (AI); oxacillin/nafcillin IV (AI), dicloxacillin PO (AI) MRSA: clindamycin (if susceptible) IV or PO, ceftaroline IV,[174] vancomycin IV, or TMP/SMX PO (AII)	For MSSA: amox/clav For CA-MRSA: linezolid IV, PO; daptomycin IV[175]
– Moderate to severe infections, treat empirically for CA-MRSA.	Pneumonia, sepsis, myositis, osteomyelitis, etc	MSSA: oxacillin/nafcillin IV (AI); a 1st-generation cephalosporin (cefazolin IV) (AI) ± gentamicin (AIII) MRSA: vancomycin (AII) OR clindamycin (if susceptible) (AII) OR ceftaroline (AII) Combination therapy with gentamicin and/or rifampin not prospectively studied	For CA-MRSA: linezolid (AII); OR daptomycin[176] for non-pulmonary infection (AII) (studies published in children); ceftaroline IV (studies published in children) Approved for adults in 2015: dalbavancin, oritavancin, tedizolid (See Chapter 4.)

Staphylococcus, coagulase negative[177,178]	Nosocomial bacteremia (neonatal bacteremia), infected intravascular catheters, CNS shunts, UTI	Empiric: vancomycin (AII) OR ceftaroline (AII)	If susceptible: nafcillin (or other anti-staph beta-lactam); rifampin (in combination); clindamycin, linezolid; ceftaroline IV; daptomycin for age >1 y (but not for pneumonia)
Stenotrophomonas maltophilia[179,180]	Sepsis	TMP/SMX (AII)	Ceftazidime, doxycycline, minocycline, tigecycline, levofloxacin
Streptobacillus moniliformis[171,181]	Rat-bite fever (Haverhill fever)	Penicillin G (AIII); ampicillin (AIII); for endocarditis, ADD gentamicin or streptomycin (AIII).	Doxycycline, ceftriaxone, carbapenems, clindamycin, vancomycin
Streptococcus, group A[182]	Pharyngitis, impetigo, adenitis, cellulitis, necrotizing fasciitis	Penicillin (AI); amoxicillin (AI)	A 1st-generation cephalosporin (cefazolin or cephalexin) (AI), clindamycin (AI), a macrolide (AI), vancomycin (AIII) For recurrent streptococcal pharyngitis, clindamycin or amox/clav, or the addition of rifampin to the last 4 days of therapy (AIII)
Streptococcus, group B[183]	Neonatal sepsis, pneumonia, meningitis	Penicillin (AII) or ampicillin (AII)	Gentamicin is used initially for presumed synergy until group B strep has been identified as the cause of infection and a clinical/microbiologic response has been documented (AIII).

D. PREFERRED THERAPY FOR SPECIFIC BACTERIAL AND MYCOBACTERIAL PATHOGENS (continued)

Organism	Clinical Illness	Drug of Choice (evidence grade)	Alternatives
Streptococcus, milleri/anginosus group (*S intermedius, anginosus,* and *constellatus;* includes some beta-hemolytic group C and group G streptococci)[184–186]	Pneumonia, sepsis, skin and soft tissue infection,[187] sinusitis,[188] arthritis, brain abscess, meningitis	Penicillin G (AIII); ampicillin (AIII); ADD gentamicin for serious infection (AIII); ceftriaxone. Many strains show decreased susceptibility to penicillin, requiring higher dosages to achieve adequate antibiotic exposure.	Clindamycin, vancomycin
Streptococcus pneumoniae[189–192] With widespread use of conjugate pneumococcal vaccines, antibiotic resistance in pneumococci has decreased.[192]	Sinusitis, otitis[189]	Amoxicillin, high-dose (90 mg/kg/day div bid) (AII); standard dose (40–45 mg/kg/day div tid) may again be effective following widespread use of PCV13 vaccines.[192]	Amox/clav, cefdinir, cefpodoxime, cefuroxime, clindamycin, OR ceftriaxone IM
	Meningitis	Ceftriaxone (AI); vancomycin is no longer required; ceftriaxone-resistant strains have not been reported to cause meningitis in the post-PCV13 era (AIII).	Penicillin G alone for pen-S strains; ceftriaxone alone for ceftriaxone-susceptible strains
	Pneumonia, osteomyelitis/arthritis,[190] sepsis	Ampicillin (AII); ceftriaxone (AI)	Penicillin G alone for pen-S strains; ceftriaxone alone for ceftriaxone-susceptible strains
Streptococcus, viridans group (alpha-hemolytic streptococci, most commonly *S sanguinis, S oralis* [*mitis*], *S salivarius, S mutans, S morbillorum*)[193]	Endocarditis; oropharyngeal, deep head/neck space infections	Penicillin G ± gentamicin (AII) OR ceftriaxone ± gentamicin (AII)	Vancomycin

Treponema pallidum[48,194]	Syphilis (See chapters 5 and 6.)	Penicillin G (AII)	Desensitize to penicillin preferred to alternate therapies. Doxycycline, ceftriaxone.
Ureaplasma urealyticum[48,195]	Genitourinary infections	Azithromycin (AII)	Erythromycin; doxycycline, ofloxacin (for adolescent genital infections)
	Neonatal pneumonia (Antibiotic therapy may not be effective.)	Azithromycin (AIII)	
Vibrio cholerae[196,197]	Cholera	Doxycycline (AI) OR azithromycin (AII)	If susceptible: ciprofloxacin, TMP/SMX
Vibrio vulnificus[198,199]	Sepsis, necrotizing fasciitis	Doxycycline AND ceftazidime (AII)	Ciprofloxacin AND ceftriaxone
Yersinia enterocolitica[200,201]	Diarrhea, mesenteric enteritis, reactive arthritis, sepsis	TMP/SMX for enteritis (AIII); ciprofloxacin or ceftriaxone for invasive infection (AIII)	Gentamicin, doxycycline
Yersinia pestis[202–204]	Plague	Gentamicin (AIII)	Levofloxacin, doxycycline, ciprofloxacin
Yersinia pseudo-tuberculosis[205,206]	Mesenteric adenitis; Far East scarlet-like fever; reactive arthritis	TMP/SMX (AIII) or ciprofloxacin (AIII)	Ceftriaxone, gentamicin, doxycycline

8. Preferred Therapy for Specific Fungal Pathogens

NOTES

- See Chapter 2 for discussion of the differences between polyenes, azoles, and echinocandins.
- **Abbreviations:** ABLC, amphotericin B lipid complex (Abelcet); AmB, amphotericin B; AmB-D, amphotericin B deoxycholate, the conventional standard AmB (original trade name Fungizone); bid, twice daily; CNS, central nervous system; CSF, cerebrospinal fluid; CT, computed tomography; div, divided; ECMO, extracorporeal membrane oxygenation; HAART, highly active antiretroviral therapy; HIV, human immunodeficiency virus; IV, intravenous; L-AmB, liposomal amphotericin B (AmBisome); PO, orally; qd, once daily; qid, 4 times daily; spp, species; TMP/SMX, trimethoprim/sulfamethoxazole.

A. OVERVIEW OF MORE COMMON FUNGAL PATHOGENS AND THEIR USUAL PATTERN OF ANTIFUNGAL SUSCEPTIBILITIES

Fungal Species	Amphotericin B Formulations	Fluconazole	Itraconazole	Voriconazole	Posaconazole	Isavuconazole	Flucytosine	Caspofungin, Micafungin, or Anidulafungin
Aspergillus calidoustus	++	–	–	–	–	–	–	++
Aspergillus fumigatus	+	–	±	++	+	++	–	+
Aspergillus terreus	–	–	+	++	+	++	–	+
Blastomyces dermatitidis	++	+	++	+	+	+	–	–
Candida albicans	+	++	+	+	+	+	+	++
Candida auris	±	–	±	±	+	+	±	++
Candida glabrata	+	–	±	±	±	±	+	±
Candida guilliermondii	+	±	+	+	+	+	+	±
Candida krusei	+	–	–	+	+	+	+	++
Candida lusitaniae	–	++	+	+	+	+	+	+
Candida parapsilosis	++	++	+	+	+	+	+	+
Candida tropicalis	+	+	+	+	+	+	+	++

Coccidioides immitis	++	++	+	+	++	+	—	—
Cryptococcus spp	++	+	+	+	+	+	++	—
Fusarium spp	±	—	—	++	+	+	—	—
Histoplasma capsulatum	++	+	++	+	+	+	—	—
Lomentospora (formerly *Scedosporium*) *prolificans*	—	—	±	±	±	±	—	±
Mucor spp	++	—	±	—	+	++	—	—
Paracoccidioides spp	+	+	++	+	+	+	—	—
Penicillium spp	±	—	++	+	+	+	—	—
Rhizopus spp	++	—	—	—	+	+	—	—
Scedosporium apiospermum	—	—	±	+	+	+	—	±
Sporothrix spp	+	+	++	+	+	+	—	—
Trichosporon spp	—	+	+	++	+	+	—	—

NOTE: **++** = preferred; **+** = acceptable; **±** = possibly effective (see text for further discussion); **—** = unlikely to be effective.

B. SYSTEMIC INFECTIONS

Infection	Therapy (evidence grade)	Comments
Prophylaxis		
Prophylaxis of invasive fungal infection in patients with hematologic malignancies[1–11]	Fluconazole 6 mg/kg/day for prevention of infection (AII). Posaconazole for prevention of infection has been well studied in adults (AI) and offers anti-mold coverage.[4]	Fluconazole is not effective against molds and some strains of *Candida*. Posaconazole PO, voriconazole PO, and micafungin IV are effective in adults in preventing yeast and mold infections but are not well studied in children for this indication.[12]
Prophylaxis of invasive fungal infection in patients with solid organ transplants[13–17]	Fluconazole 6 mg/kg/day for prevention of infection (AII)	AmB, caspofungin, micafungin, voriconazole, or posaconazole may be effective in preventing infection.
Treatment		
Aspergillosis[1,18–29]	Voriconazole (AI) 18 mg/kg/day IV div q12h for a loading dose on the first day, then 16 mg/kg/day IV div q12h as a maintenance dose for children 2–12 y or 12–14 y and weighing <50 kg. In children ≥15 y or 12–14 y and weighing >50 kg, use adult dosing (load 12 mg/kg/day IV div q12h on the first day, then 8 mg/kg/day div q12h as a maintenance dose) (AII). When stable, may switch from voriconazole IV to voriconazole PO at a dose of 18 mg/kg/day div bid for children 2–12 y and at least 400 mg/day div bid for children >12 y (AII). Dosing in children <2 y is less clear, but doses are generally higher (AIII). These are only initial dosing recommendations; it is critical to understand that continued dosing in all ages is guided by close monitoring of trough serum voriconazole concentrations in individual patients (AII). Unlike in adults, voriconazole PO bioavailability in children is only approximately 50%–60%, so trough levels are crucial when using PO.[30]	Voriconazole is the preferred primary antifungal therapy for all clinical forms of aspergillosis. Early initiation of therapy in patients with strong suspicion of disease is important while a diagnostic evaluation is conducted. Optimal voriconazole trough serum concentrations (generally thought to be 2–5 mcg/mL) are essential. Check trough level 2–5 days after initiation of therapy, and repeat the following week to verify and 4 days after a change of dose.[29] It is critical to monitor trough concentrations to guide therapy due to high inter-patient variability.[31] Low voriconazole concentrations are a leading cause of clinical failure. Younger children (especially <3 y) often have lower trough voriconazole levels and need much higher dosing. Dosing for younger children should begin as listed but will invariably need to be increased. Total treatment course is for a minimum of 6–12 wk, largely dependent on the degree and duration of immunosuppression and evidence of disease improvement.

Alternatives for primary therapy when voriconazole cannot be administered: L-AmB 5 mg/kg/day (AII) or isavuconazole (AI). Dosing of isavuconazole in children is unknown. ABLC is another possible alternative. Echinocandin primary monotherapy should not be used for treating invasive aspergillosis (CII). AmB-D should be used only in resource-limited settings in which no alternative agent is available (AII).	Salvage antifungal therapy options after failed primary therapy include a change of antifungal class (using L-AmB or an echinocandin), switching to isavuconazole, switching to posaconazole (serum trough concentrations $\geq$1 mcg/mL), or using combination antifungal therapy. Careful consideration has to be used before beginning azole therapy after a patient has failed azole prophylaxis. Combination antifungal therapy with voriconazole plus an echinocandin may be considered in select patients. The addition of anidulafungin to voriconazole as combination therapy found some statistical benefit to the combination over voriconazole monotherapy in only certain patients.[32] In vitro data suggest some synergy with 2 (but not 3) drug combinations: an azole plus an echinocandin is the most well studied. If combination therapy is employed, this is likely best done initially when voriconazole trough concentrations may not yet be appropriate. Routine antifungal susceptibility testing is not recommended but is suggested for patients suspected of having an azole-resistant isolate or who are unresponsive to therapy. Azole-resistant *Aspergillus fumigatus* is increasing. If local epidemiology suggests $>$10% azole resistance, empiric initial therapy should be voriconazole + echinocandin OR with L-AmB, and subsequent therapy guided based on antifungal susceptibilities.[33] Micafungin likely has equal efficacy to caspofungin against aspergillosis.[34] Return of immune function is paramount to treatment success; for children receiving corticosteroids, decreasing the corticosteroid dosage or changing to steroid-sparing protocols is important.

B. SYSTEMIC INFECTIONS (continued)

Infection	Therapy (evidence grade)	Comments
Bipolaris, Cladophialophora, Curvularia, Exophiala, Alternaria, and other agents of **phaeohyphomycosis** (dematiaceous, pigmented molds)[33–42]	Voriconazole (AI) 18 mg/kg/day IV div q12h for a loading dose on the first day, then 16 mg/kg/day IV div q12h as a maintenance dose for children 2–12 y or 12–14 y and weighing <50 kg. In children ≥15 y or 12–14 y and weighing >50 kg, use adult dosing (load 12 mg/kg/day IV div q12h on the first day, then 8 mg/kg/day div q12h as a maintenance dose) (AII). When stable, may switch from voriconazole IV to voriconazole PO at a dose of 18 mg/kg/day div bid for children 2–12 y and at least 400 mg/day div bid for children >12 y (AII). Dosing in children <2 y is less clear, but doses are generally higher (AIII). These are only initial dosing recommendations; continued dosing in all ages is guided by close monitoring of trough serum voriconazole concentrations in individual patients (AII). Unlike in adults, voriconazole PO bioavailability in children is only approximately 50%–60%, so trough levels are crucial.[30] Alternatives could include posaconazole (trough concentrations >1 mcg/mL) or combination therapy with an echinocandin + azole or an echinocandin + L-AmB (BIII).	Aggressive surgical debulking/excision is essential for CNS lesions. These can be highly resistant infections, so strongly recommend antifungal susceptibility testing to guide therapy and consultation with a pediatric infectious diseases expert. Antifungal susceptibilities are often variable, but empiric therapy with voriconazole is the best start. Optimal voriconazole trough serum concentrations (generally thought to be 2–5 mcg/mL) are important for success. Check trough level 2–5 days after initiation of therapy, and repeat the following week to verify and 4 days after a change of dose. It is critical to monitor trough concentrations to guide therapy due to high inter-patient variability.[31] Low voriconazole concentrations are a leading cause of clinical failure. Younger children (especially <3 y) often have lower voriconazole levels and need much higher dosing.
Blastomycosis (North American)[43–49]	For moderate–severe pulmonary disease: ABLC or L-AmB 5 mg/kg IV daily for 1–2 wk or until improvement noted, followed by itraconazole oral solution 10 mg/kg/day div bid (max 400 mg/day) PO for a total of 6–12 mo (AIII). Itraconazole loading dose (double dose for first 2 days) is recommended in adults but has not been studied in children (but likely helpful).	Itraconazole oral solution provides greater and more reliable absorption than capsules and only the oral solution should be used (on an empty stomach); serum concentrations of itraconazole should be determined 5 days after start of therapy to ensure adequate drug exposure. For blastomycosis, maintain trough itraconazole concentrations 1–2 mcg/mL

	For mild–moderate pulmonary disease: itraconazole oral solution 10 mg/kg/day div bid (max 400 mg/day) PO for a total of 6–12 mo (AIII). Itraconazole loading dose (double dose for first 2 days) recommended in adults but has not been studied in children (but likely helpful). For CNS blastomycosis: L-AmB or ABLC (preferred over AmB-D) for 4–6 wk, followed by an azole (fluconazole is preferred, at 12 mg/kg/day after a loading dose of 25 mg/kg; alternatives for CNS disease are voriconazole or itraconazole), for a total of at least 12 mo and until resolution of CSF abnormalities (AII). Some experts suggest combination therapy with L-AmB/ABLC plus high-dose fluconazole as induction therapy in CNS blastomycosis until clinical improvement (BIII).	(values for both itraconazole and hydroxyl-itraconazole are added together). If only itraconazole capsules are available, use 20 mg/kg/day div q12h and take with cola product to increase gastric acidity and bioavailability. Alternative to itraconazole: 12 mg/kg/day fluconazole (BIII) after a loading dose of 25 mg/kg/day. Patients with extrapulmonary blastomycosis should receive at least 12 mo of total therapy. If induction with L-AmB alone is failing, add itraconazole or high-dose fluconazole until clinical improvement. Lifelong itraconazole if immunosuppression cannot be reversed.
Candidiasis[50–54] (See Chapter 2.)		
– Cutaneous	Topical therapy (alphabetic order): ciclopirox, clotrimazole, econazole, haloprogin, ketoconazole, miconazole, oxiconazole, sertaconazole, sulconazole	Fluconazole 6 mg/kg/day PO qd for 5–7 days Relapse common in cases of chronic mucocutaneous disease, and antifungal susceptibilities critical to drive appropriate therapy

B. SYSTEMIC INFECTIONS (continued)

Infection	Therapy (evidence grade)	Comments
– Disseminated, acute (including catheter fungemia) infection	For neutropenic patients: An echinocandin is recommended as initial therapy. Caspofungin 70 mg/m² IV loading dose on day 1 (max dose 70 mg), followed by 50 mg/m² IV (max dose 70 mg) on subsequent days (AII); OR micafungin 2 mg/kg/day q24h (children weighing <40 kg), up to max dose 100 mg/day (AII).[55] ABLC or L-AmB 5 mg/kg/day IV q24h (BII) is an effective but less attractive alternative due to potential toxicity (AII). Fluconazole (12 mg/kg/day q24h, after a load of 25 mg/kg/day) is an alternative for patients who are not critically ill and have had no prior azole exposure (CIII). A fluconazole loading dose is standard of care in adult patients but has only been studied in infants (not yet in children)[56]—it is very likely that the beneficial effect of a loading dose extends to children. Fluconazole can be used as step-down therapy in stable neutropenic patients with susceptible isolates and documented bloodstream clearance (CIII). For children of all ages on ECMO, fluconazole is dosed as 35 mg/kg load on day 1 followed by 12 mg/kg/day (BII).[57] For non-neutropenic patients: An echinocandin is also recommended as initial therapy. Caspofungin 70 mg/m² IV loading dose on day 1 (max dose 70 mg), followed by 50 mg/m² IV (max dose 70 mg) on subsequent days (AII); OR micafungin 2 mg/kg/day q24h (children weighing <40 kg), up to max dose 100 mg/day (AI).[43] Fluconazole (12 mg/kg/day IV or PO q24h, after a load of 25 mg/kg/day) is an acceptable alternative to an	Prompt removal of infected IV catheter or any infected devices is absolutely critical to success (AII). For infections with *Candida krusei* or *Candida glabrata*, an echinocandin is preferred; however, there are increasing reports of some *C glabrata* resistance to echinocandins (treatment would, therefore, be lipid formulation L-AmB or ABLC) (BIII). There are increasing reports of some *Candida tropicalis* resistance to fluconazole. Lipid formulation AmB (5 mg/kg daily) is a reasonable alternative if there is intolerance, limited availability, or resistance to other antifungal agents (AI). Transition from a lipid AmB to fluconazole is recommended after 5–7 days among patients who have isolates that are susceptible to fluconazole, who are clinically stable, and in whom repeat cultures on antifungal therapy are negative (AI). Voriconazole (18 mg/kg/day div q12h load, followed by 16 mg/kg/day div q12h) is effective for candidemia but offers little advantage over fluconazole as initial therapy. Voriconazole is recommended as step-down oral therapy for selected cases of candidemia due to *C krusei* or if mold coverage is needed. Follow-up blood cultures should be performed every day or every other day to establish the time point at which candidemia has been cleared (AIII). Duration of therapy is for 2 wk AFTER negative cultures in pediatric patients without obvious metastatic complications and after symptom resolution (AII).

	echinocandin as initial therapy in selected patients, including those who are not critically ill and who are considered unlikely to have a fluconazole-resistant *Candida* spp (AI). For children of all ages on ECMO, fluconazole is dosed as 35 mg/kg load followed by 12 mg/kg/day (BII).[57] Transition from an echinocandin to fluconazole (usually within 5–7 days) is recommended for non-neutropenic patients who are clinically stable, have isolates that are susceptible to fluconazole (eg, *Candida albicans*), and have negative repeat blood cultures following initiation of antifungal therapy (AII). For CNS infections: L-AmB/ABLC (5 mg/kg/day), and AmB-D (1 mg/kg/day) as an alternative, combined with or without flucytosine 100 mg/kg/day PO div q6h (AII) until initial clinical response, followed by step-down therapy with fluconazole (12 mg/kg/day q24h, after a load of 25 mg/kg/day); echinocandins do not achieve therapeutic concentrations in CSF.	In neutropenic patients, ophthalmologic findings of choroidal and vitreal infection are minimal until recovery from neutropenia; therefore, dilated funduscopic examinations should be performed within the first week after recovery from neutropenia (AIII). All non-neutropenic patients with candidemia should ideally have a dilated ophthalmologic examination, preferably performed by an ophthalmologist, within the first week after diagnosis (AIII).
– Disseminated, chronic (hepatosplenic) infection	Initial therapy with lipid formulation AmB (L-AmB or ABLC, 5 mg/kg daily) OR an echinocandin (caspofungin 70 mg/m^2 IV loading dose on day 1 [max dose 70 mg], followed by 50 mg/m^2 IV [max dose 70 mg] on subsequent days OR micafungin 2 mg/kg/day q24h in children weighing <40 kg [max dose 100 mg]) for several weeks, followed by oral fluconazole in patients unlikely to have a fluconazole-resistant isolate (12 mg/kg/day q24h, after a load of 25 mg/kg/day) (AIII). Therapy should continue until lesions resolve on repeat imaging, which is usually several months. Premature discontinuation of antifungal therapy can lead to relapse (AIII).	If chemotherapy or hematopoietic cell transplantation is required, it should not be delayed because of the presence of chronic disseminated candidiasis, and antifungal therapy should be continued throughout the period of high risk to prevent relapse (AIII).

B. SYSTEMIC INFECTIONS (continued)

Infection	Therapy (evidence grade)	Comments
– Neonatal[53] (See Chapter 5.)	AmB-D (1 mg/kg/day) is recommended therapy (AII).[58] Fluconazole (12 mg/kg/day q24h, after a load of 25 mg/kg/day) is an alternative if patient has not been on fluconazole prophylaxis (AII).[59] For treatment of neonates and young infants (<120 days) on ECMO, fluconazole is loaded with 35 mg/kg on day 1, followed by 12 mg/kg/day q24h (BII). Lipid formulation AmB is an alternative but carries a theoretical risk of less urinary tract penetration compared with AmB-D (CIII). Duration of therapy for candidemia without obvious metastatic complications is for 2 wk AFTER documented clearance and resolution of symptoms (therefore, generally 3 wk total). Echinocandins should be used with caution and generally limited to salvage therapy or to situations in which resistance or toxicity preclude the use of AmB-D or fluconazole (CIII). Role of flucytosine in neonates with meningitis is questionable and not routinely recommended due to toxicity concerns. The addition of flucytosine (100 mg/kg/day div q6h) may be considered as salvage therapy in patients who have not had a clinical response to initial AmB therapy, but adverse effects are frequent (CIII).	In nurseries with high rates of candidiasis (>10%), IV or oral fluconazole prophylaxis (AI) (3–6 mg/kg twice weekly for 6 wk) in high-risk neonates (birth weight <1,000 g) is recommended. Oral nystatin, 100,000 units 3 times daily for 6 wk, is an alternative to fluconazole in neonates with birth weights <1,500 g in situations in which availability or resistance precludes the use of fluconazole (CII). Lumbar puncture and dilated retinal examination recommended in neonates with cultures positive for *Candida* spp from blood and/or urine (AIII). Same recommended for all neonates with birth weight <1,500 g with candiduria with or without candidemia (AIII). CT or ultrasound imaging of genitourinary tract, liver, and spleen should be performed if blood cultures are persistently positive (AIII). Meningoencephalitis in the neonate occurs at a higher rate than in older children/adults. Central venous catheter removal is strongly recommended. Infected CNS devices, including ventriculostomy drains and shunts, should be removed if possible.
– Oropharyngeal, esophageal[50]	Mild oropharyngeal disease: clotrimazole 10 mg troches PO 5 times daily OR nystatin 100,000 U/mL, 4–6 mL qid for 7–14 days.	For fluconazole-refractory oropharyngeal or esophageal disease: itraconazole oral solution OR posaconazole OR AmB IV OR an echinocandin for up to 28 days (AII).

	Alternatives also include miconazole mucoadhesive buccal 50-mg tablet to the mucosal surface over the canine fossa once daily for 7–14 days OR 1–2 nystatin pastilles (200,000 U each) qid for 7–14 days (AII). Moderate–severe oropharyngeal disease: fluconazole 6 mg/kg PO qd for 7–14 days (AII). Esophageal candidiasis: oral fluconazole (6–12 mg/kg/day, after a loading dose of 25 mg/kg/day) for 14–21 days (AI). If cannot tolerate oral therapy, use fluconazole IV OR ABLC/L-AmB/AmB-D OR an echinocandin (AI).	Esophageal disease always requires systemic antifungal therapy. A diagnostic trial of antifungal therapy for esophageal candidiasis is appropriate before performing an endoscopic examination (AI). Chronic suppressive therapy (3 times weekly) with fluconazole is recommended for recurrent infections (AI).
– Urinary tract infection	Cystitis: fluconazole 6 mg/kg qd IV or PO for 2 wk (AII). For fluconazole-resistant *C glabrata* or *C krusei*, AmB-D for 1–7 days (AIII). Pyelonephritis: fluconazole 12 mg/kg qd IV or PO for 2 wk (AIII) after a loading dose of 25 mg/kg/day. For fluconazole-resistant *C glabrata* or *C krusei*, AmB-D with or without flucytosine for 1–7 days (AIII).	Treatment is NOT recommended in asymptomatic candiduria unless high risk for dissemination; neutropenic, low birth weight neonate ($<$1,500 g); or patient will undergo urologic manipulation (AIII). Neutropenic patients and low birth weight neonates should be treated as recommended for candidemia (AIII). Removing Foley catheter, if present, may lead to a spontaneous cure in the normal host; check for additional upper urinary tract disease. AmB-D bladder irrigation is not generally recommended due to high relapse rate (an exception may be in fluconazole-resistant *Candida*) (CIII). For renal collecting system fungus balls, surgical debridement may be required in non-neonates (BIII). Echinocandins have poor urinary concentrations. AmB-D has greater urinary penetration that L-AmB/ABLC.

B. SYSTEMIC INFECTIONS (continued)

Infection	Therapy (evidence grade)	Comments
– Vulvovaginal[59]	Topical vaginal cream/tablets/suppositories (alphabetic order): butoconazole, clotrimazole, econazole, fenticonazole, miconazole, sertaconazole, terconazole, or tioconazole for 3–7 days (AI) OR fluconazole 10 mg/kg (max 150 mg) as a single dose (AII)	For uncomplicated vulvovaginal candidiasis, no topical agent is clearly superior. Avoid azoles during pregnancy. For severe disease, fluconazole 150 mg given every 72 h for 2–3 doses (AI). For recurring disease, consider 10–14 days of induction with topical agent or fluconazole, followed by fluconazole once weekly for 6 mo (AI).
Chromoblastomycosis (subcutaneous infection by dematiaceous fungi)[60–64]	Itraconazole oral solution 10 mg/kg/day PO div bid for 12–18 mo, in combination with surgical excision or repeated cryotherapy (AII). Itraconazole oral solution provides greater and more reliable absorption than capsules and only the oral solution should be used (on an empty stomach); serum concentrations of itraconazole should be determined 5 days after start of therapy to ensure adequate drug exposure. Maintain trough itraconazole concentrations 1–2 mcg/mL (values for both itraconazole and hydroxyl-itraconazole are added together).	Alternative: terbinafine plus surgery; heat and potassium iodide; posaconazole. Lesions are recalcitrant and difficult to treat.
Coccidioidomycosis[65–73]	For moderate infections: fluconazole 12 mg/kg IV/PO q24h (AII) after loading dose of 25 mg/kg/day. For severe pulmonary disease: AmB-D 1 mg/kg/day IV q24h OR ABLC/L-AmB 5 mg/kg/day IV q24h (AIII) as initial therapy for several weeks until clear improvement, followed by an oral azole for total therapy of at least 12 mo, depending on genetic or immunocompromised risk factors.	Mild pulmonary disease does not require routine therapy in the normal host and only requires periodic reassessment. There is experience with posaconazole for disease in adults but little experience in children. Isavuconazole experience in adults is increasing. Treat until serum cocci complement fixation titers drop to 1:8 or 1:4, about 3–6 mo.

	For meningitis: fluconazole 12 mg/kg/day IV q24h (AII) after loading dose of 25 mg/kg/day (AII). Itraconazole has also been effective (BIII). If no response to azole, use intrathecal AmB-D (0.1–1.5 mg/dose) with or without fluconazole (AIII). Lifelong azole suppressive therapy required due to high relapse rate. Adjunctive corticosteroids in meningitis has resulted in less secondary cerebrovascular events.[74] For extrapulmonary (non-meningeal), particularly for osteomyelitis, an oral azole such as fluconazole or itraconazole solution 10 mg/kg/day div bid for at least 12 mo (AIII), and L-AmB/ABLC as an alternative (less toxic than AmB-D) for severe disease or if worsening. Itraconazole oral solution provides greater and more reliable absorption than capsules and only the oral solution should be used (on an empty stomach); serum concentrations of itraconazole should be determined 5 days after start of therapy to ensure adequate drug exposure. Maintain trough itraconazole concentrations 1–2 mcg/mL (values for both itraconazole and hydroxyl-itraconazole are added together).	Disease in immunocompromised hosts may need to be treated longer, including potentially lifelong azole secondary prophylaxis. Watch for relapse up to 1–2 y after therapy.

B. SYSTEMIC INFECTIONS (continued)

Infection	Therapy (evidence grade)	Comments
Cryptococcosis[75–79]	For mild–moderate pulmonary disease: fluconazole 12 mg/kg/day (max 400 mg) IV/PO q24h after loading dose of 25 mg/kg/day for 6–12 mo (AII). Itraconazole is alternative if cannot tolerate fluconazole. For meningitis or severe pulmonary disease: induction therapy with AmB-D 1 mg/kg/day IV q24h OR ABLC/L-AmB 5 mg/kg/day q24h; AND flucytosine 100 mg/kg/day PO div q6h for a minimum of 2 wk and a repeat CSF culture is negative, followed by consolidation therapy with fluconazole (12 mg/kg/day with max dose 400 mg after a loading dose of 25 mg/kg/day) for a minimum of 8 more wk (AI). Then use maintenance therapy with fluconazole (6 mg/kg/day) for 6–12 mo (AI). Alternative induction therapies for meningitis or severe pulmonary disease (listed in order of preference): AmB product for 4–6 wk (AII); AmB product plus fluconazole for 2 wk, followed by fluconazole for 8 wk (BII); fluconazole plus flucytosine for 6 wk (BII).	Serum flucytosine concentrations should be obtained after 3–5 days to achieve a 2-h post-dose peak <100 mcg/mL (ideally 30–80 mcg/mL) to prevent neutropenia. For HIV-positive patients, continue maintenance therapy with fluconazole (6 mg/kg/day) indefinitely. Initiate HAART 2–10 wk after commencement of antifungal therapy to avoid immune reconstitution inflammatory syndrome. In organ transplant recipients, continue maintenance fluconazole (6 mg/kg/day) for 6–12 mo after consolidation therapy with higher dose fluconazole. For cryptococcal relapse, restart induction therapy (this time for 4–10 wk), repeat CSF analysis every 2 wk until sterile, and determine antifungal susceptibility of relapse isolate. Successful use of voriconazole, posaconazole, and isavuconazole for cryptococcosis has been reported in adult patients.
Fusarium, Lomentospora (formerly ***Scedosporium***) ***prolificans, Pseudallescheria boydii*** (and its asexual form, ***Scedosporium apiospermum***),[35,80–84] and other agents of hyalohyphomycosis	Voriconazole (AII) 18 mg/kg/day IV div q12h for a loading dose on the first day, then 16 mg/kg/day IV div q12h as a maintenance dose for children 2–12 y or 12–14 y and weighing <50 kg. In children ≥15 y or 12–14 y and weighing >50 kg, use adult dosing (load 12 mg/kg/day IV div q12h on the first day, then 8 mg/kg/day div q12h as a maintenance dose) (AII).	These can be highly resistant infections, so strongly recommend antifungal susceptibility testing against a wide range of agents to guide specific therapy and consultation with a pediatric infectious diseases expert. Optimal voriconazole trough serum concentrations (generally thought to be 2–5 mcg/mL) are important for success. Check trough level 2–5 days after initiation of therapy, and repeat the following week to verify and 4 days after a change of dose. It is critical to

When stable, may switch from voriconazole IV to voriconazole PO at a dose of 18 mg/kg/day div bid for children 2–12 y and at least 400 mg/day div bid for children >12 y (AII). Dosing in children <2 y is less clear, but doses are generally higher (AIII). These are only initial dosing recommendations; continued dosing in all ages is guided by close monitoring of trough serum voriconazole concentrations in individual patients (AII). Unlike in adults, voriconazole PO bioavailability in children is only approximately 50%–60%, so trough levels are crucial at this stage.[30]

monitor trough concentrations to guide therapy due to high inter-patient variability.[31] Low voriconazole concentrations are a leading cause of clinical failure. Younger children (especially <3 y) often have lower voriconazole levels and need much higher dosing.

Often resistant to AmB in vitro.

Alternatives: posaconazole (trough concentrations >1 mcg/mL) can be active; echinocandins have been reportedly successful as salvage therapy in combination with azoles; while there are reports of promising in vitro combinations with terbinafine, terbinafine does not obtain good tissue concentrations for these disseminated infections; miltefosine (for leishmaniasis) use has been reported.

B. SYSTEMIC INFECTIONS (continued)

Infection	Therapy (evidence grade)	Comments
Histoplasmosis[85–87]	For severe acute pulmonary disease: ABLC/L-AmB 5 mg/kg/day q24h for 1–2 wk, followed by itraconazole 10 mg/kg/day div bid (max 400 mg daily) to complete a total of 12 wk (AIII). Add methylprednisolone (0.5–1.0 mg/kg/day) for first 1–2 wk in patients with hypoxia or significant respiratory distress. For mild–moderate acute pulmonary disease: if symptoms persist for >1 mo, itraconazole 10 mg/kg/day PO solution div bid for 6–12 wk (AIII). For progressive disseminated histoplasmosis: ABLC/L-AmB 5 mg/kg/day q24h for 4–6 wk; alternative treatment is lipid AmB for 1–2 wk followed by itraconazole 10 mg/kg/day div bid (max 400 mg daily) to complete a total of 12 wk (AIII).	Mild pulmonary disease may not require therapy and, in most cases, resolves in 1 mo. CNS histoplasmosis requires initial L-AmB/ABLC (less toxic than AmB-D) therapy for 4–6 wk, followed by itraconazole for at least 12 mo and until CSF antigen resolution. Itraconazole oral solution provides greater and more reliable absorption than capsules and only the oral solution should be used (on an empty stomach); serum concentrations of itraconazole should be determined 5 days after start of therapy to ensure adequate drug exposure. Maintain trough itraconazole concentrations at >1–2 mcg/mL (values for both itraconazole and hydroxyl-itraconazole are added together). If only itraconazole capsules are available, use 20 mg/kg/day div q12h and take with cola product to increase gastric acidity and bioavailability. Potential lifelong suppressive itraconazole if cannot reverse immunosuppression. Corticosteroids recommended for 2 wk for pericarditis with hemodynamic compromise. Voriconazole and posaconazole use has been reported. Fluconazole is inferior to itraconazole.
Mucormycosis (previously known as zygomycosis)[28,88–94]	Aggressive surgical debridement combined with induction antifungal therapy: L-AmB at 5–10 mg/kg/day q24h (AII) for 3 wk. Lipid formulations of AmB are preferred to AmB-D due to increased penetration and decreased toxicity. Some experts advocate induction or salvage combination therapy with L-AmB plus an echinocandin (although data are largely in diabetic	Following clinical response with AmB, long-term oral step-down therapy with posaconazole (trough concentrations ideally for mucormycosis at >2 mcg/mL) can be attempted for 2–6 mo. No pediatric dosing exists for isavuconazole. Voriconazole has NO activity against mucormycosis or other *Zygomycetes*.

	patients with rhinocerebral disease) (CIII)[95] or combination of L-AmB plus posaconazole.[96] For salvage therapy, isavuconazole (AII)[97] or posaconazole (AIII). Following successful induction antifungal therapy (for at least 3 wk), can continue consolidation therapy with posaconazole (or use intermittent L-AmB) (BII).	Return of immune function is paramount to treatment success; for children receiving corticosteroids, decreasing the corticosteroid dosage or changing to steroid-sparing protocols is also important. Antifungal susceptibility is key if can be obtained. CNS disease likely benefits from higher doses such as L-AmB at 10 mg/kg/day q24h.
Paracoccidioido-mycosis[98–101]	Itraconazole 10 mg/kg/day (max 400 mg daily) PO solution div bid for 6 mo (AIII) OR voriconazole (dosing listed under Aspergillosis) (BI)	Alternatives: fluconazole; isavuconazole; sulfadiazine or TMP/SMX for 3–5 y. AmB is another alternative and may be combined with sulfa or azole antifungals.
Pneumocystis jiroveci (formerly ***carinii***) pneumonia[102–104]	Severe disease: preferred regimen is TMP/SMX 15–20 mg TMP component/kg/day IV div q8h (AI) OR, for TMP/SMX intolerant or TMP/SMX treatment failure, pentamidine isethionate 4 mg base/kg/day IV daily (BII), for 3 wk. Mild–moderate disease: start with IV therapy, then after acute pneumonitis is resolved, TMP/SMX 20 mg TMP component/kg/day PO div qid for 3 wk total treatment course (AII).	Alternatives: TMP AND dapsone; OR primaquine AND clindamycin; OR atovaquone. Prophylaxis: preferred regimen is TMP/SMX (5 mg TMP component/kg/day) PO div bid 3 times/wk on consecutive days; OR same dose, given qd, every day; OR atovaquone: 30 mg/kg/day for infants 1–3 mo; 45 mg/kg/day for infants/children 4–24 mo; and 30 mg/kg/day for children >24 mo; OR dapsone 2 mg/kg (max 100 mg) PO qd, OR dapsone 4 mg/kg (max 200 mg) PO once weekly. Use steroid therapy for more severe disease.
Sporotrichosis[105,106]	For cutaneous/lymphocutaneous: itraconazole 10 mg/kg/day PO solution div bid for 2–4 wk after all lesions gone (generally total of 3–6 mo) (AII) For serious pulmonary or disseminated infection or disseminated sporotrichosis: ABLC/L-AmB at 5 mg/kg/day q24h until favorable response, then step-down therapy with itraconazole PO for at least a total of 12 mo (AIII) For less severe disease, itraconazole for 12 mo	If no response for cutaneous disease, treat with higher itraconazole dose, terbinafine, or saturated solution of potassium iodide. Fluconazole is less effective. Obtain serum concentrations of itraconazole after 2 wk of therapy; want serum trough concentration >1 mcg/mL. For meningeal disease, initial L-AmB/ABLC (less toxic than AmB-D) should be 4–6 wk before change to itraconazole for at least 12 mo of therapy. Surgery may be necessary in osteoarticular or pulmonary disease.

C. LOCALIZED MUCOCUTANEOUS INFECTIONS

Infection	Therapy (evidence grade)	Comments
Dermatophytoses		
– Scalp (tinea capitis, including kerion)[107–112]	Griseofulvin ultramicrosize 10–15 mg/kg/day or microsize 20–25 mg/kg/day PO qd for 6–12 wk (AII) (taken with milk or fatty foods to augment absorption). For kerion, treat concurrently with prednisone (1–2 mg/kg/day for 1–2 wk) (AIII). Terbinafine can be used for only 2–4 wk. Terbinafine dosing is 62.5 mg/day (<20 kg), 125 mg/day (20–40 kg), or 250 mg/day (>40 kg) (AII).	Griseofulvin is superior for *Microsporum* infections, but terbinafine is superior for *Trichophyton* infections. *Trichophyton tonsurans* predominates in United States. No need to routinely follow liver function tests in normal healthy children taking griseofulvin. Alternatives: itraconazole oral solution 5 mg/kg qd or fluconazole. 2.5% selenium sulfide shampoo, or 2% ketoconazole shampoo, 2–3 times/wk should be used concurrently to prevent recurrences.
– Tinea corporis (infection of trunk/limbs/face) – Tinea cruris (infection of the groin) – Tinea pedis (infection of the toes/feet)	Alphabetic order of topical agents: butenafine, ciclopirox, clotrimazole, econazole, haloprogin, ketoconazole, miconazole, naftifine, oxiconazole, sertaconazole, sulconazole, terbinafine, and tolnaftate (AII); apply daily for 4 wk.	For unresponsive tinea lesions, use griseofulvin PO in dosages provided for scalp (tinea capitis, including kerion); fluconazole PO; itraconazole PO; OR terbinafine PO. For tinea pedis: terbinafine PO or itraconazole PO are preferred over other oral agents. Keep skin as clean and dry as possible, particularly for tinea cruris and tinea pedis.
– Tinea unguium (onychomycosis)[109,113,114]	Terbinafine 62.5 mg/day (<20 kg), 125 mg/day (20–40 kg), or 250 mg/day (>40 kg). Use for at least 6 wk (fingernails) or 12–16 wk (toenails) (AII).	Recurrence or partial response common. Alternative: itraconazole pulse therapy with 10 mg/kg/day div q12h for 1 wk per mo. Two pulses for fingernails and 3 pulses for toenails. Alternatives: fluconazole, griseofulvin.
– Tinea versicolor (also pityriasis versicolor)[109,115,116]	Apply topically: selenium sulfide 2.5% lotion or 1% shampoo daily, leave on 30 min, then rinse; for 7 days, then monthly for 6 mo (AIII); OR ciclopirox 1% cream for 4 wk (BII); OR terbinafine 1% solution (BII); OR ketoconazole 2% shampoo daily for 5 days (BII) For small lesions, topical clotrimazole, econazole, haloprogin, ketoconazole, miconazole, or naftifine	For lesions that fail to clear with topical therapy or for extensive lesions: fluconazole PO or itraconazole PO are equally effective. Recurrence common.

9. Preferred Therapy for Specific Viral Pathogens

NOTE

- **Abbreviations:** AASLD, American Association for the Study of Liver Diseases; AIDS, acquired immunodeficiency syndrome; ART, antiretroviral therapy; ARV, antiretroviral; bid, twice daily; BSA, body surface area; CDC, Centers for Disease Control and Prevention; CLD, chronic lung disease; CMV, cytomegalovirus; CrCl, creatinine clearance; DAA, direct-acting antiviral; div, divided; EBV, Epstein-Barr virus; FDA, US Food and Drug Administration; G-CSF, granulocyte-colony stimulating factor; HAART, highly active antiretroviral therapy; HBeAg, hepatitis B e antigen; HBV, hepatitis B virus; HCV, hepatitis C virus; HHS, US Department of Health and Human Services; HIV, human immunodeficiency virus; HSV, herpes simplex virus; IFN, interferon; IG, immune globulin; IM, intramuscular; IV, intravenous; PO, orally; postmenstrual age, weeks of gestation since last menstrual period PLUS weeks of chronologic age since birth; PTLD, posttransplant lymphoproliferative disorder; PREP, preexposure prophylaxis; qd, once daily; qid, 4 times daily; RSV, respiratory syncytial virus; SQ, subcutaneous; tab, tablet; TAF, tenofovir alafenamide; tid, 3 times daily; WHO, World Health Organization.

A. OVERVIEW OF NON-HIV, NON-HEPATITIS B OR C VIRAL PATHOGENS AND USUAL PATTERN OF SUSCEPTIBILITY TO ANTIVIRALS

Virus	Acyclovir	Baloxavir	Cidofovir	Famciclovir	Foscarnet	Ganciclovir
Cytomegalovirus			+		+	+
Herpes simplex virus	++			+	+	+
Influenza A and B		+				
Varicella-zoster virus	++			+	+	+

Virus	Letermovir	Oseltamivir	Peramivir	Valacyclovir	Valganciclovir	Zanamivir
Cytomegalovirus	+				++	
Herpes simplex virus				++	+	
Influenza A and B		++	+			+
Varicella-zoster virus				++		

NOTE: ++ = preferred; + = acceptable; [blank cell]= untested.

B. OVERVIEW OF HEPATITIS B OR C VIRAL PATHOGENS AND USUAL PATTERN OF SUSCEPTIBILITY TO ANTIVIRALS

Virus	Daclatasvir Plus Sofosbuvir	Elbasvir/ Grazoprevir (Zepatier)	Entecavir	Glecaprevir/ Pibrentasvir (Mavyret)	Interferon alfa-2b
Hepatitis B virus			++		+
Hepatitis C virus[a]	+[b,c,d]	+[b,d,e]		++[f,g]	

Virus	Lamivudine	Ombitasvir/ Paritaprevir/ Ritonavir Co-packaged With Dasabuvir (Viekira Pak)	Pegylated Interferon alfa-2a	Ribavirin	Sofosbuvir/ Ledipasvir (Harvoni)
Hepatitis B virus	+		+		
Hepatitis C virus[a]		+[b,d]	+[h]	+[h]	++[b,e,i,j]

Virus	Sofosbuvir Plus Ribavirin	Sofosbuvir/ Velpatasvir (Epclusa)	Sofosbuvir/ Velpatasvir/ Voxilaprevir (Vosevi)	Telbivudine	Tenofovir
Hepatitis B virus				+	++
Hepatitis C virus[a]	++[c,j,k]	+[d,f]	+[d,f]		

NOTE: ++ = preferred for patients <18 y; + = acceptable; [blank cell]= untested.

[a] HCV treatment guidelines from the Infectious Diseases Society of America and the AASLD available at www.hcvguidelines.org (accessed October 1, 2019).

[b] Treatment-naive patients with HCV genotype 1a or 1b infection who do not have cirrhosis.

[c] Treatment-naive patients with HCV genotype 3 infection who do not have cirrhosis.

[d] Not approved in patients <18 y.

[e] Treatment-naive patients with HCV genotype 4 infection who do not have cirrhosis.

[f] Active against all genotypes of HCV (1 through 6).

[g] Approved in patients ≥12 y.

[h] Likely to be replaced in pediatric patients as studies of newer molecules are performed in children. Treatment of children 3–11 y with chronic HCV infection should be deferred until IFN-free regimens are available.

[i] Treatment-naive patients with HCV genotype 5 and 6 infection who do not have cirrhosis.

[j] Approved in patients ≥3 y.

[k] Treatment-naive patients with HCV genotype 2 infection who do not have cirrhosis.

C. PREFERRED THERAPY FOR SPECIFIC VIRAL PATHOGENS

Infection	Therapy (evidence grade)	Comments
Adenovirus (pneumonia or disseminated infection in immunocompromised hosts)[1]	Cidofovir and ribavirin are active in vitro, but no prospective clinical data exist and both have significant toxicity. Two cidofovir dosing schedules have been employed in clinical settings: (1) 5 mg/kg/dose IV once weekly or (2) 1–1.5 mg/kg/dose IV 3 times/wk. If parenteral cidofovir is utilized, IV hydration and oral probenecid should be used to reduce renal toxicity.	Brincidofovir, the orally bioavailable lipophilic derivative of cidofovir also known as CMX001, is under investigation for the treatment of adenovirus in immunocompromised hosts. It is not yet commercially available.
Cytomegalovirus		
– Neonatal[2]	See Chapter 5.	
– Immunocompromised (HIV, chemotherapy, transplant-related)[3–15]	For induction: ganciclovir 10 mg/kg/day IV div q12h for 14–21 days (AII) (may be increased to 15 mg/kg/day IV div q12h). For maintenance: 5 mg/kg IV q24h for 5–7 days per week. Duration dependent on degree of immunosuppression (AII). CMV hyperimmune globulin may decrease morbidity in bone marrow transplant patients with CMV pneumonia (AII).	Use foscarnet or cidofovir for ganciclovir-resistant strains; for HIV-positive children on HAART, CMV may resolve without anti-CMV therapy. Also used for prevention of CMV disease posttransplant for 100–120 days. Data on valganciclovir dosing in young children for treatment of retinitis are unavailable, but consideration can be given to transitioning from IV ganciclovir to oral valganciclovir after improvement of retinitis is noted. Limited data on oral valganciclovir in infants[16,17] (32 mg/kg/day PO div bid) and children (dosing by BSA [dose (mg) = 7 × BSA × CrCl]).[5]
– Prophylaxis of infection in immunocompromised hosts[4,18]	Ganciclovir 5 mg/kg IV daily (or 3 times/wk) (started at engraftment for stem cell transplant patients) (BII) Valganciclovir at total dose in milligrams = 7 × BSA × CrCl (use maximum CrCl 150 mL/min/1.73 m^2) orally once daily with	Neutropenia is a complication with ganciclovir and valganciclovir prophylaxis and may be addressed with G-CSF. Prophylaxis and preemptive treatment strategies are effective, but preemptive treatment in high-risk adult liver transplant recipients is superior to prophylaxis.[9]

	food for children 4 mo–16 y (max dose 900 mg/day) for primary prophylaxis in HIV patients[19] who are CMV antibody positive and have severe immunosuppression (CD4 count <50 cells/mm^3 in children ≥ 6 y; CD4 percentage $<5\%$ in children <6 y) (CIII) Letermovir (adults ≥ 18 y, CMV-seropositive recipients [R+] of an allogeneic hematopoietic stem cell transplant) 480 mg administered PO qd or as IV infusion over 1 h through 100 days posttransplant (BI).[20]	
Enterovirus	Supportive therapy; no antivirals currently FDA approved	Pocapavir PO is currently under investigation for enterovirus (poliovirus). As of November 2019, pocapavir may be available for compassionate use. Pleconaril PO is currently under consideration for submission to FDA for approval for treatment of neonatal enteroviral sepsis syndrome.[21] As of November 2019, it is not available for compassionate use.
Epstein-Barr virus		
– Mononucleosis, encephalitis[22–24]	Limited data suggest small clinical benefit of valacyclovir in adolescents for mononucleosis (3 g/day div tid for 14 days) (CIII). For EBV encephalitis: ganciclovir IV OR acyclovir IV (AIII).	No prospective data on benefits of acyclovir IV or ganciclovir IV in EBV clinical infections of normal hosts. Patients suspected to have infectious mononucleosis should not be given ampicillin or amoxicillin, which cause nonallergic morbilliform rashes in a high proportion of patients with active EBV infection (AII). Therapy with short-course corticosteroids (prednisone 1 mg/kg per day PO [maximum 20 mg/day] for 7 days with subsequent tapering) may have a beneficial effect on acute symptoms in patients with marked tonsillar inflammation with impending airway obstruction, massive splenomegaly, myocarditis, hemolytic anemia, or hemophagocytic lymphohistiocytosis (BIII).

C. PREFERRED THERAPY FOR SPECIFIC VIRAL PATHOGENS (continued)

Infection	Therapy (evidence grade)	Comments
– Posttransplant lymphoproliferative disorder[25,26]	Ganciclovir (AIII)	Decrease immune suppression if possible, as this has the most effect on control of EBV; rituximab, methotrexate have been used but without controlled data. Preemptive treatment with ganciclovir may decrease PTLD in solid organ transplants.
Hepatitis B virus (chronic)[27–45]	AASLD preferred treatments for children and adolescents[46]: IFN-alfa-2b for children 1–18 y: 3 million U/m² BSA SQ 3 times/wk for 1 wk, followed by dose escalation to 6 million U/m² BSA (max 10 million U/dose); OR entecavir for children ≥2 y (optimum duration of therapy unknown [BII]) Entecavir dosing IF no prior nucleoside therapy: ≥16 y: 0.5 mg qd 2–15 y: 10–11 kg: 0.15 mg oral solution qd >11–14 kg: 0.2 mg oral solution qd >14–17 kg: 0.25 mg oral solution qd >17–20 kg: 0.3 mg oral solution qd >20–23 kg: 0.35 mg oral solution qd >23–26 kg: 0.4 mg oral solution qd >26–30 kg: 0.45 mg oral solution qd >30 kg: 0.5 mg oral solution or tab qd If prior nucleoside therapy: Double the dosage in each weight bracket for entecavir listed previously; OR tenofovir dipivoxil fumarate for adolescents ≥12 y and adults 300 mg qd.	AASLD nonpreferred treatments for children and adults: Lamivudine 3 mg/kg/day (max 100 mg) PO q24h for 52 wk for children ≥2 y (children coinfected with HIV and HBV should use the approved dose for HIV) (AII). Lamivudine approved for children ≥2 y, but antiviral resistance develops on therapy in 30%; OR adefovir for children ≥12 y (10 mg PO q24h for a minimum of 12 mo; optimum duration of therapy unknown) (BII); OR telbivudine (adult dose 600 mg qd). There are not sufficient clinical data to identify the appropriate dose for use in children. Indications for treatment of chronic HBV infection, with or without HIV coinfection, are (1) evidence of ongoing HBV viral replication, as indicated by serum HBV DNA (>20,000 without HBeAg positivity or >2,000 IU/mL with HBeAg positivity) for >6 mo and persistent elevation of serum transaminase levels for >6 mo, or (2) evidence of chronic hepatitis on liver biopsy (BII). Antiviral therapy is not warranted in children without necroinflammatory liver disease (BIII). Treatment is not recommended for children with immunotolerant chronic HBV infection (ie, normal serum transaminase levels despite detectable HBV DNA) (BII).

	NOTE: TAF also is a preferred treatment for adults (25 mg daily) but has not been studied in children.	All patients with HBV and HIV coinfection should initiate ART, regardless of CD4 count. This should include 2 drugs that have HBV activity as well, specifically tenofovir (dipivoxil fumarate or alafenamide) plus lamivudine or emtricitabine.[46] Patients who are already receiving effective ART that does not include a drug with HBV activity should have treatment changed to include tenofovir (dipivoxil fumarate or alafenamide) plus lamivudine or emtricitabine; alternatively, entecavir is reasonable if patients are receiving a fully suppressive ART regimen.

C. PREFERRED THERAPY FOR SPECIFIC VIRAL PATHOGENS (continued)

Infection	Therapy (evidence grade)	Comments
Hepatitis C virus (chronic)[47–54]	Genotype 1: Daily fixed-dose combination of ledipasvir (90 mg)/sofosbuvir (400 mg) (Harvoni) for patients with genotype 1 who are treatment-naive without cirrhosis or with compensated cirrhosis, or treatment-experienced with or without cirrhosis Genotype 2: Daily sofosbuvir (400 mg) plus weight-based ribavirin (see later in table) for patients with genotype 2 who are treatment-naive or treatment-experienced without cirrhosis or with compensated cirrhosis Genotype 3: Daily sofosbuvir (400 mg) plus weight-based ribavirin (see later in table) for patients with genotype 3 who are treatment-naive or treatment-experienced without cirrhosis or with compensated cirrhosis Genotypes 4, 5, or 6: Daily fixed-dose combination of ledipasvir (90 mg)/sofosbuvir (400 mg) (Harvoni) for patients with genotype 4, 5, or 6 who are treatment-naive or treatment-experienced without cirrhosis or with compensated cirrhosis Genotypes 1–6: Daily fixed-dose combination of glecaprevir (300 mg)/pibrentasvir (120 mg) (Mavyret) for patients ≥12 y with genotype 1–6 who are treatment-naive or treatment-experienced without cirrhosis or with compensated cirrhosis	Treatment of HCV infections in adults has been revolutionized in recent years with the licensure of numerous highly effective DAAs for use in adults, adolescents, and children as young as 3 y. Ledipasvir/sofosbuvir has been found to be safe and effective in children 6–11 y,[54] and Harvoni and sofosbuvir are now approved down to 3 y. Given the efficacy of these new treatment regimens in adults (AI),[55–70] treatment of children should consist only of IFN-free regimens. The following treatment is recommended, based on viral genotype[71]: Sofosbuvir (Sovaldi) and sofosbuvir in a fixed dose combination tab with ledipasvir (Harvoni) are now approved for patients ≥3 y, and glecaprevir/pibrentasvir (Mavyret) is now approved for patients ≥12 y. Treatment should be considered for all HIV/HCV-coinfected children >3 y who have no contraindications to treatment (BIII).

	Dosing for ribavirin in combination therapy with sofosbuvir for adolescents ≥12 y or ≥35 kg: <47 kg: 15 mg/kg/day in 2 div doses 47–49 kg: 600 mg/day in 2 div doses 50–65 kg: 800 mg/day in 2 div doses 66–80 kg: 1,000 mg/day in 2 div doses >80 kg: 1,200 mg/day in 2 div doses	
Herpes simplex virus		
– Third trimester maternal suppressive therapy[72–74]	Acyclovir or valacyclovir maternal suppressive therapy in pregnant women reduces HSV recurrences and viral shedding at the time of delivery but does not fully prevent neonatal HSV[73] (BIII).	
– Neonatal	See Chapter 5.	
– Mucocutaneous (normal host)	Acyclovir 80 mg/kg/day PO div qid (max dose 800 mg) for 5–7 days, or 15 mg/kg/day IV as 1–2 h infusion div q8h (AII) Valacyclovir 20 mg/kg/dose (max dose 1 g) PO bid[75] for 5–7 days (BII) Suppressive therapy for frequent recurrence (no pediatric data): acyclovir 20 mg/kg/dose bid or tid (max dose 400 mg) for 6–12 mo, then reevaluate need (AIII)	Foscarnet for acyclovir-resistant strains. Immunocompromised hosts may require 10–14 days of therapy. Topical acyclovir not efficacious and therefore is not recommended.
– Genital	Adult doses: acyclovir 400 mg PO tid for 7–10 days; OR valacyclovir 1 g PO bid for 10 days; OR famciclovir 250 mg PO tid for 7–10 days (AI)	All 3 drugs have been used as prophylaxis to prevent recurrence. Topical acyclovir not efficacious and therefore is not recommended.

C. PREFERRED THERAPY FOR SPECIFIC VIRAL PATHOGENS (continued)

Infection	Therapy (evidence grade)	Comments
– Encephalitis	Acyclovir 60 mg/kg/day IV as 1–2 h infusion div q8h; for 21 days for infants ≤4 mo. For older infants and children, 45 mg/kg/day IV as 1–2 h infusion div q8h (AIII).	Safety of high-dose acyclovir (60 mg/kg/day) not well defined beyond the neonatal period; can be used but monitor for neurotoxicity and nephrotoxicity.
– Keratoconjunctivitis	1% trifluridine or 0.15% ganciclovir ophthalmic gel (AII)	Consultation with ophthalmologist required for assessment and management (eg, concomitant use of topical steroids in certain situations)
Human herpesvirus 6		
– Immunocompromised children[76]	No prospective comparative data; ganciclovir 10 mg/kg/day IV div q12h used in case report (AIII)	May require high dose to control infection; safety and efficacy not defined at high doses.
Human immunodeficiency virus		
Current information on HIV treatment and opportunistic infections for children[77] is posted at http://aidsinfo.nih.gov/ContentFiles/PediatricGuidelines.pdf (accessed October 1, 2019); other information on HIV programs is available at www.cdc.gov/hiv/policies/index.html (accessed October 1, 2019). Consult with an HIV expert, if possible, for current recommendations, as treatment options are complicated and constantly evolving.		
– Therapy of HIV infection		
State-of-the-art therapy is rapidly evolving with introduction of new agents and combinations; currently there are 16 individual ARV agents approved for use by the FDA that have pediatric indications and that continue to be actively used, as well as multiple combinations;	Effective therapy (HAART) consists of ≥3 agents, including 2 nucleoside reverse transcriptase inhibitors, plus either a protease inhibitor, a non-nucleoside reverse transcriptase inhibitor, or an integrase inhibitor; many different combination regimens give similar treatment outcomes; choice of agents depends on the age of the child, viral load, consideration of potential	Assess drug toxicity (based on the agents used) and virologic/immunologic response to therapy (quantitative plasma HIV and CD4 count) initially monthly and then every 3–6 mo during the maintenance phase.

guidelines for children and adolescents are continually updated on the AIDSinfo and CDC websites given previously.	viral resistance, and extent of immune depletion, in addition to judging the child's ability to adhere to the regimen.	
– Children of any age	Any child with AIDS or significant HIV-related symptoms (clinical category C and most B conditions) should be treated (AI). Recent guidance from the WHO and HHS guidelines committees now recommends treatment for **all children** regardless of age, CD4 count, or clinical status, with situation-specific levels of urgency.	Adherence counseling and appropriate ARV formulations are critical for successful implementation.
– First 3 y after birth	HAART with ≥3 drugs is now recommended for **all infants** ≤36 mo, regardless of clinical status or laboratory values (AI).	Preferred therapy in the first 2 wk after birth is zidovudine and lamivudine PLUS either nevirapine or raltegravir. Preferred therapy from 2 wk–3 y: zidovudine and lamivudine or abacavir and lamivudine (>3 mo) PLUS either lopinavir/ritonavir (toxicity concerns preclude its use until a postmenstrual age of 42 wk and a postnatal age of at least 14 days is reached) or raltegravir.
– HIV-infected children ≥3–<12 y	**Treat all** with any CD4 count (AI).	Preferred regimens comprise: Weight <25 kg: zidovudine and lamivudine (at any age) or abacavir and either lamivudine or emtricitabine PLUS either atazanavir/ritonavir or darunavir/ritonavir or raltegravir Weight ≥25 kg: zidovudine and lamivudine (at any age), or abacavir or TAF and either lamivudine or emtricitabine, PLUS either dolutegravir or elvitegravir/cobicistat

C. PREFERRED THERAPY FOR SPECIFIC VIRAL PATHOGENS (continued)

Infection	Therapy (evidence grade)	Comments
– HIV-infected youth ≥12 y	**Treat all** regardless of CD4 count (AI).	Preferred regimens comprise TAF or tenofovir (adolescents/Tanner stage 4 or 5) plus emtricitabine OR abacavir plus lamivudine PLUS dolutegravir, raltegravir, or bictegravir. **NOTE:** A recent report suggests the possibility of neural tube defects developing in offspring of women who become pregnant while on dolutegravir and/or use it during the first trimester. Caution should be exercised, including pregnancy testing and counseling, before initiating dolutegravir (and other integrase inhibitors). Further data and advice are anticipated as more data become available.
– Antiretroviral-experienced child	Consult with HIV specialist.	Consider treatment history and drug resistance testing and assess adherence.
– HIV exposures, nonoccupational	Therapy recommendations for exposures available on the CDC website at www.cdc.gov/hiv/guidelines/preventing.html (accessed October 1, 2019)	Postexposure prophylaxis remains unproven but substantial evidence supports its use; consider individually regarding risk, time from exposure, and likelihood of adherence; prophylactic regimens administered for 4 wk.
– Negligible exposure risk (urine, nasal secretions, saliva, sweat, or tears—no visible blood in secretions) OR >72 h since exposure	Prophylaxis not recommended (BIII)	
– Significant exposure risk (blood, semen, vaginal, or rectal secretions from a known HIV-infected individual) AND <72 h since exposure	Prophylaxis recommended (BIII) Preferred regimens 4 wk–<2 y: zidovudine PLUS lamivudine PLUS either raltegravir or lopinavir/ritonavir 2–12 y: tenofovir PLUS emtricitabine PLUS raltegravir ≥13 y: tenofovir PLUS emtricitabine PLUS either raltegravir or dolutegravir	Consultation with a pediatric HIV specialist is advised.

– Significant exposure risk **preexposure prophylaxis**	Truvada (tenofovir 300 mg/emtricitabine 200 mg): 1 tab daily	Daily PREP has proven efficacy for prevention of HIV infection in individuals at high risk. It is FDA approved for adolescents/youth (13–24 y; ≥35 kg). Strategies for use include both episodic and continuous administration. Baseline HIV and renal function testing is indicated, and it is recommended to evaluate HIV infection status and renal function approximately every 3 mo while on PREP.
– HIV exposure, occupational[78]	See guidelines on CDC website at www.cdc.gov/hiv/guidelines/preventing.html (accessed October 1, 2019).	

C. PREFERRED THERAPY FOR SPECIFIC VIRAL PATHOGENS (continued)

Infection	Therapy (evidence grade)	Comments
Influenza virus Recommendations for the treatment of influenza can vary from season to season; access the American Academy of Pediatrics website (www.aap.org) and the CDC website (www.cdc.gov/flu/professionals/antivirals/summary-clinicians.htm; accessed October 1, 2019) for the most current, accurate information.		
Influenza A and B		
– Treatment[79–81]	Oseltamivir Preterm, <38 wk postmenstrual age: 1 mg/kg/dose PO bid[79] Preterm, 38–40 wk postmenstrual age: 1.5 mg/kg/dose PO bid[79] Preterm, >40 wk postmenstrual age: 3.0 mg/kg/dose PO bid Term, birth–8 mo: 3.0 mg/kg/dose PO bid 9–11 mo: 3.5 mg/kg/dose PO bid[80] 12–23 mo: 30 mg/dose PO bid 2–12 y: ≤15 kg: 30 mg bid; 16–23 kg: 45 mg bid; 24–40 kg: 60 mg bid; >40 kg: 75 mg bid ≥13 y: 75 mg bid OR Zanamivir ≥7 y: 10 mg by inhalation bid for 5 days OR Peramivir (BII) 2–12 y: single IV dose 12 mg/kg, up to 600 mg max 13–17 y: single IV dose 600 mg OR Baloxavir (BII) ≥12 y: 40–79 kg: single PO dose 40 mg ≥80 kg: single PO dose 80 mg	Oseltamivir currently is drug of choice for treatment of influenza infections. For patients 12–23 mo, the original FDA-approved unit dose of 30 mg/dose may provide inadequate drug exposure; 3.5 mg/kg/dose PO bid has been studied,[80] but study population sizes were small. Studies of parenteral zanamivir have been completed in children.[82] However, this formulation of the drug is not approved in the United States and is not available for compassionate use. The adamantanes, amantadine and rimantadine, currently are not effective for treatment due to near-universal resistance of influenza A. Resistance to baloxavir is being monitored carefully across the world. Problems with resistance are beginning to limit use of baloxavir in Japan.

– Chemoprophylaxis	Oseltamivir 3 mo–12 y: The mg dose given for prophylaxis is the same as for the treatment dose for all ages, but it is given qd for prophylaxis instead of bid for treatment. Zanamivir ≥5 y: 10 mg by inhalation qd for as long as 28 days (community outbreaks) or 10 days (household setting).	Oseltamivir currently is drug of choice for chemoprophylaxis of influenza infection. Unless the situation is judged critical, oseltamivir chemoprophylaxis is not routinely recommended for patients <3 mo because of limited safety and efficacy data in this age group. The adamantanes, amantadine and rimantadine, currently are not effective for chemoprophylaxis due to near-universal resistance of influenza A.
Measles[83]	No prospective data on antiviral therapy. Ribavirin is active against measles virus in vitro. Vitamin A is beneficial in children with measles and is recommended by WHO for all children with measles regardless of their country of residence (qd dosing for 2 days): for children ≥1 y: 200,000 IU; for infants 6–12 mo: 100,000 IU; for infants <6 mo: 50,000 IU (BII). Even in countries where measles is not usually severe, vitamin A should be given to all children with severe measles (eg, requiring hospitalization). Parenteral and oral formulations are available in the United States.	IG prophylaxis for exposed, unimmunized children: 0.5 mL/kg (max 15 mL) IM
Respiratory syncytial virus[84,85]		
– Therapy (severe disease in compromised host)	Ribavirin (6-g vial to make 20 mg/mL solution in sterile water), aerosolized over 18–20 h daily for 3–5 days (BII)	Aerosol ribavirin provides only a small benefit and should only be considered for use for life-threatening infection with RSV. Airway reactivity with inhalation precludes routine use.

C. PREFERRED THERAPY FOR SPECIFIC VIRAL PATHOGENS (continued)

Infection	Therapy (evidence grade)	Comments
– Prophylaxis (palivizumab, Synagis for high-risk infants) (BI)[84,85]	Prophylaxis: palivizumab (a monoclonal antibody) 15 mg/kg IM monthly (max 5 doses) for the following high-risk infants (AI): In first year after birth, palivizumab prophylaxis is recommended for infants born before 29 wk 0 days' gestation. Palivizumab prophylaxis is not recommended for otherwise healthy infants born at ≥29 wk 0 days' gestation. In first year after birth, palivizumab prophylaxis is recommended for preterm infants with CLD of prematurity, defined as birth at <32 wk 0 days' gestation and a requirement for >21% oxygen for at least 28 days after birth. Clinicians may administer palivizumab prophylaxis in the first year after birth to certain infants with hemodynamically significant heart disease.	Palivizumab does not provide benefit in the treatment of an active RSV infection. Palivizumab prophylaxis may be considered for children <24 mo who will be profoundly immunocompromised during the RSV season. Palivizumab prophylaxis is not recommended in the second year after birth except for children who required at least 28 days of supplemental oxygen after birth and who continue to require medical support (supplemental oxygen, chronic corticosteroid therapy, or diuretic therapy) during the 6-mo period before the start of the second RSV season. Monthly prophylaxis should be discontinued in any child who experiences a breakthrough RSV hospitalization. Children with pulmonary abnormality or neuromuscular disease that impairs the ability to clear secretions from the upper airways may be considered for prophylaxis in the first year after birth. Insufficient data are available to recommend palivizumab prophylaxis for children with cystic fibrosis or Down syndrome. The burden of RSV disease and costs associated with transport from remote locations may result in a broader use of palivizumab for RSV prevention in Alaska Native populations and possibly in selected other American Indian populations. Palivizumab prophylaxis is not recommended for prevention of health care–associated RSV disease.

Varicella-zoster virus[86]		
– Infection in a normal host	Acyclovir 80 mg/kg/day (max single dose 800 mg) PO div qid for 5 days (AI)	The sooner antiviral therapy can be started, the greater the clinical benefit.
– Severe primary chickenpox, disseminated infection (cutaneous, pneumonia, encephalitis, hepatitis); immunocompromised host with primary chickenpox or disseminated zoster	Acyclovir 30 mg/kg/day IV as 1–2 h infusion div q8h for 10 days (acyclovir doses of 45–60 mg/kg/day in 3 div doses IV should be used for disseminated or central nervous system infection). Dosing also can be provided as 1,500 mg/m^2/day IV div q8h. Duration in immunocompromised children: 7–14 days, based on clinical response (AI).	Oral valacyclovir, famciclovir, foscarnet also active

10. Preferred Therapy for Specific Parasitic Pathogens

NOTES

- For some parasitic diseases, therapy may be available only from the Centers for Disease Control and Prevention (CDC), as noted. The CDC provides up-to-date information about parasitic diseases and current treatment recommendations at www.cdc.gov/parasites (accessed September 30, 2019). Consultation is available from the CDC for parasitic disease diagnostic services (www.cdc.gov/dpdx; accessed September 30, 2019); parasitic disease testing and experimental therapy at 404/639-3670; for malaria, 770/488-7788 or 855/856-4713 toll-free, Monday through Friday, 9:00 am to 5:00 pm ET, and the emergency number 770/488-7100 for after hours, weekends, and holidays (correct as of September 30, 2019). Antiparasitic drugs available from the CDC Drug Service can be reviewed and requested at www.cdc.gov/laboratory/drugservice/formulary.html (accessed September 30, 2019).
- Additional information about many of the organisms and diseases mentioned here, along with treatment recommendations, can be found in the appropriate sections in the American Academy of Pediatrics *Red Book* and the CDC website for parasitic diseases, www.cdc.gov/parasites (accessed September 30, 2019)
- **Abbreviations:** AmB, amphotericin B; A-P, atovaquone/proguanil; ASTMH, American Society of Tropical Medicine and Hygiene; bid, twice daily; CDC, Centers for Disease Control and Prevention; CNS, central nervous system; CrCl, creatinine clearance; CSF, cerebrospinal fluid; CT, computed tomography; DEC, diethylcarbamazine; div, divided; DS, double strength; FDA, US Food and Drug Administration; G6PD, glucose-6-phosphate dehydrogenase; GI, gastrointestinal; HIV, human immunodeficiency virus; IDSA, Infectious Diseases Society of America; IM, intramuscular; IND, investigational new drug; IV, intravenous; MF, microfilariae; MRI, magnetic resonance imaging; PAIR, puncture, aspiration, injection, re-aspiration; PHMB, polyhexamethylene biguanide; PO, orally; qd, once daily; qid, 4 times daily; qod, every other day; spp, species; SQ, subcutaneous; tab, tablet; TB, tuberculosis; TD, traveler's diarrhea; tid, 3 times daily; TMP/SMX, trimethoprim/sulfamethoxazole.

A. SELECTED COMMON PATHOGENIC PARASITES AND SUGGESTED AGENTS FOR TREATMENT

	Albendazole/ Mebendazole	Triclabendazole	Metronidazole/ Tinidazole	Praziquantel	Ivermectin	Nitazoxanide	DEC	Pyrantel Pamoate	Paromomycin	TMP/SMX
Ascariasis	++				+	+		+		
Blastocystis spp			+			+			+	+
Cryptosporidiosis						+			+	
Cutaneous larva migrans	++				++					
Cyclosporiasis			–			+				++
Cystoisospora spp						+				++
Dientamoebiasis	–		++			+			+	
Liver fluke *Clonorchis* and *Opisthorchis*	+			++						
Fasciola hepatica and *Fasciola gigantica*		++								
Lung fluke	–			++						
Giardia spp	+		++			++			+	
Hookworm	++				–			+		
Loiasis	+						++			
Mansonella ozzardi	–				+		–			
Mansonella perstans	±			–	–		±			

Onchocerciasis				++			
Pinworm	++						++
Schistosomiasis			++				
Strongyloides spp	+			++			
Tapeworm			++		+		
Toxocariasis	++					+	
Trichinellosis	++						
Trichomoniasis		++					
Trichuriasis	++						
Wuchereria bancrofti	+					++	

NOTE: **++** = preferred; **+** = acceptable; **±** = possibly effective (see text for further discussion); **—** = unlikely to be effective; [blank cell] = untested.

B. PREFERRED THERAPY FOR SPECIFIC PARASITIC PATHOGENS

Disease/Organism	Treatment (evidence grade)	Comments
Acanthamoeba	See Amebic meningoencephalitis.	
Amebiasis[1–5]		
Entamoeba histolytica		
– Asymptomatic intestinal colonization	Paromomycin 25–30 mg/kg/day PO div tid for 7 days; OR iodoquinol 30–40 mg/kg/day (max 650 mg/dose) PO div tid for 20 days; OR diloxanide furoate (not commercially available in the United States) 20 mg/kg/day PO div tid (max 500 mg/dose) for 10 days (CII)	Follow-up stool examination to ensure eradication of carriage; screen/treat positive close contacts. *Entamoeba dispar* and *Entamoeba moshkovskii* do not require treatment.
– Colitis	Metronidazole 35–50 mg/kg/day PO div tid for 10 days; OR tinidazole (age >3 y) 50 mg/kg/day PO (max 2 g) qd for 3 days FOLLOWED BY paromomycin or iodoquinol, as above, to eliminate cysts (BII)	Avoid antimotility drugs, steroids. Take tinidazole with food to decrease GI side effects; if unable to take tabs, pharmacists can crush tabs and mix with syrup. Avoid alcohol ingestion with metronidazole and tinidazole. Preliminary data support use of nitazoxanide to treat clinical infection, but it may not prevent parasitological failure: age ≥12 y, 500 mg bid for 3 days; ages 4–11 y, 200 mg bid for 3 days; ages 1–3 y, 100 mg bid for 3 days.
– Liver abscess, extraintestinal disease	Metronidazole 35–50 mg/kg/day IV q8h, switch to PO when tolerated, for 7-10 days; OR tinidazole (age >3 y) 50 mg/kg/day PO (max 2 g) qd for 5 days FOLLOWED BY paromomycin or iodoquinol, as above, to eliminate cysts (BII).	Nitazoxanide 500 mg bid for 10 days (≥12 y) (or doses as above for <12 y) is an alternative. Serologic assays >95% positive in extraintestinal amebiasis. Percutaneous or surgical drainage may be indicated for large liver abscesses or inadequate response to medical therapy. Avoid alcohol ingestion with metronidazole and tinidazole.

		Take tinidazole with food to decrease GI side effects; if unable to take tabs, pharmacists can crush tabs and mix with syrup.
Amebic meningoencephalitis[6–10]		
Naegleria fowleri	AmB 1.5 mg/kg/day IV div 2 doses for 3 days, then 1 mg/kg/day qd for 11 days; PLUS AmB intrathecally 1.5 mg qd for 2 days, then 1 mg/day qod for 8 days; PLUS azithromycin 10 mg/kg/day IV or PO (max 500 mg/day) for 28 days; PLUS fluconazole 10 mg/kg/day IV or PO qd (max 600 mg/day) for 28 days; PLUS rifampin 10 mg/kg/day qd IV or PO (max 600 mg/day) for 28 days; PLUS miltefosine $<$45 kg 50 mg PO bid; $\geq$45 kg 50 mg PO tid (max 2.5 mg/kg/day) for 28 days PLUS dexamethasone 0.6 mg/kg/day div qid for 4 days	Treatment recommendations based on regimens used for 5 known survivors; available at https://www.cdc.gov/parasites/naegleria/treatment-hcp.html (accessed September 30, 2019). Conventional amphotericin preferred; liposomal AmB is less effective in animal models. Treatment outcomes usually unsuccessful; early therapy (even before diagnostic confirmation if indicated) may improve survival. Miltefosine is available commercially (contact www.impavido.com for help in obtaining the drug); CDC provides expertise in management of patients with *N fowleri* infection (770/488-7100).
Acanthamoeba	Combination regimens including miltefosine, fluconazole, and pentamidine favored by some experts; TMP/SMX, metronidazole, and a macrolide may be added. Other drugs that have been used alone or in combination include rifampin, other azoles, sulfadiazine, flucytosine, and caspofungin. Keratitis: topical therapies include PHMB (0.02%) or biguanide chlorhexidine, combined with propamidine isethionate (0.1%) or hexamidine (0.1%) (topical therapies not approved in United States but available at compounding pharmacies).	Optimal treatment regimens uncertain; combination therapy favored. Miltefosine is available commercially (contact www.impavido.com for help in obtaining the drug); CDC is available for consultation about use of this drug (770/488-7100). Keratitis should be evaluated by an ophthalmologist. Prolonged treatment often needed.

B. PREFERRED THERAPY FOR SPECIFIC PARASITIC PATHOGENS (continued)

Disease/Organism	Treatment (evidence grade)	Comments
Balamuthia mandrillaris	Combination regimens preferred. Drugs that have been used alone or in combination include pentamidine, 5-flucytosine, fluconazole, macrolides, sulfadiazine, miltefosine, thioridazine, AmB, itraconazole, and albendazole.	Optimal treatment regimen uncertain; regimens based on case reports; prolonged treatment often needed. Surgical resection of CNS lesions may be beneficial.
Ancylostoma braziliense	See Cutaneous larva migrans.	
Ancylostoma caninum	See Cutaneous larva migrans.	
Ancylostoma duodenale	See Hookworm.	
Angiostrongyliasis[11–14]		
Angiostrongylus cantonensis (cerebral disease)	Supportive care	Most patients recover without antiparasitic therapy; treatment may provoke severe neurologic symptoms. Corticosteroids, analgesics, and repeat lumbar puncture may be of benefit. Prednisolone (1–2 mg/kg/day, up to 60 mg qd, in 2 div doses, for 2 wk) may shorten duration of headache and reduce need for repeat lumbar puncture. Ocular disease may require surgery or laser treatment.
Angiostrongylus costaricensis (eosinophilic enterocolitis)	Supportive care	Surgery may be pursued to exclude another diagnosis such as appendicitis or to remove inflamed intestine.
Ascariasis (*Ascaris lumbricoides*)[15]	First line: albendazole 400 mg PO once OR mebendazole 500 mg once or 100 mg bid for 3 days (BII) Pregnant women: pyrantel pamoate 11 mg/kg max 1 g once Alternatives: ivermectin 150–200 mcg/kg PO once (CII); nitazoxanide	Follow-up stool ova and parasite examination after therapy not essential. Take albendazole with food (bioavailability increases with food, especially fatty meals). Albendazole has theoretical risk of causing seizures in patients coinfected with cysticercosis.

	Age 1–3 y: 100 mg PO bid for 3 days Age 4–11 y: 200 mg PO bid for 3 days Age ≥12 y: 500 mg PO bid for 3 days	
Babesiosis (*Babesia* spp)[16–20]	Mild to moderate disease: azithromycin 10 mg/kg/day (max 500 mg/dose) PO on day 1; 5 mg/kg/day from day 2 on (max 250 mg/dose) for 7–10 days PLUS atovaquone 40 mg/kg/day (max 750 mg/dose) PO div bid (preferred due to more favorable adverse event profile) OR clindamycin 20-40 mg/kg/day IV div tid or qid (max 600 mg per dose), PLUS quinine 25 mg/kg/day PO (max 650 mg/dose) div tid for 7–10 days Severe disease: azithromycin 10 mg/kg/day (max 500 mg/dose) IV for 7–10 days PLUS atovaquone 40 mg/kg/day (max 750 mg/dose) PO div bid; OR clindamycin 20-40 mg/kg/day IV div tid or qid (max 600 mg per dose), PLUS quinine 25 mg/kg/day PO (max 650 mg/dose) div tid for 7–10 days	Most asymptomatic infections with *Babesia microti* in immunocompetent individuals do not require treatment. Daily monitoring of hematocrit and percentage of parasitized red blood cells (until <5%) is helpful in guiding management. Exchange blood transfusion may be of benefit for severe disease and *Babesia divergens* infection. Higher doses of medications and prolonged therapy may be needed for asplenic or immunocompromised individuals. Clindamycin and quinine remains the regimen of choice for *Babesia divergens*.
Balantidium coli[21]	Tetracycline (patients >7 y) 40 mg/kg/day PO div qid for 10 days (max 2 g/day) (CII); OR metronidazole 35–50 mg/kg/day PO div tid for 5 days; OR iodoquinol 30–40 mg/kg/day PO (max 2 g/day) div tid for 20 days	Optimal treatment regimen uncertain. Prompt stool examination may increase detection of rapidly degenerating trophozoites. None of these medications are approved for this indication. Nitazoxanide may also be effective.
Baylisascaris procyonis (raccoon roundworm)[22,23]	Albendazole 25–50 mg/kg/day PO for 10–20 days given as soon as possible (<3 days) after exposure (eg, ingestion of raccoon feces or contaminated soil) might prevent clinical disease (CIII).	Therapy generally unsuccessful to prevent fatal outcome or severe neurologic sequelae once CNS disease present. Steroids may be of value in decreasing inflammation in CNS or ocular infection. Albendazole bioavailability increased with food, especially fatty meals.

B. PREFERRED THERAPY FOR SPECIFIC PARASITIC PATHOGENS (continued)

Disease/Organism	Treatment (evidence grade)	Comments
Blastocystis spp[24,25]	Metronidazole 30 mg/kg/day (max 750 mg per dose) PO div tid for 5–10 days (BII); OR tinidazole 50 mg/kg (max 2 g) once (age >3 y) (BII)	Pathogenesis debated. Asymptomatic individuals do not need treatment; diligent search for other pathogenic parasites recommended for symptomatic individuals with *B hominis*. Paromomycin, nitazoxanide (500 mg PO bid for ages ≥12 y; 200 mg PO bid for 3 days for age 4–11 y; 100 mg PO bid for 3 days for age 1–3 y), and TMP/SMX also may be effective. Metronidazole resistance may occur. Take tinidazole with food; tabs may be crushed and mixed with flavored syrup.
Brugia malayi, Brugia timori	See Filariasis.	
Chagas disease (*Trypanosoma cruzi*)[26–28]	See Trypanosomiasis.	
Clonorchis sinensis	See Flukes.	
Cryptosporidiosis (*Cryptosporidium parvum*)[29–32]	Nitazoxanide, age 12–47 mo, 5 mL (100 mg) bid for 3 days; age 4–11 y, 10 mL (200 mg) bid for 3 days; age ≥12 y, 500 mg (tab or suspension) PO bid for 3 days (BII). Paromomycin 30 mg/kg/day div bid–qid (CII); OR azithromycin 10 mg/kg/day for 5 days (CII); OR paromomycin AND azithromycin given as combination therapy may yield initial response but may not result in sustained cure in immunocompromised individuals.	Recovery depends largely on the immune status of the host; treatment not required in all immunocompetent individuals. Medical therapy may have limited efficacy in HIV-infected patients not receiving effective antiretroviral therapy. Longer courses (>2 wk) may be needed in solid organ transplant patients.

Cutaneous larva migrans or creeping eruption[33,34] (dog and cat hookworm) (*Ancylostoma caninum, Ancylostoma braziliense, Uncinaria stenocephala*)	Ivermectin 200 mcg/kg PO for 1 day (CII); OR albendazole 15 mg/kg/day (max 400 mg) PO qd for 3 days (CII)	Albendazole bioavailability increased with food, especially fatty meals
Cyclospora spp[35,36] (cyanobacterium-like agent)	TMP/SMX 8–10 mg TMP/kg/day (max 1 DS tab bid) PO div bid for 7–10 days (BIII); nitazoxanide may be an alternative for TMP/SMX-allergic patients 500 mg bid for 7 days (adult dose).	HIV-infected patients may require higher doses/longer therapy. Ciprofloxacin 30 mg/kg/day div bid for 7 days may be an alternative; treatment failures have been reported.
Cysticercosis[37–40] (*Cysticercus cellulosae;* larva of *Taenia solium*)	Neurocysticercosis. Patients with 1–2 viable parenchymal cysticerci: albendazole 15 mg/kg/day PO div bid (max 1,200 mg/day) for 10–14 days (CII) OR praziquantel 50 mg/kg/day PO div tid for 10–14 days; PLUS steroids (prednisone 1.0 mg/kg/day or dexamethasone 0.1 mg/kg/day) begun at least 1 day before antiparasitic therapy, continued during antiparasitic treatment followed by rapid taper (to reduce inflammation associated with dying organisms) Patients with >2 viable parenchymal cysticerci: albendazole 15 mg/kg/day PO div bid (max 1,200 mg/day) for 10–14 days PLUS praziquantel 50 mg/kg/day PO div tid (CII) for 10–14 days plus steroids (prednisone 1.0 mg/kg/day or dexamethasone 0.1 mg/kg/day) begun at least 1 day before antiparasitic therapy, continued during antiparasitic treatment followed by rapid taper (to reduce inflammation associated with dying organisms).	Collaboration with a specialist with experience treating this condition is recommended. See IDSA/ASTMH guidelines.[40] For infection caused by only 1–2 cysts, some do not use steroid therapy routinely with active treatment. Management of seizures, cerebral edema, intracranial hypertension, or hydrocephalus, when present, is the focus of initial therapy and may require antiepileptic drugs, neuroendoscopy, or surgical approaches before considering antiparasitic therapy. Imaging with both CT and MRI is recommended for classifying disease in patients newly diagnosed with neurocysticercosis. Optimal dose and duration of steroid therapy is uncertain. Screening for TB infection and *Strongyloides* is recommended for patients likely to require prolonged steroid therapy. Take albendazole with food (bioavailability increases with food, especially fatty meals).

B. PREFERRED THERAPY FOR SPECIFIC PARASITIC PATHOGENS (continued)

Disease/Organism	Treatment (evidence grade)	Comments
Cystoisospora belli (formerly *Isospora belli*)[41]	TMP/SMX 8–10 mg TMP/kg/day PO (or IV) div bid for 7–10 days (max 160 mg TMP/800 mg SMX bid); OR ciprofloxacin 500 mg PO div bid for 7 days	Infection often self-limited in immunocompetent hosts; consider treatment if symptoms do not resolve by 5–7 days or are severe. Pyrimethamine plus leucovorin and nitazoxanide are alternatives. Immunocompromised patients should be treated; longer courses or suppressive therapy may be needed for severely immunocompromised patients.
Dientamoebiasis[42,43] (*Dientamoeba fragilis*)	Metronidazole 35–50 mg/kg/day PO div tid for 10 days (max 500–750 mg/dose); OR paromomycin 25–35 mg/kg/day PO div tid for 7 days; OR iodoquinol 30–40 mg/kg/day (max 650 mg/dose) PO div tid for 20 days (BII)	Routine treatment of asymptomatic individuals not indicated. Treatment indicated when no other cause except *Dientamoeba* found for abdominal pain or diarrhea lasting >1 wk. Take paromomycin with meals and iodoquinol after meals. Tinidazole, nitazoxanide, tetracycline, and doxycycline also may be effective. Albendazole and mebendazole have no activity against *Dientamoeba.*
Diphyllobothrium latum	See Tapeworms.	
Dipylidium caninum	See Tapeworms.	
Echinococcosis[44,45]		
Echinococcus granulosus	Albendazole 10–15 mg/kg/day PO div bid (max 800 mg/day) for 1–6 mo alone (CIII) or as adjunctive therapy with surgery or percutaneous treatment; initiate 4–30 days before and continue for at least 1 mo after surgery.	Involvement with specialist with experience treating this condition recommended. Surgery is the treatment of choice for management of complicated cysts. PAIR technique effective for appropriate cysts. Mebendazole is an alternative if albendazole is unavailable; if used, continue for 3 mo after PAIR. Take albendazole with food (bioavailability increases with food, especially fatty meals).

Echinococcus multilocularis	Surgical treatment generally the treatment of choice; postoperative albendazole 10–15 mg/kg/day PO div bid (max 800 mg/day) should be administered to reduce relapse; duration uncertain (at least 2 y with long-term monitoring for relapse). Benefit of preoperative albendazole unknown.	Involvement with specialist with experience treating this condition recommended. Take albendazole with food (bioavailability increases with food, especially fatty meals).
Entamoeba histolytica	See Amebiasis.	
Enterobius vermicularis	See Pinworms.	
Fasciola hepatica	See Flukes.	
Fasciolopsis buski	See Flukes.	
Eosinophilic meningitis	See Angiostrongyliasis.	
Filariasis[46–49]		
– River blindness (*Onchocerca volvulus*)	Ivermectin 150 mcg/kg PO once (AII); repeat q3–6mo until asymptomatic and no ongoing exposure; OR if no ongoing exposure, doxycycline 4 mg/kg/day PO (max 200 mg/day div bid) for 6 wk followed by a single dose of ivermectin; provide 1 dose of ivermectin for symptomatic relief 1 wk before beginning doxycycline.	Doxycycline targets *Wolbachia,* the endosymbiotic bacteria associated with *O volvulus.* Assess for *L loa* coinfection before using ivermectin if exposure occurred in settings where both *Onchocerca* and *L loa* are endemic. Treatment of onchocerciasis in the setting of *L loa* infection is uncertain and consultation with a specialist familiar with these diseases is recommended. Moxidectin was approved for treatment of onchocerciasis (to kill MF) in 2018 for children age ≥12 y; not yet available commercially in the US. Screening for loiasis recommended before use. Safety and efficacy of repeat doses have not been studied. Safety and efficacy in children age <12 y have not been established.

B. PREFERRED THERAPY FOR SPECIFIC PARASITIC PATHOGENS (continued)

Disease/Organism	Treatment (evidence grade)	Comments
– Tropical pulmonary eosinophilia[50]	DEC (from CDC) 6 mg/kg/day PO div tid for 12–21 days; antihistamines/corticosteroids for allergic reactions (CII)	DEC is available from the CDC Physicians' Hotlines for Parasitic Disease Cases at 404/718-4745; https://www.cdc.gov/parasites/lymphaticfilariasis/health_professionals/dxtx.html (accessed September 30, 2019); the CDC Drug Service number is 404/639-3670.
Loa loa	Symptomatic loiasis with MF of *L loa*/mL <8,000: DEC (from CDC) 8–10 mg/kg/day PO div tid for 21 days Symptomatic loiasis, with MF/mL ≥8,000: apheresis followed by DEC Albendazole (symptomatic loiasis, with MF/mL <8,000 and failed 2 rounds of DEC, OR symptomatic loiasis, with MF/mL ≥8,000 to reduce level to <8,000 prior to treatment with DEC) 200 mg PO bid for 21 days	Involvement with specialist with experience treating this condition recommended. Quantification of microfilarial levels is essential before treatment. Do not use DEC if onchocerciasis is present. Apheresis or albendazole may be used to reduce microfilarial levels before treatment with DEC.
Mansonella ozzardi	Ivermectin 200 mcg/kg PO once	DEC and albendazole not effective
Mansonella perstans	Combination therapy with DEC and albendazole 400 mg PO bid for 21 days may be effective.	Relatively resistant to DEC, ivermectin, albendazole, and mebendazole; doxycycline 4 mg/kg/day PO (max 200 mg/day div bid) for 6 wk beneficial for clearing microfilaria in Mali
Wuchereria bancrofti, Brugia malayi, Brugia timori, Mansonella streptocerca	DEC (from CDC) 6 mg/kg/day div tid for 12 days OR 6 mg/kg/day PO as a single dose (AII). Consider adding doxycycline 4 mg/kg/day PO (max 200 mg/day div bid) for 4–6 wk.	Avoid DEC with *Onchocerca* and *L loa* coinfection; doxycycline (4 mg/kg/day PO, max 200 mg/day div bid, for 4–6 wk) may be used; albendazole has activity against adult worms. Effectiveness of doxycycline in *Mansonella streptocerca* unknown. DEC is available from CDC (404/639-3670).

Flukes		
Liver flukes[51] (*Clonorchis sinensis, Opisthorchis* spp)	Praziquantel 75 mg/kg PO div tid for 2 days (BII); OR albendazole 10 mg/kg/day PO for 7 days (CIII). Single 40 mg/kg dose praziquantel may be effective for *Opisthorchis viverrini*.[52]	Take praziquantel with liquids and food. Take albendazole with food (bioavailability increases with food, especially fatty meals).
Lung fluke[53,54] (*Paragonimus westermani* and other *Paragonimus* lung flukes)	Praziquantel 75 mg/kg PO div tid for 2 days (BII) Triclabendazole 10 mg/kg, orally, once or twice (approved for children age ≥6 y for fascioliasis)	Triclabendazole should be taken with food to facilitate absorption.
Sheep liver fluke[55] (*Fasciola hepatica, Fasciola gigantica*)	Triclabendazole 10 mg/kg/dose PO bid for 1–2 days (approved for ages ≥6 y) (BII) OR nitazoxanide PO (take with food), age 12–47 mo, 100 mg/dose bid for 7 days; age 4–11 y, 200 mg/dose bid for 7 days; age ≥12 y, 1 tab (500 mg)/dose bid for 7 days (CII)	Responds poorly to praziquantel; albendazole and mebendazole ineffective. Triclabendazole should be taken with food to facilitate absorption.
Intestinal fluke (*Fasciolopsis buski*)	Praziquantel 75 mg/kg PO div tid for 1 day (BII)	

B. PREFERRED THERAPY FOR SPECIFIC PARASITIC PATHOGENS (continued)

Disease/Organism	Treatment (evidence grade)	Comments
Giardiasis (*Giardia intestinalis* [formerly *lamblia*])[56–58]	Tinidazole 50 mg/kg/day (max 2 g) PO for 1 day (approved for age >3 y) (BII); OR nitazoxanide PO (take with food), age 1–3 y, 100 mg/dose bid for 3 days; age 4–11 y, 200 mg/dose bid for 3 days; age ≥12 y, 500 mg/dose bid for 3 days (BII)	Alternatives: metronidazole 15 mg/kg/day (max 250 mg/dose) PO div tid for 5–7 days (BII); albendazole 10–15 mg/kg/day (max 400 mg/dose) PO for 5 days (CII) OR mebendazole 200 mg PO tid for 5 days; OR paromomycin 30 mg/kg/day div tid for 5–10 days; furazolidone 8 mg/kg/day (max 100 mg/dose) in 4 doses for 7–10 days (not available in United States); quinacrine (refractory cases) 6 mg/kg/day PO div tid (max 100 mg/dose) for 5 days. If therapy ineffective, may try a higher dose or longer course of the same agent, or an agent in a different class; combination therapy may be considered for refractory cases. Prolonged courses may be needed for immunocompromised patients (eg, hypogammaglobulinemia). Treatment of asymptomatic carriers not usually indicated.
Hookworm[59–61] *Necator americanus*, *Ancylostoma duodenale*	Albendazole 400 mg once (repeat dose may be necessary) (BII); OR mebendazole 100 mg PO for 3 days OR 500 mg PO once; OR pyrantel pamoate 11 mg/kg (max 1 g/day) (BII) PO qd for 3 days	
Hymenolepis nana	See Tapeworms.	
Isospora belli	See *Cytoisospora belli*.	
Leishmaniasis[62–69] (including kala-azar) *Leishmania* spp	Visceral: liposomal AmB 3 mg/kg/day on days 1–5, day 14, and day 21 (AI); OR sodium stibogluconate (from CDC) 20 mg/kg/day IM or IV for 28 days (or longer) (BIII); OR miltefosine 2.5 mg/kg/day PO (max 150 mg/day) for 28 days (BII) (FDA-approved	Consultation with a specialist familiar with management of leishmaniasis is advised strongly, especially when treating patients with HIV coinfection. See IDSA/ASTMH guidelines.[62]

regimen: 50 mg PO bid for 28 days for weight 30–44 kg; 50 mg PO tid for 28 days for weight ≥45 kg); other AmB products available but not approved for this indication. Cutaneous and mucosal disease: There is no generally accepted treatment of choice; treatment decisions should be individualized. Uncomplicated cutaneous: combination of debridement of eschars, cryotherapy, thermotherapy, intralesional pentavalent antimony, and topical paromomycin (not available in United States). Complicated cutaneous: oral or parenteral systemic therapy with miltefosine 2.5 mg/kg/day PO (max 150 mg/day) for 28 days (FDA-approved regimen: 50 mg PO bid for 28 days for weight 30–44 kg; 50 mg PO tid for 28 days for weight ≥45 kg) (BII); OR sodium stibogluconate 20 mg/kg/day IM or IV for 20 days (BIII); OR pentamidine isethionate 2–4 mg/kg/day IV or IM qod for 4–7 doses; OR amphotericin (various regimens); OR azoles (fluconazole 200–600 mg PO qd for 6 wk; or ketoconazole or itraconazole); also intralesional and topical alternatives. Mucosal: sodium stibogluconate 20 mg/kg/day IM or IV for 28 days; OR AmB (Fungizone) 0.5–1 mg/kg/day IV qd or qod for cumulative total of approximately 20–45 mg/kg; OR liposomal AmB approximately 3 mg/kg/day IV qd for cumulative total of approximately 20–60 mg/kg; OR miltefosine 2.5 mg/kg/day PO (max 150 mg/day) for 28 days (FDA-approved regimen: 50 mg PO bid for 28 days for weight 30–44 kg; 50 mg PO tid for 28 days for weight ≥45 kg); OR pentamidine isethionate 2–4 mg/kg/day IV or IM qod or 3 times/wk for ≥15 doses (considered a lesser alternative).	Region where infection acquired, spp of *Leishmania*, skill of practitioner with some local therapies, and drugs available in the United States affect therapeutic choices. For immunocompromised patients with visceral disease, FDA-approved dosing of liposomal amphotericin is 4 mg/kg on days 1–5, 10, 17, 24, 31, and 38, with further therapy on an individual basis.

B. PREFERRED THERAPY FOR SPECIFIC PARASITIC PATHOGENS (continued)

Disease/Organism	Treatment (evidence grade)	Comments
Lice *Pediculosis capitis* or *humanus*, *Phthirus pubis*[70,71]	Follow manufacturer's instructions for topical use: permethrin 1% (≥2 mo) OR pyrethrin (children aged ≥2 y) (BII); OR 0.5% ivermectin lotion (≥6 mo) (BII); OR spinosad 0.9% topical suspension (≥6 mo) (BII); OR benzyl alcohol lotion 5% (≥6 mo) (BIII); OR malathion 0.5% (children aged ≥2 y) (BIII); OR topical or oral ivermectin 200 mcg/kg PO once (400 mcg/kg for ≥15 kg); repeat 7–10 days later.	Launder bedding and clothing; for eyelash infestation, use petrolatum; for head lice, remove nits with comb designed for that purpose. Benzyl alcohol can be irritating to skin; parasite resistance unlikely to develop. Consult health care professional before re-treatment with ivermectin lotion; re-treatment with spinosad topical suspension usually not needed unless live lice seen 1 wk after treatment. Administration of 3 doses of ivermectin (1 dose/wk separately by weekly intervals) may be needed to eradicate heavy infection.
Malaria[72,73]		
Plasmodium falciparum, *Plasmodium vivax*, *Plasmodium ovale*, *Plasmodium malariae*	CDC Malaria Hotline 770/488-7788 or 855/856-4713 toll-free (Monday–Friday, 9:00 am–5:00 pm ET) or emergency consultation after hours 770/488-7100; online information at https://www.cdc.gov/malaria/diagnosis_treatment/index.html (accessed September 30, 2019). Consult infectious diseases or tropical medicine specialist if unfamiliar with malaria.	Consultation with a specialist familiar with management of malaria is advised, especially for severe malaria. No antimalarial drug provides absolute protection against malaria; fever after return from an endemic area should prompt an immediate evaluation. Emphasize personal protective measures (insecticides, bed nets, clothing, and avoidance of dusk–dawn mosquito exposures).
Prophylaxis		See https://wwwnc.cdc.gov/travel/yellowbook/2018/infectious-diseases-related-to-travel/malaria#5217 (accessed September 30, 2019).
For areas with chloroquine-resistant *P falciparum* or *P vivax*	A-P: 5–8 kg, ½ pediatric tab/day; ≥9–10 kg, ¾ pediatric tab/day; ≥11–20 kg, 1 pediatric tab (62.5 mg atovaquone/25 mg proguanil); ≥21–30 kg, 2 pediatric tabs; ≥31–40 kg, 3 pediatric tabs;	Avoid mefloquine for persons with a history of seizures or psychosis, active depression, or cardiac conduction abnormalities; see black box warning. Avoid A-P in severe renal impairment (CrCl <30).

	≥40 kg, 1 adult tab (250 mg atovaquone/100 mg proguanil) PO qd starting 1–2 days before travel and continuing 7 days after last exposure; for children <5 kg, data on A-P limited (BII); OR mefloquine: for children <5 kg, 5 mg/kg; ≥5–9 kg, ⅛ tab; ≥10–19 kg, ¼ tab; ≥20–30 kg, ½ tab; ≥31–45 kg, ¾ tab; ≥45 kg (adult dose), 1 tab PO once weekly starting the wk before arrival in area and continuing for 4 wk after leaving area (BII); OR doxycycline (patients >7 y): 2 mg/kg (max 100 mg) PO qd starting 1–2 days before arrival in area and continuing for 4 wk after leaving area (BIII); OR primaquine (check for G6PD deficiency before administering): 0.5 mg/kg base qd starting 1 day before travel and continuing for 5 days after last exposure (BII)	*P falciparum* resistance to mefloquine exists along the borders between Thailand and Myanmar and Thailand and Cambodia, Myanmar and China, and Myanmar and Laos; isolated resistance has been reported in southern Vietnam. Take doxycycline with adequate fluids to avoid esophageal irritation and food to avoid GI side effects; use sunscreen and avoid excessive sun exposure. Tafenoquine approved August 2018 for use in those ≥18 y; must test for G6PD deficiency before use; pregnancy testing recommended before use. Loading dose 200 mg daily for 3 days before travel; 200 mg weekly during travel; after return, 200 mg once 7 days after last maintenance dose; tabs must be swallowed whole. May also be used to prevent malaria in areas with chloroquine-resistant malaria.
For areas without chloroquine-resistant *P falciparum* or *P vivax*	Chloroquine phosphate 5 mg base/kg (max 300 mg base) PO once weekly, beginning the wk before arrival in area and continuing for 4 wk after leaving area (available in suspension outside the United States and Canada and at compounding pharmacies) (AII). After return from heavy or prolonged (months) exposure to infected mosquitoes: consider treatment with primaquine (check for G6PD deficiency before administering) 0.5 mg base/kg PO qd with final 2 wk of chloroquine for prevention of relapse with *P ovale* or *P vivax*.	
Treatment of disease		See https://www.cdc.gov/malaria/resources/pdf/treatmenttable.pdf (accessed September 30, 2019).

B. PREFERRED THERAPY FOR SPECIFIC PARASITIC PATHOGENS (continued)

Disease/Organism	Treatment (evidence grade)	Comments
– Chloroquine-resistant *P falciparum* or *P vivax*	Oral therapy: artemether/lumefantrine 6 doses over 3 days at 0, 8, 24, 36, 48, and 60 h; <15 kg, 1 tab/dose; ≥15–25 kg, 2 tabs/dose; ≥25–35 kg, 3 tabs/dose; >35 kg, 4 tabs/dose (BII); A-P: for children <5 kg, data limited; ≥5–8 kg, 2 pediatric tabs (62.5 mg atovaquone/25 mg proguanil) PO qd for 3 days; ≥9–10 kg, 3 pediatric tabs qd for 3 days; ≥11–20 kg, 1 adult tab (250 mg atovaquone/100 mg proguanil) qd for 3 days; >20–30 kg, 2 adult tabs qd for 3 days; >30–40 kg, 3 adult tabs qd for 3 days; >40 kg, 4 adult tabs qd for 3 days (BII); OR quinine 30 mg/kg/day (max 2 g/day) PO div tid for 3–7 days AND doxycycline 4 mg/kg/day div bid for 7 days OR clindamycin 30 mg/kg/day div tid (max 900 mg tid) for 7 days. Parenteral therapy: artesunate (available from CDC). Children > 20 kg: 2.4 mg/kg/dose IV at 0, 12, 24, and 48 h. Children < 20 kg: 3.0 mg/kg/dose IV at 0, 12, 24, and 48 h (from CDC) (BI) AND follow artesunate by one of the following: artemether/lumefantrine, A-P, doxycycline (clindamycin in pregnant women), or, if no other options, mefloquine, all dosed as above. If needed, give interim treatment until artesunate arrives. See CDC website for details: https://www.cdc.gov/malaria/resources/pdf/treatmenttable.pdf (accessed September 30, 2019). For prevention of relapse with *P vivax, P ovale:* primaquine (check for G6PD deficiency before administering) 0.5 mg base/kg/day PO for 14 days.	Mild disease may be treated with oral antimalarial drugs; severe disease (impaired level of consciousness, convulsion, hypotension, or parasitemia >5%) should be treated parenterally. Avoid mefloquine for treatment of malaria, if possible, given higher dose and increased incidence of adverse events. Take clindamycin and doxycycline with plenty of liquids. Do not use primaquine or tafenoquine during pregnancy. Avoid artemether/lumefantrine and mefloquine in patients with cardiac arrhythmias, and avoid concomitant use of drugs that prolong QT interval. Take A-P and artemether/lumefantrine with food or milk. Aretsunate must be requested from CDC; see www.cdc.gov/malaria/resources/pdf/treatmenttable.pdf (accessed September 30, 2019). For relapses of primaquine-resistant *P vivax* or *P ovale*, consider retreating with primaquine 30 mg (base) for 28 days. Tafenoquine approved July 2018 for prevention of relapse with *P vivax* malaria in those ≥16 y. 300 mg on the first or second day of appropriate therapy for acute malaria. Must test for G6PD deficiency before use; pregnancy testing recommended before use; tabs must be swallowed whole.

– Chloroquine-susceptible *P falciparum*, chloroquine-susceptible *P vivax*, *P ovale*, *P malariae*	Oral therapy: chloroquine 10 mg/kg base (max 600 mg base) PO then 5 mg/kg 6, 24, and 48 h after initial dose. Parenteral therapy: artesunate, as above. After return from heavy or prolonged (months) exposure to infected mosquitoes: consider treatment with primaquine (check for G6PD deficiency before administering) 0.5 mg base/kg PO qd with final 2 wk of chloroquine for prevention of relapse with *P ovale* or *P vivax*.	Alternative if chloroquine not available: hydroxychloroquine 10 mg base/kg PO immediately, followed by 5 mg base/kg PO at 6, 24, and 48 h. For relapses of primaquine-resistant *P vivax* or *P ovale*, consider retreating with primaquine 30 mg (base) for 28 days.
Mansonella ozzardi, *Mansonella perstans*, *Mansonella streptocerca*	See Filariasis.	
Naegleria	See Amebic meningoencephalitis.	
Necator americanus	See Hookworm.	
Onchocerca volvulus	See Filariasis.	
Opisthorchis spp	See Flukes.	
Paragonimus westermani	See Flukes.	
Pinworms (*Enterobius vermicularis*)	Mebendazole 100 mg once, repeat in 2 wk; OR albendazole 400 mg PO once (age ≥2 y); 200 mg PO once <2 y; ≥20 kg, 400 mg PO once; repeat in 2 wk (BII); OR pyrantel pamoate 11 mg/kg (max 1 g) PO once (BII); repeat in 2 wk.	Treat entire household (and if this fails, consider treating close child care/school contacts); re-treatment of contacts after 2 wk may be needed to prevent reinfection. Safety of mebendazole in children has not been established. There are limited data in children ≤2 y; some studies suggest it is safe in children as young as 1 y.
Plasmodium spp	See Malaria.	
Pneumocystis	See Chapter 8, Table 8B, *Pneumocystis jiroveci* (formerly *carinii*) pneumonia.	

B. PREFERRED THERAPY FOR SPECIFIC PARASITIC PATHOGENS (continued)

Disease/Organism	Treatment (evidence grade)	Comments
Scabies (*Sarcoptes scabiei*)[74]	Permethrin 5% cream applied to entire body (including scalp in infants), left on for 8–14 h then bathe, repeat in 1 wk (BII); OR ivermectin 200 mcg/kg PO once weekly for 2 doses (BII); OR crotamiton 10% applied topically overnight on days 1, 2, 3, and 8, bathe in am (BII).	Launder bedding and clothing. Crotamiton treatment failure has been observed. Ivermectin safety not well established in children <15 kg and pregnant women. Reserve lindane for patients >10 y who do not respond to other therapy; concern for toxicity. Itching may continue for weeks after successful treatment; can be managed with antihistamines.
Schistosomiasis (*Schistosoma haematobium, Schistosoma japonicum, Schistosoma mansoni, Schistosoma mekongi, Schistosoma intercalatum*)[75–77]	Praziquantel 40 (for *S haematobium, S mansoni,* and *S intercalatum*) or 60 (for *S japonicum* and *S mekongi*) mg/kg/day PO div bid (if 40 mg/day) or tid (if 60 mg/day) for 1 day (AI)	Take praziquantel with food and liquids. Oxamniquine (not available in United States) 20 mg/kg PO div bid for 1 day (Brazil) or 40–60 mg/kg/day for 2–3 days (most of Africa) (BII). Re-treat with the same dose if eggs still present 6–12 wk after initial treatment.
Strongyloidiasis (*Strongyloides stercoralis*)[78,79]	Ivermectin 200 mcg/kg PO qd for 1–2 days (BI); OR albendazole 400 mg PO bid for 7 days (or longer for disseminated disease) (BII)	Albendazole is less effective but may be adequate if longer courses used. For immunocompromised patients (especially with hyperinfection syndrome), veterinary SQ formulations may be lifesaving. The SQ formulation may be used under a single-patient IND protocol request to the FDA. Ivermectin safety not well established in children <15 kg and pregnant women.
Tapeworms – *Taenia saginata, Taenia solium, Hymenolepis nana, Diphyllobothrium latum, Dipylidium caninum*	Praziquantel 5–10 mg/kg PO once (25 mg/kg once; may repeat 10 days later; for *H nana*) (BII); OR niclosamide (not available in United States) 50 mg/kg (max 2 g) PO once, chewed thoroughly	Nitazoxanide may be effective (published clinical data limited) 500 mg PO bid for 3 days for age >11 y; 200 mg PO bid for 3 days for age 4–11 y; 100 mg PO bid for 3 days for age 1–3 y.

	Weight 11–34 kg: 1 g in a single dose on day 1 then 500 mg/day PO for 6 days Weight >34 kg: 1.5 g in a single dose on day 1 then 1 g/day PO for 6 days; for *H nana*	
Toxocariasis[80] (*Toxocara canis* [dog roundworm] and *Toxocara cati* [cat roundworm])	Visceral larval migrans: albendazole 400 mg PO bid for 5 days (BII) Ocular larva migrants: albendazole 400 mg PO, 15 mg/kg/day div bid, max 800 mg/day (800 mg div bid for adults) for 2–4 wk with prednisone (0.5–1 mg/kg/day with slow taper)	Mild disease often resolves without treatment. Corticosteroids may be used for severe symptoms in visceral larval migrans. Mebendazole (100–200 mg/day PO bid for 5 days) is an alternative.
Toxoplasmosis (*Toxoplasma gondii*)[81–83]	Pyrimethamine 2 mg/kg/day PO div bid for 2 days (max 100 mg) then 1 mg/kg/day (max 25 mg/day) PO qd AND sulfadiazine 120 mg/kg/day PO div qid (max 6 g/day); with supplemental folinic acid and leucovorin 10–25 mg with each dose of pyrimethamine (AI) for 3–6 wk. See Chapter 5 for congenital infection. For treatment in pregnancy, spiramycin 50–100 mg/kg/day PO div qid (available as investigational therapy through the FDA at 301/796-0563) (CII).	Experienced ophthalmologic consultation encouraged for treatment of ocular disease. Treatment continued for 2 wk after resolution of illness (approximately 3–6 wk); concurrent corticosteroids given for ocular or CNS infection. Prolonged therapy if HIV positive. Take pyrimethamine with food to decrease GI adverse effects; sulfadiazine should be taken on an empty stomach with water. Clindamycin, azithromycin, or atovaquone plus pyrimethamine may be effective for patients intolerant of sulfa-containing drugs. Consult expert advice for treatment during pregnancy and management of congenital infection.

B. PREFERRED THERAPY FOR SPECIFIC PARASITIC PATHOGENS (continued)

Disease/Organism	Treatment (evidence grade)	Comments
Traveler's diarrhea[84–87]	Azithromycin 10 mg/kg qd for 1–3 days (AII); OR rifaximin 200 mg PO tid for 3 days (ages ≥12 y) (BIII); OR ciprofloxacin (BII)	See TD guidelines: https://academic.oup.com/jtm/article/24/suppl_1/S63/3782742 (accessed October 14, 2019). Azithromycin preferable to ciprofloxacin for travelers to Southeast Asia and India given high prevalence of fluoroquinolone-resistant *Campylobacter.* Do not use rifaximin for *Campylobacter, Salmonella, Shigella*, and other causes of invasive diarrhea. Antibiotic regimens may be combined with loperamide (≥2 y). Rifamycin approved in adults >18 y for treatment of TD caused by noninvasive strains of *Escherichia coli* (388 mg [2 tabs] bid for 3 days).
Trichinellosis (*Trichinella spiralis*)[88]	Albendazole 400 mg PO bid for 8–14 days (BII) OR mebendazole 200–400 mg PO tid for 3 days, then 400–500 mg PO tid for 10 days	Therapy ineffective for larvae already in muscles. Anti-inflammatory drugs, steroids for CNS or cardiac involvement or severe symptoms.
Trichomoniasis (*Trichomonas vaginalis*)[89]	Tinidazole 50 mg/kg (max 2 g) PO for 1 dose (BII) OR metronidazole 2 g PO for 1 dose OR metronidazole 500 mg PO bid for 7 days (BII)	Treat sex partners simultaneously. Metronidazole resistance occurs and may be treated with higher-dose metronidazole or tinidazole.
Trichuris trichiura	See Whipworm (Trichuriasis).	
Trypanosomiasis		
– Chagas disease[26–28] (*Trypanosoma cruzi*)	Benznidazole PO: age <12 y, 5–8 mg/kg/day div bid for 60 days; ≥12 y, 5–7 mg/kg/day div bid for 60 days (BIII); OR nifurtimox PO (from CDC): age 1–10 y, 15–20 mg/kg/day div tid or qid for 90 days; 11–16 y, 12.5–15 mg/kg/day div tid or qid for 90 days; ≥17 y, 8–10 mg/kg/day div tid–qid for 90 days (BIII)	Therapy recommended for acute and congenital infection, reactivated infection, and chronic infection in children aged <18 y; consider in those up to age 50 y with chronic infection without advanced cardiomyopathy. Benznidazole has been approved by the FDA for use in children ages 2–12 y.

		Side effects are common but occur less often in younger patients. Both drugs contraindicated in pregnancy.
Sleeping sickness[90–93] – Acute (hemolymphatic) stage (*Trypanosoma brucei gambiense* [West African]; *T brucei rhodesiense* [East African])	*Tb gambiense:* pentamidine isethionate 4 mg/kg/day (max 300 mg) IM or IV for 7–10 days (BII) *Tb rhodesiense:* suramin (from CDC) 2 mg test dose IV, then 20 mg/kg (max 1 g) IV on days 1, 3, 7, 14, and 21 (BII)	CSF examination required for all patients to assess CNS involvement. Consult with infectious diseases or tropical medicine specialist if unfamiliar with trypanosomiasis. Examination of the buffy coat of peripheral blood may be helpful. *Tb gambiense* may be found in lymph node aspirates.
– Late (CNS) stage (*Trypanosoma brucei gambiense* [West African]; *T brucei rhodesiense* [East African])	*Tb gambiense:* eflornithine 400 mg/kg/day IV div qid for 14 days; OR eflornithine (from CDC) 400 mg/kg/day IV div bid for 7 days PLUS nifurtimox 15 mg/kg/day for 10 days (BIII). *Tb rhodesiense:* melarsoprol, 2–3.6 mg/kg/day IV for 3 days; after 7 days, 3.6 mg/kg/day for 3 days; after 7 days, 3.6 mg/kg/day for 3 days; corticosteroids often given with melarsoprol to decrease risk of CNS toxicity.	CSF examination needed for management (double-centrifuge technique recommended); perform repeat CSF examinations every 6 mo for 2 y to detect relapse.
Uncinaria stenocephala	See Cutaneous larva migrans.	
Whipworm (Trichuriasis) *Trichuris trichiura*	Mebendazole 100 mg PO bid for 3 days OR 500 mg PO qd for 3 days; OR albendazole 400 mg PO for 3 days; OR ivermectin 200 mcg/kg/day PO qd for 3 days (BII)	Treatment can be given for 5–7 days for heavy infestation.
Wuchereria bancrofti	See Filariasis.	
Yaws	Azithromycin 30 mg/kg max 2 g once (also treats bejel and pinta)	Alternative regimens include IM benzathine penicillin and second-line agents doxycycline, tetracycline, and erythromycin.

11. Alphabetic Listing of Antimicrobials

NOTES

- Higher dosages in a dose range are generally indicated for more serious infections. For pathogens with higher minimal inhibitory concentrations against beta-lactam antibiotics, a more prolonged infusion of the antibiotic will allow increased antibacterial effect (see Chapter 3).
- Maximum dosages for adult-sized children (eg, ≥40 kg) are based on US Food and Drug Administration (FDA)-approved product labeling or post-marketing data.
- Antiretroviral medications are not listed in this chapter. See Chapter 9.
- Drugs with FDA-approved dosage, or dosages based on randomized clinical trials, are given a Level of Evidence I. Dosages for which data are collected from noncomparative trials or small comparative trials are given a Level of Evidence II. Dosages based on expert or consensus opinion or case reports are given a Level of Evidence III.
- If no oral liquid form is available, round the child's dose to a combination of available solid dosage forms. Consult a pediatric pharmacist for recommendations on mixing with food (eg, crushing tablets, emptying capsule contents) and the availability of extemporaneously compounded liquid formulations.
- Cost estimates are in US dollars per course, or per month for maintenance regimens. Estimates are based on wholesale acquisition costs at the editor's institution. These may differ from that of the reader. Legend: $ = <$100, $$ = $100–$400, $$$ = $401–$1,000, $$$$ = >$1,000, $$$$$ = >$10,000.
- There are some agents that we do not recommend even though they may be available. We believe they are significantly inferior to those we do recommend (see chapters 5–10) and could possibly lead to poor outcomes if used. Such agents are not listed.
- **Abbreviations:** AOM, acute otitis media; AUC:MIC, area under the curve–minimum inhibitory concentration; bid, twice daily; BSA, body surface area; CABP, community-acquired bacterial pneumonia; CA-MRSA, community-associated methicillin-resistant *Staphylococcus aureus*; cap, capsule or caplet; CF, cystic fibrosis; CMV, cytomegalovirus; CNS, central nervous system; CrCl, creatinine clearance; div, divided; DR, delayed release; EC, enteric coated; ER, extended release; FDA, US Food and Drug Administration; GI, gastrointestinal; hs, bedtime; HSV, herpes simplex virus; IBW, ideal body weight; IM, intramuscular; INH, isoniazid; IV, intravenous; IVesic, intravesical; IVPB, intravenous piggyback (premixed bag); LD, loading dose; MAC, *Mycobacterium avium* complex; MIC, minimum inhibitory concentration; MRSA, methicillin-resistant *S aureus;* NS, normal saline (physiologic saline solution); oint, ointment; OPC, oropharyngeal candidiasis; ophth, ophthalmic; PEG, pegylated; PIP, piperacillin; PJP, *Pneumocystis* jiroveci; PMA, post-menstrual age; PO, oral; pwd, powder; qd, once daily; qhs, every bedtime; qid, 4 times daily; RSV, respiratory

syncytial virus; RTI, respiratory tract infection; SIADH, syndrome of inappropriate antidiuretic hormone; SMX, sulfamethoxazole; soln, solution; SPAG-2, small particle aerosol generator model-2; SQ, subcutaneous; SSSI, skin and skin structure infection; STI, sexually transmitted infection; susp, suspension; tab, tablet; TB, tuberculosis; TBW, total body weight; tid, 3 times daily; TMP, trimethoprim; top, topical; UTI, urinary tract infection; vag, vaginal; VZV, varicella-zoster virus.

A. SYSTEMIC ANTIMICROBIALS WITH DOSAGE FORMS AND USUAL DOSAGES

Generic and Trade Names	Dosage Form (cost estimate)	Route	Dose (evidence level)	Interval
Acyclovir,[a] Zovirax (See Valacyclovir as another oral formulation to achieve therapeutic acyclovir serum concentrations.)	500-, 1,000-mg vials ($)	IV	15–45 mg/kg/day (I) (See chapters 5 and 9.) Max 1,500 mg/m²/day (II) (See Chapter 12.)	q8h
	200-mg/5-mL susp ($$) 200-mg cap ($) 400-, 800-mg tab ($)	PO	900 mg/m²/day (I) 60–80 mg/kg/day, max 3,200 mg/day (I) Adult max 4 g/day for VZV (I) (See chapters 5 and 9.)	q8h q6–8h
Albendazole,[a] Albenza	200-mg tab ($$-$$$$)	PO	15 mg/kg/day for cysticercosis or echinococcosis (I). See Chapter 10 for max doses and other indications.	q12h
Amikacin,[a] Amikin	500-, 1,000-mg vials ($)	IV, IM	15–22.5 mg/kg/day[b] (I) (See Chapter 1.) 30–35 mg/kg/day[b] for CF (II)	q8–24h q24h
		IVesic	50–100 mL of 0.5 mg/mL in NS (III)	q12h
Amoxicillin,[a] Amoxil	125-, 200-, 250-, 400-mg/5-mL susp ($) 125-, 250-mg chew tab ($) 250-, 500-mg cap ($) 500-, 875-mg tab ($)	PO	Standard dose: 40–45 mg/kg/day (I) High dose: 80–90 mg/kg/day (I) 150 mg/kg/day for penicillin-resistant *Streptococcus pneumoniae* otitis media (III) Max 4,000 mg/day (III)	q8–12h q12h q8h

A. SYSTEMIC ANTIMICROBIALS WITH DOSAGE FORMS AND USUAL DOSAGES (continued)

Generic and Trade Names	Dosage Form (cost estimate)	Route	Dose (evidence level)	Interval
Amoxicillin/clavulanate,[a] Augmentin	16:1 Augmentin XR: 1,000/62.5-mg tab ($$)	PO	16:1 formulation: ≥40 kg and adults 4,000-mg amoxicillin/day (not per kg) (I)	q12h
	14:1 Augmentin ES: 600/42.9-mg/5-mL susp ($)	PO	14:1 formulation: 90-mg amoxicillin/kg/day (I), max 4,000 mg/day (III)	q12h
	7:1 Augmentin ($): 875/125-mg tab 200/28.5-, 400/57-mg chew tab 200/28.5-, 400/57-mg/5-mL susp	PO	7:1 formulation: 25- or 45-mg amoxicillin/kg/day, max 1,750 mg/day (I)	q12h
	4:1 Augmentin: 500/125-mg tab ($) 125/31.25-mg/5-mL susp ($$$) 250/62.5-mg/5-mL susp ($)	PO	20- or 40-mg amoxicillin component/kg/day (max 1,500 mg/day) (I)	q8h
	2:1 Augmentin: 250 mg/125-mg tab ($)	PO	2:1 formulation: ≥40 kg: 750-mg amoxicillin/day (not per kg) (I)	q8h
Amphotericin B deoxycholate,[a] Fungizone	50-mg vial ($$)	IV	1–1.5 mg/kg pediatric and adults (I), no max 0.5 mg/kg for *Candida* esophagitis or cystitis (II)	q24h
		IVesic	50–100 mcg/mL in sterile water × 50–100 mL (III)	q8h
Amphotericin B, lipid complex, Abelcet	100-mg/20-mL vial ($$$)	IV	5 mg/kg pediatric and adult dose (I) No max	q24h
Amphotericin B, liposomal, AmBisome	50-mg vial ($$$$)	IV	5 mg/kg pediatric and adult dose (I) No max	q24h
Ampicillin sodium[a]	125-, 250-, 500-mg vial ($) 1-, 2-, 10-g vial ($)	IV, IM	50–200 mg/kg/day, max 8 g/day (I) 300–400 mg/kg/day, max 12 g/day endocarditis/meningitis (III)	q6h q4–6h

Ampicillin trihydrate[a]	500-mg cap ($)	PO	50–100 mg/kg/day if <20 kg (I) ≥20 kg and adults 1–2 g/day (I)	q6h
Ampicillin/sulbactam,[a] Unasyn	1/0.5-, 2/1-, 10/5-g vial ($$)	IV, IM	200-mg ampicillin component/kg/day (I) ≥40 kg and adults 4–max 8 g/day (I)	q6h
Anidulafungin, Eraxis	50-, 100-mg vial ($$)	IV	1.5–3 mg/kg LD, then 0.75–1.5 mg/kg (II) Max 200-mg LD, then 100 mg (I)	q24h
Artemether and lumefantrine, Coartem	20/120-mg tab ($-$$)	PO	5–<15 kg: 1 tab/dose (I) ≥15–<25 kg: 2 tabs/dose (I) ≥25–<35 kg: 3 tabs/dose (I) ≥35 kg: 4 tabs/dose (I)	6 doses over 3 days at 0, 8, 24, 36, 48, 60 h
Atovaquone,[a] Mepron	750-mg/5-mL susp ($$-$$$)	PO	30 mg/kg/day if 1–3 mo or >24 mo (I) 45 mg/kg/day if >3–24 mo (I) Max 1,500 mg/day (I)	q12h q24h for prophylaxis
Atovaquone and proguanil,[a] Malarone	62.5/25-mg pediatric tab ($-$$) 250/100-mg adult tab ($-$$)	PO	Prophylaxis for malaria: 11–20 kg: 1 pediatric tab, 21–30 kg: 2 pediatric tabs, 31–40 kg: 3 pediatric tabs, >40 kg: 1 adult tab (I) Treatment: 5–8 kg: 2 pediatric tabs, 9–10 kg: 3 pediatric tabs, 11–20 kg: 1 adult tab, 21–30 kg: 2 adult tabs, 31–40 kg: 3 adult tabs, >40 kg: 4 adult tabs (I)	q24h

A. SYSTEMIC ANTIMICROBIALS WITH DOSAGE FORMS AND USUAL DOSAGES (continued)

Generic and Trade Names	Dosage Form (cost estimate)	Route	Dose (evidence level)	Interval
Azithromycin,[a] Zithromax	250-, 500-, 600-mg tab ($) 100-, 200-mg/5-mL susp ($) 1-g packet for susp ($)	PO	Otitis: 10 mg/kg/day for 1 day, then 5 mg/kg for 4 days; or 10 mg/kg/day for 3 days; or 30 mg/kg once (I). Pharyngitis: 12 mg/kg/day for 5 days, max 2,500-mg total dose (I). Sinusitis: 10 mg/kg/day for 3 days, max 1.5-g total dose (I). CABP: 10 mg/kg for 1 day, then 5 mg/kg/day for 4 days (max 1.5-g total dose), or 60 mg/kg once of ER (Zmax) susp, max 2 g (I). MAC prophylaxis: 5 mg/kg/day, max 250 mg (I), or 20 mg/kg, max 1.2 g weekly. Adult dosing for RTI: 500 mg day 1, then 250 mg daily for 4 days or 500 mg for 3 days. Adult dosing for STI: non-gonorrhea: 1 g once. Gonorrhea: 2 g once. See other indications in chapters 6 and 10.	q24h
	500-mg vial ($)	IV	10 mg/kg, max 500 mg (II)	q24h
Aztreonam,[a] Azactam	1-, 2-g vial ($$-$$$)	IV, IM	90–120 mg/kg/day, max 8 g/day (I)	q6–8h
Baloxavir (Xofluza)	20-, 40-mg tab ($-$$)	PO	≥12 y (I): 40–<80 kg: 40 mg (not per kg), ≥80 kg: 80 mg (not per kg)	One time
Benznidazole	12.5-, 100-mg tab Only available at www.benznidazoletablets.com	PO	2–12 y: 5–8 mg/kg/day (I) See also Chapter 10, Trypanosomiasis.	q12h
Bezlotoxumab, Zinplava	1-g vial ($$$$)	IV	Adults: 10 mg/kg	One time
Capreomycin, Capastat	1-g vial ($$$$)	IV, IM	15–30 mg/kg (III), max 1 g (I)	q24h

Caspofungin,[a] Cancidas	50-, 70-mg vial ($$$)	IV	Load with 70 mg/m² once, then 50 mg/m², max 70 mg (I)	q24h
Cefaclor,[a] Ceclor	250-, 500-mg cap ($) 500-mg ER tab ($$)	PO	20–40 mg/kg/day, max 1 g/day (I)	q12h
Cefadroxil,[a] Duricef	250-, 500-mg/5-mL susp ($) 500-mg cap ($) 1-g tab ($)	PO	30 mg/kg/day, max 2 g/day (I)	q12–24h
Cefazolin,[a] Ancef	0.5-, 1-, 10-g vial ($)	IV, IM	25–100 mg/kg/day (I)	q8h
			100–150 mg/kg/day for serious infections (III), max 12 g/day	q6h
Cefdinir,[a] Omnicef	125-, 250-mg/5-mL susp ($) 300-mg cap ($)	PO	14 mg/kg/day, max 600 mg/day (I)	q12–24h
Cefepime,[a] Maxipime	1-, 2-g vial ($)	IV, IM	100 mg/kg/day, max 4 g/day (I)	q12h
			150 mg/kg/day empiric therapy of fever with neutropenia, max 6 g/day (I)	q8h
Cefixime, Suprax	100-, 200-mg/5-mL susp[a] ($$) 100-, 200-mg chew tab ($$) 400-mg cap ($$)	PO	8 mg/kg/day, max 400 mg/day (I)	q24h
			For convalescent oral therapy of serious infections, up to 20 mg/kg/day (III)	q12h
Cefotaxime,[a] Claforan	0.5-, 1-, 2-, 10-g vial ($) Not being manufactured in the United States (verified June 25, 2019)	IV, IM	150–180 mg/kg/day, max 8 g/day (I)	q8h
			200–225 mg/kg/day for meningitis, max 12 g/day (I)	q6h
Cefotetan,[a] Cefotan	1-, 2-g vial ($-$$) 1-, 2-g IVPB ($-$$)	IV, IM	60–100 mg/kg/day (II), max 6 g/day (I)	q12h
Cefoxitin,[a] Mefoxin	1-, 2-, 10-g vial ($)	IV, IM	80–160 mg/kg/day, max 12 g/day (I)	q6–8h

A. SYSTEMIC ANTIMICROBIALS WITH DOSAGE FORMS AND USUAL DOSAGES (continued)

Generic and Trade Names	Dosage Form (cost estimate)	Route	Dose (evidence level)	Interval
Cefpodoxime,[a] Vantin	100-mg/5-mL susp ($) 100-, 200-mg tab ($)	PO	10 mg/kg/day, max 400 mg/day (I)	q12h
Cefprozil,[a] Cefzil	125-, 250-mg/5-mL susp ($) 250-, 500-mg tab ($)	PO	15–30 mg/kg/day, max 1 g/d (I)	q12h
Ceftaroline, Teflaro	400-, 600-mg vial ($$$$)	IV	≥2 mo–<2 y: 24 mg/kg/day (I) ≥2 y: 36 mg/kg/day (I) >33 kg: 1.2 g/day (I) Adults: 1.2 g/day (I) 45–60 mg/kg/day, max 3 g/day ± prolonged infusion for CF (II)	q8h q8–12h q12h q8h
Ceftazidime,[a] Tazicef, Fortaz	0.5-, 1-, 2-, 6-g vial ($) 1-, 2-g IVPB ($$)	IV, IM	90–150 mg/kg/day, max 6 g/day (I)	q8h
		IV	200–300 mg/kg/day for serious *Pseudomonas* infection, max 12 g/day (II)	q8h
Ceftazidime/avibactam, Avycaz	2-g/0.5-g vial ($$$$)	IV	3–5 mo: 120 mg ceftazidime/kg/day (I) ≥6 mo: 150 mg ceftazidime/kg/day, max 6 g (not per kg)/day (I)	q8h infused over 2 h
Ceftolozane/tazobactam, Zerbaxa	1.5-g (1-g/0.5-g) vial ($$$$)	IV	Adults 4.5 g (3 g/1.5 g)/day (I) Investigational in children	q8h
Ceftriaxone,[a] Rocephin	0.25-, 0.5-, 1-, 2-, 10-g vial ($)	IV, IM	50–75 mg/kg/day, max 2 g/day (I) Meningitis: 100 mg/kg/day, max 4 g/day (I) 50 mg/kg, max 1 g, 1–3 doses q24h for AOM (II)	q24h q12h
Cefuroxime,[a] Ceftin	250-, 500-mg tab ($)	PO	20–30 mg/kg/day, max 1 g/day (I) For bone and joint infections, up to 100 mg/kg/day, max 3 g/day (III)	q12h q8h
Cefuroxime,[a] Zinacef	0.75-, 1.5-g vial ($)	IV, IM	100–150 mg/kg/day, max 6 g/day (I)	q8h

Cephalexin,[a] Keflex	125-, 250-mg/5-mL susp ($) 250-, 500-mg cap, tab ($) 750-mg cap ($$)	PO	25–50 mg/kg/day (I)	q12h
			75–100 mg/kg/day for bone and joint, or severe infections (II), max 4 g/day (I)	q6–8h
Chloroquine phosphate,[a] Aralen	250-, 500-mg (150-, 300-mg base) tabs ($-$$)	PO	See Chapter 10, Malaria.	
Cidofovir,[a] Vistide	375-mg vial ($$$)	IV	5 mg/kg (III); see Chapter 9, Adenovirus.	Weekly
Ciprofloxacin,[a] Cipro	250-, 500-mg/5-mL susp ($-$$) 250-, 500-, 750-mg tab ($)	PO	20–40 mg/kg/day, max 1.5 g/day (I) Do not administer susp via feeding tubes.	q12h
	100-mg tab ($)	PO	Adult women with uncomplicated acute cystitis: 200 mg/day for 3 days (I)	
	200-, 400-mg IVPB ($)	IV	20–30 mg/kg/day, max 1.2 g/day (I)	q12h
Clarithromycin,[a] Biaxin	125-, 250-mg/5-mL susp ($) 250-, 500-mg tab ($)	PO	15 mg/kg/day, max 1 g/day (I)	q12h
Clarithromycin extended release,[a] Biaxin XL	500-mg ER tab ($)	PO	Adults 1 g (I)	q24h
Clindamycin,[a] Cleocin	75 mg/5-mL soln ($) 75-, 150-, 300-mg cap ($)	PO	10–25 mg/kg/day, max 1.8 g/day (I) 30–40 mg/kg/day for CA-MRSA, intra-abdominal infection, or AOM (III)	q8h
	0.3-, 0.6-, 0.9-, 9-g vial ($) 0.3-, 0.6-, 0.9-g IVPB ($)	IV, IM	20–40 mg/kg/day, max 2.7 g/day (I)	q8h
Clotrimazole,[a] Mycelex	10-mg lozenge ($)	PO	≥3 y: dissolve lozenge in mouth (I).	5 times daily
Colistimethate,[a] Coly-Mycin M	150-mg (colistin base) vial ($-$$) 1-mg base = 2.7-mg colistimethate	IV, IM	2.5- to 5-mg base/kg/day based on IBW (I) Up to 5- to 7-mg base/kg/day (III)	q8h
Cycloserine, Seromycin	250-mg cap ($$$$)	PO	10–20 mg/kg/day (III) Adults max 1 g/day (I)	q12h

A. SYSTEMIC ANTIMICROBIALS WITH DOSAGE FORMS AND USUAL DOSAGES (continued)

Generic and Trade Names	Dosage Form (cost estimate)	Route	Dose (evidence level)	Interval
Daclatasvir, Daklinza	30-, 60-, 90-mg tab ($$$$$)	PO	Adults: 30–90 mg + sofosbuvir ± ritonavir (I). See Chapter 9, Hepatitis C virus.	q24h
Dalbavancin, Dalvance	500-mg vial ($$$$)	IV	Adults 1,500 mg (I) 6–<18 y: 18 mg/kg (max 1,500 mg) (II) 3 mo–< 6 y: 22.5 mg/kg (II)	One time
Dapsone[a]	25-, 100-mg tab ($)	PO	2 mg/kg, max 100 mg (I)	q24h
			4 mg/kg, max 200 mg (I)	Once weekly
Daptomycin,[a] Cubicin	350-, 500-mg vial ($$-$$$)	IV	For SSSI (I): 1–2 y: 10 mg/kg, 2–6 y: 9 mg/kg, 7–11 y: 7 mg/kg,12–17 y: 5 mg/kg. For *Staphylococcus aureus* bacteremia (I):1–6 y: 12 mg/kg, 7–11 y: 9 mg/kg, 12–17 y: 7 mg/kg. For other indications, see Chapter 6. Adults: 4–6 mg/kg TBW (I).	q24h
Dasabuvir + ombitasvir/paritaprevir/ritonavir, Viekira PAK	250-mg tab + 12.5-/75-/50-mg tab ($$$$$)	PO	Adults: 1 dasabuvir tab q12h + 2 combo tabs every morning ± ribavirin (I). See Chapter 9, Hepatitis C virus.	
Delafloxacin, Baxdela	450-mg tab ($$$$)	PO	Adults 450 mg (I)	q12h
	300-mg vial ($$$$)	IV	Adults 300 mg (I)	
Demeclocycline,[a] Declomycin	150-, 300-mg tab ($-$$)	PO	≥8 y: 7–13 mg/kg/day, max 600 mg/day (I). Dosage differs for SIADH.	q6–12h
Dicloxacillin,[a] Dynapen	250-, 500-mg cap ($)	PO	12–25 mg/kg/day (adults 0.5–1 g/day) (I) For bone and joint infections, up to 100 mg/kg/day, max 2 g/day (III)	q6h

Doxycycline, Vibramycin	25-mg/5-mL susp[a] ($) 50-mg/5-mL syrup ($$) 20-, 40-, 50-, 75-, 100-, 150-mg tab/cap[a] ($-$$) 200-mg tab[a] ($$$)	PO	≥8 y: 4.4 mg/kg/day LD on day 1, then 2.2–4.4 mg/kg/day, max 200 mg/day (I)	q12–24h
	100-mg vial[a] ($$)	IV		
LymePak (not yet commercially available as of November 2019)[c]	100-mg tab	PO	≥8 y and ≥45 kg: 100 mg (not per kg)	q12h
Elbasvir/Grazoprevir, Zepatier	50-mg/100-mg tab ($$$$)	PO	Adults 1 tab	q24h
Entecavir, Baraclude See Chapter 9, Hepatitis B virus.	0.05-mg/mL soln ($$$) 0.5-, 1-mg tab[a] ($$)	PO	2–<16 y (I) (Double the following doses if previous lamivudine exposure.): 10–11 kg: 0.15 mg >11–14 kg: 0.2 mg >14–17 kg: 0.25 mg >17–20 kg: 0.3 mg >20–23 kg: 0.35 mg >23–26 kg: 0.4 mg >26–30 kg: 0.45 mg >30 kg: 0.5 mg ≥16 y: 0.5 mg (I)	q24h
Eravacycline, Xerava	50-mg vial ($$$)	IV	≥18 y: 1 mg/kg	q12h
Ertapenem,[a] Invanz	1-g vial ($$-$$$)	IV, IM	30 mg/kg/day, max 1 g/day (I) ≥13 y and adults: 1 g/day (I)	q12h q24h
Erythromycin base	250-, 500-mg tab[a] ($$) 250-mg EC cap[a] ($) 250-, 333-, 500-mg DR tab (Ery-Tab) ($$)	PO	50 mg/kg/day, max 4 g/day (I). Dose differs for GI prokinesis.	q6–8h

A. SYSTEMIC ANTIMICROBIALS WITH DOSAGE FORMS AND USUAL DOSAGES (continued)

Generic and Trade Names	Dosage Form (cost estimate)	Route	Dose (evidence level)	Interval
Erythromycin ethylsuccinate,[a] EES, EryPed	200-, 400-mg/5-mL susp ($$-$$$) 400-mg tab ($$$)	PO	50 mg/kg/day, max 4 g/day (I). Dose differs for GI prokinesis.	q6–8h
Erythromycin lactobionate, Erythrocin	0.5-g vial ($$$)	IV	20 mg/kg/day, max 4 g/day (I)	q6h
Erythromycin stearate	250-mg tab ($$-$$$)	PO	50 mg/kg/day, max 4 g/day (I)	q6–8h
Ethambutol,[a] Myambutol	100-, 400-mg tab ($)	PO	15–25 mg/kg, max 2.5 g (I)	q24h
Ethionamide, Trecator	250-mg tab ($$)	PO	15–20 mg/kg/day, max 1 g/day (I)	q12–24h
Famciclovir,[a] Famvir	125-, 250-, 500-mg tab ($)	PO	Adults 0.5–2 g/day (I)	q8–12h
Fidaxomicin, Dificid	200-mg tab ($$$$)	PO	≥6 y: 400 mg (not per kg)/day (II) Adults ≥18 y: 400 mg/day (I)	q12h
Fluconazole,[a] Diflucan	50-, 100-, 150-, 200-mg tab ($) 50-, 200-mg/5-mL susp ($)	PO	6–12 mg/kg, max 800 mg (I). 800–1,000 mg/day may be used for some CNS fungal infections. See Chapter 8.	q24h
	200-, 400-mg IVPB ($)	IV		
Flucytosine,[a] Ancobon	250-, 500-mg cap ($$$$)	PO	100 mg/kg/day (I)[b]	q6h
Foscarnet, Foscavir	6-g vial ($$$$)	IV	CMV/VZV: 180 mg/kg/day (I)	q8–12h
			CMV suppression: 90–120 mg/kg (I)	q24h
			HSV: 120 mg/kg/day (I)	q8–12h
Fosfomycin, Monurol	3-g oral granules ($)	PO	Adult women with uncomplicated acute cystitis: 3 g	Once
Fosfomycin, Contepo	6-g vial (not yet commercially available as of November 2019)	IV	Adults: 18 g/day Investigational in children	q8h

Ganciclovir,[a] Cytovene	500-mg vial ($$)	IV	CMV treatment: 10 mg/kg/day (I)	q12h
			CMV suppression: 5 mg/kg (I)	q24h
			VZV: 10 mg/kg/day (III)	q12h
Gentamicin[a]	10-mg/mL vial ($) 40-mg/mL vial ($)	IV, IM	3–7.5 mg/kg/day (I), CF and oncology 7–10 mg/kg/day (II).[b] See Chapter 1 for q24h dosing.	q8–24h
		IVesic	0.5 mg/mL in NS x 50–100 mL (III)	q12h
Glecaprevir/Pibrentasvir, Mavyret	100-mg/40-mg tab ($$$$$)	PO	Adults 300 mg/120 mg (I)	q24h
Griseofulvin microsize,[a] Grifulvin V	125-mg/5-mL susp ($) 500-mg tab ($$)	PO	20–25 mg/kg (II), max 1 g (I)	q24h
Griseofulvin ultramicrosize,[a] Gris-PEG	125-, 250-mg tab ($)	PO	10–15 mg/kg (II), max 750 mg (I)	q24h
Imipenem/cilastatin,[a] Primaxin	250/250-, 500/500-mg vial ($$)	IV, IM	60–100 mg/kg/day, max 4 g/day (I) IM form not approved for <12 y	q6h
Interferon-PEG Alfa-2a, Pegasys Alfa-2b, PegIntron	All ($$$$) 180-mcg vials, prefilled syringes 50-mcg vial	SQ	See Chapter 9, Hepatitis B virus and Hepatitis C virus.	Weekly
Isavuconazonium (isavuconazole), Cresemba	186-mg cap (100-mg base) ($$$$)	PO	Adults 200 mg base per *dose* PO/IV (base = isavuconazole)	q8h x 6 doses, then q24h
	372-mg vial (200-mg base) ($$$$)	IV		

A. SYSTEMIC ANTIMICROBIALS WITH DOSAGE FORMS AND USUAL DOSAGES (continued)

Generic and Trade Names	Dosage Form (cost estimate)	Route	Dose (evidence level)	Interval
Isoniazid,[a] Nydrazid	50-mg/5-mL soln ($$) 100-, 300-mg tab ($) 1,000-mg vial ($$)	PO IV, IM	10–15 mg/kg/day, max 300 mg/day (I)	q12–24h
			With directly observed biweekly therapy, dosage is 20–30 mg/kg, max 900 mg/dose (I).	Twice weekly
			In combination with rifapentine (see Rifapentine, Priftin): >12 y: 15 mg/kg rounded up to the nearest 50 or 100 mg; 900 mg max 2–<12 y: 25 mg/kg; 900 mg max	Once weekly
Itraconazole, Sporanox	50-mg/5-mL soln ($$) (Preferred over capsules; see Chapter 8.) 100-mg cap[a] ($)	PO	10 mg/kg/day (II), max 200 mg/day	q12h
			5 mg/kg/day for chronic mucocutaneous *Candida* (II)	q24h
Ivermectin,[a] Stromectol	3-mg tab ($)	PO	0.15-0.2 mg/kg, no max (I)	1 dose
Ketoconazole,[a] Nizoral	200-mg tab ($)	PO	≥2 y: 3.3–6.6 mg/kg, max 400 mg (I)	q24h
Letermovir, Prevymis	240-, 480-mg tab ($$$$)	PO	Adults 480 mg (I), 240 mg if concomitant cyclosporine therapy (I). See Chapter 9, Cytomegalovirus.	q24h
	240-, 480-mg vial ($$$$)	IV		
Levofloxacin,[a] Levaquin	125-mg/5-mL soln ($) 250-, 500-, 750-mg tab ($) 500-, 750-mg vial ($) 250-, 500-, 750-mg IVPB ($)	PO, IV	For postexposure anthrax prophylaxis (I): <50 kg: 16 mg/kg/day, max 500 mg/day ≥50 kg: 500 mg For respiratory infections: <5 y: 20 mg/kg/day (II) ≥5 y: 10 mg/kg/day, max 500 mg/day (II)	 q12h q24h q12h q24h
Linezolid,[a] Zyvox	100-mg/5-mL susp ($$$) 600-mg tab ($) 200-, 600-mg IVPB ($$)	PO, IV	Pneumonia, complicated SSSI (I): Birth–11 y: 30 mg/kg/day >11 y: 1.2 g/day	 q8h q12h

			Uncomplicated SSSI (I): Birth–<5 y: 30 mg/kg/day 5–11 y: 20 mg/kg/day >11–18 y: 1.2 g/day	 q8h q12h q12h
Mebendazole, Emverm	100-mg chew tab ($$$$)	PO	≥2y: 100 mg (not per kg) (I) See Chapter 10, Hookworm, Pinworms, Roundworm, Whipworm (Trichuriasis), and other indications.	See Chapter 10.
Mefloquine,[a] Lariam	250-mg tab ($)	PO	See Chapter 10, Malaria.	
Meropenem,[a] Merrem	0.5-, 1-g vial ($)	IV	60 mg/kg/day, max 3 g/day (I) 120 mg/kg/day meningitis, max 6 g/day (I)	q8h q8h
Meropenem/Vaborbactam, Vabomere	2-g vial (contains 1-g each meropenem + vaborbactam) ($$$$)	IV	Adults 6 g meropenem/day (I) Investigational in children	q8h
Methenamine hippurate,[a] Hiprex	1-g tab ($)	PO	6–12 y: 1–2 g/day (I) >12 y: 2 g/day (I)	q12h
Methenamine mandelate[a]	0.5-, 1-g tab ($)		<6 y: 75 mg/kg/day (I) 6–12 y: 2 g/day (I) >12 y: 4 g/day (I)	q6h
Metronidazole,[a] Flagyl	250-, 500-mg tab ($) 250-, 500-mg/5-mL susp ($) 375-mg cap ($$)	PO	30–50 mg/kg/day, max 2,250 mg/day (I)	q8h
	500-mg IVPB ($)	IV	22.5–40 mg/kg/day (II), max 4 g/day (I)	q6–8h
Micafungin,[a] Mycamine	50-, 100-mg vial ($$$)	IV	2–4 mg/kg, max 150 mg (I)	q24h

A. SYSTEMIC ANTIMICROBIALS WITH DOSAGE FORMS AND USUAL DOSAGES (continued)

Generic and Trade Names	Dosage Form (cost estimate)	Route	Dose (evidence level)	Interval
Miltefosine, Impavido	50-mg cap Only available at www.impavido.com	PO	<12 y: 2.5 mg/kg/day (II) ≥12 y (I): 30–44 kg: 50 mg (not per kg) ≥45 kg: 50 mg (not per kg) See Chapter 10, Leishmaniasis, Amebic meningoencephalitis.	bid bid tid
Minocycline, Minocin	50-, 75-, 100-mg cap[a] ($) 50-, 75-, 100-mg tab[a] ($) 100-mg vial ($$$$)	PO, IV	≥8 y: 4 mg/kg/day, max 200 mg/day (I)	q12h
Minocycline ER, Solodyn,[a] Ximino[a]	55-, 65-, 80-, 105-, 115-mg ER tab[a] ($$) 45-, 90-, 135-mg ER cap ($$$)	PO	≥12 y: 1 mg/kg/day for acne (I). Round dose to nearest strength tab or cap.	q24h
Moxidectin[b]	2-mg tab	PO	≥12 y: 8 mg (I)	Once
Moxifloxacin,[a] Avelox	400-mg tab ($) 400-mg IVPB ($$)	PO, IV	Adults 400 mg/day (I)	q24h
			Studied but not FDA approved in children (II) IV: 3 mo–<2 y: 12 mg/kg/day 2–<6 y: 10 mg/kg/day ≥6–<12 y: 8 mg/kg/day (max 400 mg/day) ≥12–<18 y (weight <45 kg): 8 mg/kg/day	q12h
			≥12–<18 y (weight >45 kg): 400 mg	q24h
Nafcillin,[a] Nallpen	1-, 2-, 10-g vial ($$)	IV, IM	150–200 mg/kg/day (II) Max 12 g/day div q4h (I)	q6h
Neomycin sulfate[a]	500-mg tab ($)	PO	50–100 mg/kg/day (II), max 12 g/day (I)	q6–8h

Nitazoxanide, Alinia	100-mg/5-mL susp ($$$) 500-mg tab ($$$)	PO	1–3 y: 200 mg/day (I) 4–11 y: 400 mg/day (I) ≥12 y: 1 g/day (I)	q12h
Nitrofurantoin,[a] Furadantin	25-mg/5-mL susp ($$$)	PO	5–7 mg/kg/day, max 400 mg/day (I)	q6h
			1–2 mg/kg for UTI prophylaxis (I)	q24h
Nitrofurantoin macrocrystals,[a] Macrodantin	25-, 50-, 100-mg cap ($)	PO	Same as susp	
Nitrofurantoin monohydrate and macrocrystalline,[a] Macrobid	100-mg cap ($)	PO	>12 y: 200 mg/day (I)	q12h
Nystatin,[a] Mycostatin	500,000-U/5-mL susp ($) 500,000-U tabs ($)	PO	Infants 2 mL/dose, children 4–6 mL/dose, to coat oral mucosa Tabs: 3–6 tabs/day	q6h
Obiltoxaximab, Anthim	600-mg/6-mL vial Available from the Strategic National Stockpile	IV	≤15 kg: 32 mg/kg (I) >15–40 kg: 24 mg/kg (I) >40 kg and adults: 16 mg/kg (I)	Once
Omadacycline, Nuzyra	150-mg tab ($$$$)	PO	Adults: 450 mg qd for 2 days, then 300 mg (not per kg)	q24h
	100-mg vial ($$$$)	IV	Adults: 200 mg once, then 100 mg (not per kg)	
Oritavancin, Orbactiv	400-mg vial ($$$)	IV	Adults 1.2 g/day (I) Investigational in children	One time

A. SYSTEMIC ANTIMICROBIALS WITH DOSAGE FORMS AND USUAL DOSAGES (continued)

Generic and Trade Names	Dosage Form (cost estimate)	Route	Dose (evidence level)	Interval
Oseltamivir,[a] Tamiflu (See chapters 5 and 9, Influenza.)	30-mg/5-mL susp ($) 30-, 45-, 75-mg cap[a] ($)	PO	Preterm <38 wk PMA (II): 2 mg/kg/day Preterm 38–40 wk PMA (II): 3 mg/kg/day Preterm >40 wk PMA (II), and term, birth–8 mo (I): 6 mg/kg/day 9–11 mo (II): 7 mg/kg/day ≥12 mo (I): (not per kg) ≤15 kg: 60 mg/day >15–23 kg: 90 mg/day >23–40 kg: 120 mg/day >40 kg: 150 mg/day	q12h
			Prophylaxis: Give half the daily dose q24h.	q24h
Oxacillin,[a] Bactocill	1-, 2-, 10-g vial ($$)	IV, IM	100 mg/kg/day, max 12 g/day (I) 150–200 mg/kg/day for meningitis (III)	q4–6h
Palivizumab, Synagis	50-, 100-mg vial ($$$$)	IM	15 mg/kg (I). See Chapter 9 for indications.	Monthly during RSV season, max 5 doses
Paromomycin,[a] Humatin	250-mg cap ($)	PO	25–35 mg/kg/day, max 4 g/day (I)	q8h
Penicillin G intramuscular				
– Penicillin G benzathine, Bicillin L-A	600,000 U/mL in 1-, 2-, 4-mL prefilled syringes ($-$$)	IM	Infants: 50,000 U/kg Children <60 lb: 300,000–600,000 U, ≥60 lb: 900,000 U (not per kg) (I) (FDA approved in 1952 for dosing by pounds) Adults 1.2–2.4 million U (I) See also chapters 5 and 6, Syphilis.	1 dose

– Penicillin G procaine	600,000 U/mL in 1-, 2-mL prefilled syringes ($$)	IM	Infants: 50,000 U/kg See also Chapter 5, Syphilis. Children (I): <60 lb: 300,000 U (not per kg) ≥60 lb or >12 y: 600,000 U Adults 600,000–1,200,000 U (I).	q24h
Penicillin G intravenous				
– Penicillin G K,[a] Pfizerpen	5-, 20-million U vial ($)	IV, IM	100,000–300,000 U/kg/day (I). Max daily dose is 24 million U.	q4–6h
– Penicillin G sodium[a]	5-million U vial ($-$$)	IV, IM	100,000–300,000 U/kg/day (I). Max daily dose is 24 million U.	q4–6h
Penicillin V oral				
– Penicillin V K[a]	125-, 250-mg/5-mL soln ($) 250-, 500-mg tab ($)	PO	25–50 mg/kg/day, max 2 g/day (I)	q6h
Pentamidine, Pentam, Nebupent	300-mg vial ($$$)	IV, IM	4 mg/kg/day (I), max 300 mg	q24h
	300-mg vial ($$)	Inhaled	300 mg for prophylaxis (I)	Monthly
Peramivir, Rapivab	200-mg vial ($$-$$$)	IV	12 mg/kg, max 600 mg (I)	One time
Piperacillin/tazobactam,[a] Zosyn	2/0.25-, 3/0.375-, 4/0.5-, 12/1.5-, 36/4.5-g vial ($)	IV	<40 kg: 240–300 mg PIP/kg/day, max 16 g PIP/day (I) Adults 8–12 g/day	q8h
Plazomicin, Zemdri	500-mg vial ($$$$)	IV	Adults 15 mg/kg (I)	q24h
Polymyxin B[a]	500,000 U vial ($) 1 mg = 10,000 U	IV	2.5 mg/kg/day (I) Adults 2 mg/kg LD, then 2.5–3 mg/kg/day, dose based on TBW, no max (II)	q12h

A. SYSTEMIC ANTIMICROBIALS WITH DOSAGE FORMS AND USUAL DOSAGES (continued)

Generic and Trade Names	Dosage Form (cost estimate)	Route	Dose (evidence level)	Interval
Posaconazole, Noxafil	200-mg/5-mL susp ($$$$)	PO	<13 y: under investigation, 18 mg/kg/day with serum trough monitoring. See Chapter 8.	q8h
			≥13 y and adults (I):	
			Candida or *Aspergillus* prophylaxis: 600 mg/day	q8h
			OPC treatment: 100 mg q12h for 1 day, then 100 mg/day	q24h
			Refractory OPC: 800 mg/day	q12h
	100-mg DR tab ($$$-$$$$)	PO	≥13 y and adults (I): *Candida* or *Aspergillus* prophylaxis: 300 mg (not per kg) q12h for 1 day, then 300 mg per day	q24h
	300-mg/16.7-mL vial ($$$$)	IV		
Praziquantel,[a] Biltricide	600-mg tab ($-$$)	PO	20–25 mg/kg/dose, no max (I) Round dose to nearest 200 mg (1/3 tab)	q4–6h for 3 doses
Primaquine phosphate[a]	15-mg base tab ($) (26.3-mg primaquine phosphate)	PO	0.5 mg base/kg, max 30 mg (III) See Chapter 10, Malaria.	q24h
Pyrantel pamoate[a]	250-mg base/5-mL susp ($) (720-mg pyrantel pamoate/5-mL)	PO	11 mg (base)/kg, max 1 g (I)	Once
Pyrazinamide[a]	500-mg tab ($)	PO	30 mg/kg/day, max 2 g/day (I)	q24h
			Directly observed biweekly therapy, 50 mg/kg (I), no max.	Twice weekly
Quinupristin/dalfopristin, Synercid	150/350-mg vial (500-mg total) ($$$$)	IV	22.5 mg/kg/day (II) Adults 15–22.5 mg/kg/day, no max (I)	q8h q8–12h

Raxibacumab	1,700-mg/35-mL vial Available from the Strategic National Stockpile for a bioterrorism event	IV	≤15 kg: 80 mg/kg (I) >15–50 kg: 60 mg/kg (I) >50 kg: 40 mg/kg (I)	Once
Ribavirin, Rebetol, Ribasphere	200-mg/5-mL soln ($$) 200-mg cap/tab[a] ($) 400-, 600-mg tab ($$$$) 600-, 800-, 1,000-, 1,200-mg dose paks ($$$$)	PO	15 mg/kg/day (I). 12–17 y (I): 40–49 kg: 600 mg/day 50–65 kg: 800 mg/day 66–80 kg: 1,000 mg/day 81–105 kg: 1,200 mg/day >105 kg: 1,400 mg/day Given as combination therapy with other agents; see Chapter 9, Hepatitis C virus.	q12h
Ribavirin,[a] Virazole	6-g vial ($$$$$)	Inhaled	1 vial by SPAG-2; see Chapter 9, Respiratory syncytial virus.	q24h
Rifabutin,[a] Mycobutin	150-mg cap ($$$)	PO	5 mg/kg for MAC prophylaxis (II) 10–20 mg/kg for MAC or TB treatment (I) Max 300 mg/day	q24h
Rifampin,[a] Rifadin	150-, 300-mg cap ($) 600-mg vial ($$-$$$)	PO, IV	10–20 mg/kg, max 600 mg for active TB (in combination) (I) or as single drug therapy for latent TB (4 mo).	q24h
			With directly observed biweekly therapy, dosage is still 10–20 mg/kg/dose (max 600 mg).	Twice weekly
			20 mg/kg/day for 2 days for meningococcus prophylaxis, max 1.2 g/day (I)	q12h
Rifampin/isoniazid/ pyrazinamide, Rifater	120-/50-/300-mg tab ($$)	PO	≥15 y and adults (I): ≤44 kg: 4 tab 45–54 kg: 5 tab ≥55 kg: 6 tab	q24h

A. SYSTEMIC ANTIMICROBIALS WITH DOSAGE FORMS AND USUAL DOSAGES (continued)

Generic and Trade Names	Dosage Form (cost estimate)	Route	Dose (evidence level)	Interval
Rifamycin, Aemcolo	194-mg tab ($$)	PO	Adults: 2 tabs for traveler's diarrhea	q12h for 3 days
Rifapentine, Priftin	150-mg tab ($)	PO	≥12 y and adults: 600 mg/dose (I)	Twice weekly
			>2 y, with INH (see Isoniazid), for treatment of latent TB: 10–14 kg: 300 mg 14.1–25 kg: 450 mg 25.1–32 kg: 600 mg 32.1–50 kg: 750 mg >50 kg: 900 mg max	Once weekly
Rifaximin, Xifaxan	200-mg tab ($$$)	PO	≥12 y and adults: 600 mg/day (I) 20–30 mg/kg/day, max 1.6 g/day (III)	q8h
Sarecycline, Seysara	60-, 100-, 150 mg tabs ($$$)	PO	For acne ≥9 y: 60 mg (not per kg) 55–84 kg: 100 mg >84 kg: 150 mg	q24h
Secnidazole, Solosec	2-g granules ($$)	PO	Adults 2 g (I)	Once
Sofosbuvir, Sovaldi	400-mg tab ($$$$$)	PO	≥12 y and adults: 400 mg (I). See Chapter 9, Hepatitis C virus.	q24h
Sofosbuvir/Ledipasvir,[a] Harvoni	400-/90-mg tab ($$$$$)	PO	≥12 y and adults: 1 tab (I). See Chapter 9, Hepatitis C virus.	q24h
Sofosbuvir/Velpatasvir,[a] Epclusa	400-/100-mg tab ($$$$)	PO	Adults 1 tab (I). See Chapter 9, Hepatitis C virus.	q24h
Sofosbuvir/Velpatasvir/Voxilaprevir, Vosevi	400-/100-/100-mg tab ($$$$$)	PO	Adults 1 tab (I). See Chapter 9, Hepatitis C virus.	q24h

Streptomycin[a]	1-g vial ($$)	IM, IV	20–40 mg/kg/day, max 1 g/day[b] (I)	q12–24h
Sulfadiazine[a]	500-mg tab ($$)	PO	120–150 mg/kg/day, max 4–6 g/day (I). See Chapter 10.	q6h
			Rheumatic fever secondary prophylaxis 500 mg qd if ≤27 kg, 1,000 mg qd if >27 kg (II)	q24h
Tecovirimat, Tpoxx	200-mg cap Available from the Strategic National Stockpile for a bioterrorism event	PO	13–<25 kg: 1 cap (I) 25–<40 kg: 2 caps (I) ≥40 kg: 3 caps (I)	q12h
Tedizolid, Sivextro	200-mg tab ($$$$) 200-mg vial ($$$$)	PO, IV	Adults 200 mg (I) 12–17 y: 200 mg (II) Investigational in younger children	q24h
Telavancin, Vibativ	250-, 750-mg vial ($$$$)	IV	Adults 10 mg/kg (I)	q24h
Tenofovir, Viread	40 mg per scoop powder for mixing with soft food ($$$) 150-, 200-, 250-mg tabs ($$$$) 300-mg tabs[a] ($)	PO	≥2 y: 8 mg/kg (round to nearest 20 mg [½ scoop]) 17–<22 kg: 150 mg (not per kg) 22–<28 kg: 200 mg 28–<35 kg: 250 mg ≥35 kg: 300 mg See Chapter 9, Hepatitis B virus.	q24h
Terbinafine, Lamisil	250-mg tab[a] ($)	PO	Adults 250 mg (I)	q24h
Tetracycline[a]	250-, 500-mg cap ($)	PO	≥8 y: 25–50 mg/kg/day (I)	q6h
Tinidazole,[a] Tindamax	250-, 500-mg tab ($$)	PO	50 mg/kg, max 2 g (I). See Chapter 10.	q24h
Tobramycin,[a] Nebcin	10-mg/mL vial ($) 40-mg/mL vial ($)	IV, IM	3–7.5 mg/kg/day (CF 7–10)[b]; see Chapter 1 regarding q24h dosing.	q8–24h
Tobramycin inhalation, Tobi,[a] Bethkis	300-mg ampule ($$$$)	Inhaled	≥6 y: 600 mg/day (I)	q12h

A. SYSTEMIC ANTIMICROBIALS WITH DOSAGE FORMS AND USUAL DOSAGES (continued)

Generic and Trade Names	Dosage Form (cost estimate)	Route	Dose (evidence level)	Interval
Tobi Podhaler	28-mg cap for inhalation ($$$$$)	Inhaled	≥6 y: 224 mg/day via Podhaler device (I)	q12h
Triclabendazole, Egaten (not yet commercially available as of November 2019)[c]	250-mg scored tab	PO	≥6 y: 20 mg/kg/day, given as 2 doses in one day See Chapter 10, Flukes.	q12h
Trimethoprim/ sulfamethoxazole,[a] Bactrim, Septra	80-mg TMP/400-mg SMX tab (single strength) ($) 160-mg TMP/800-mg SMX tab (double strength) ($) 40-mg TMP/200-mg SMX per 5-mL oral susp ($) 16-mg TMP/80-mg SMX per mL injection soln in 5-, 10-, 30-mL vial ($$)	PO, IV	8–10 mg TMP/kg/day (I) Higher dosing for MIC 1 (II) 0–<6 y: 15 mg/kg/day 6–21 y: 12 mg/kg/day	q12h
			2 mg TMP/kg/day for UTI prophylaxis (I)	q24h
			15–20 mg TMP/kg/day for PJP treatment (I), no max	q6–8h
			150 mg TMP/m²/day, OR 5 mg TMP/kg/day for PJP prophylaxis (I), max 160 mg TMP/day	q12h 3 times a wk OR q24h
Valacyclovir,[a] Valtrex	500-mg, 1-g tab ($)	PO	VZV: ≥3 mo: 60 mg/kg/day (I, II) HSV: ≥3 mo: 40 mg/kg/day (II) Max single dose 1 g (I)	q8h q12h
Valganciclovir,[a] Valcyte	250-mg/5-mL soln ($$$) 450-mg tab ($$)	PO	Congenital CMV treatment: 32 mg/kg/day (II). See Chapter 5. CMV prophylaxis (in mg, not mg/kg): 7 mg × BSA (m²) x CrCl (mL/min/1.73 m² using the modified Schwartz formula), max 900 mg (I). See also Chapter 9.	q12h q24h

Vancomycin, Vancocin	125-, 250-mg/5-mL susp ($-$$) 125-, 250-mg cap[a] ($$)	PO	40 mg/kg/day (I), max 500 mg/day (III)	q6h
	0.5-, 0.75-, 1-, 5-, 10-g vial[a] ($)	IV	30–40 mg/kg/day[b] (I) For invasive MRSA infection, 60–70 mg/kg/day adjusted to achieve an AUC:MIC of >400 mg/L x h or trough ≥10 mg/L (II)	q6–8h
Voriconazole,[a,b] Vfend See Chapter 8, Aspergillosis.	200-mg/5-mL susp ($$$) 50-, 200-mg tab ($$)	PO	≥2 y and <50 kg: 18 mg/kg/day, max 700 mg/day (I) ≥50 kg: 400–600 mg/day (I)	q12h
	200-mg vial ($$)	IV	≥2 y and <50 kg: 18 mg/kg/day LD for 1 day, then 16 mg/kg/day (I) ≥50 kg: 12 mg/kg/day LD for 1 day, then 8 mg/kg/day (I)	q12h
Zanamivir, Relenza	5-mg blister cap for inhalation ($)	Inhaled	Prophylaxis: ≥5 y: 10 mg/day (I)	q24h
			Treatment: ≥7 y: 20 mg/day (I)	q12h

[a] Available in a generic formulation.

[b] Monitor serum concentrations.

B. TOPICAL ANTIMICROBIALS (SKIN, EYE, EAR, MUCOSA)

Generic and Trade Names	Dosage Form	Route	Dose	Interval
Acyclovir, Sitavig	50-mg tab	Buccal	Adults 50 mg, for herpes labialis	One time
Azithromycin, AzaSite	1% ophth soln	Ophth	1 drop	bid for 2 days then qd for 5 days
Bacitracin[a]	Ophth oint	Ophth	Apply to affected eye.	q3–4h
	Oint[b]	Top	Apply to affected area.	bid–qid
Benzyl alcohol, Ulesfia	5% lotion	Top	Apply to scalp and hair.	Once; repeat in 7 days.
Besifloxacin, Besivance	0.6% ophth susp	Ophth	≥1 y: 1 drop to affected eye	tid
Butenafine, Mentax, Lotrimin-Ultra	1% cream	Top	≥12 y: apply to affected area.	qd
Butoconazole, Gynazole-1	2% prefilled cream	Vag	Adults 1 applicatorful	One time
Ciclopirox,[a] Loprox, Penlac	0.77% cream, gel, lotion	Top	≥10 y: apply to affected area.	bid
	1% shampoo		≥16 y: apply to scalp.	Twice weekly
	8% nail lacquer		≥12 y: apply to infected nail.	qd
Ciprofloxacin,[a] Cetraxal	0.2% otic soln	Otic	≥1 y: apply 3 drops to affected ear.	bid for 7 days
Ciprofloxacin, Ciloxan	0.3% ophth soln[a]	Ophth	Apply to affected eye.	q2h for 2 days then q4h for 5 days
	0.3% ophth oint			q8h for 2 days then q12h for 5 days
Ciprofloxacin, Otiprio	6% otic susp	Otic	≥6 mo: 0.1 mL each ear intratympanic, 0.2 mL to external ear canal for otitis externa	One time

Ciprofloxacin + dexamethasone, Ciprodex	0.3% + 0.1% otic soln	Otic	≥6 mo: apply 4 drops to affected ear.	bid for 7 days
Ciprofloxacin + fluocinolone, Otovel	0.3% + 0.025% otic soln	Otic	≥6 mo: instill 0.25 mL to affected ear.	bid for 7 days
Ciprofloxacin + hydrocortisone, Cipro HC	0.2% + 1% otic soln	Otic	≥1 y: apply 3 drops to affected ear.	bid for 7 days
Clindamycin				
Cleocin	100-mg ovule	Vag	1 ovule	qhs for 3 days
	2% vaginal cream[a]		1 applicatorful	qhs for 3–7 days
Cleocin-T[a]	1% soln, gel, lotion	Top	Apply to affected area.	qd–bid
Clindesse	2% cream	Vag	Adolescents and adults 1 applicatorful	One time
Evoclin[a]	1% foam			qd
Clindamycin + benzoyl peroxide, BenzaClin	1% gel[a]	Top	≥12 y: apply to affected area.	bid
Acanya	1.2% gel	Top	Apply small amount to face.	q24h
Clindamycin + tretinoin, Ziana, Veltin	1.2% gel	Top	Apply small amount to face.	hs
Clotrimazole,[a,b] Lotrimin	1% cream, lotion, soln	Top	Apply to affected area.	bid
Gyne-Lotrimin-3[a,b]	2% cream	Vag	≥12 y: 1 applicatorful	qhs for 7–14 days
Gyne-Lotrimin-7[a,b]	1% cream			qhs for 3 days
Clotrimazole + betamethasone,[a] Lotrisone	1% + 0.05% cream, lotion	Top	≥12 y: apply to affected area.	bid
Colistin + neomycin + hydrocortisone, Coly-Mycin S, Cortisporin TC otic	0.3% otic susp	Otic	Apply 3–4 drops to affected ear canal; may use with wick.	q6–8h

B. TOPICAL ANTIMICROBIALS (SKIN, EYE, EAR, MUCOSA) (continued)

Generic and Trade Names	Dosage Form	Route	Dose	Interval
Cortisporin; bacitracin + neomycin + polymyxin B + hydrocortisone	Oint	Top	Apply to affected area.	bid–qid
Cortisporin; neomycin + polymyxin B + hydrocortisone	Otic soln[a]	Otic	3 drops to affected ear	bid–qid
	Cream	Top	Apply to affected area.	bid–qid
Dapsone, Aczone	5% gel	Top	≥12 y: Apply to affected area.	bid
	7.5% gel			qd
Econazole,[a] Spectazole	1% cream	Top	Apply to affected area.	qd–bid
Efinaconazole, Jublia	10% soln	Top	Apply to toenail.	qd for 48 wk
Erythromycin[a]	0.5% ophth oint	Ophth	Apply to affected eye.	q4h
Akne-Mycin	2% oint	Top	Apply to affected area.	bid
Ery Pads	2% pledgets[a]			
Eryderm,[a] Erygel[a]	2% soln, gel			
Erythromycin + benzoyl peroxide,[a] Benzamycin	3% gel	Top	≥12 y: apply to affected area.	qd–bid
Ganciclovir, Zirgan	0.15% ophth gel	Ophth	≥2 y: 1 drop in affected eye	q3h while awake (5 times/day) until healed then tid for 7 days
Gatifloxacin, Zymar	0.3% ophth soln	Ophth	1 drop in affected eye	q2h for 2 days then q6h
Gatifloxacin,[a] Zymaxid	0.5% ophth soln	Ophth	≥1 y: 1 drop in affected eye	q2h for 1 day then q6h

Gentamicin,[a] Garamycin	0.1% cream, oint	Top	Apply to affected area.	tid–qid
	0.3% ophth soln, oint	Ophth	Apply to affected eye.	q1–4h (soln) q4–8h (oint)
Gentamicin + prednisolone, Pred-G	0.3% ophth soln, oint	Ophth	Adults: apply to affected eye.	q1–4h (soln) qd–tid (oint)
Imiquimod,[a] Aldara	5% cream	Top	≥12y: to perianal or external genital warts	3 times per wk
Ivermectin, Sklice	0.5% lotion	Top	≥6 mo: thoroughly coat hair and scalp, rinse after 10 minutes.	Once
Ivermectin, Soolantra	1% cream	Top	Adults: apply to face.	qd
Ketoconazole,[a] Nizoral	2% shampoo	Top	≥12 y: apply to affected area.	qd
	2% cream			qd–bid
Extina, Xolegel	2% foam, gel			bid
Nizoral A-D	1% shampoo			bid
Levofloxacin,[a] Quixin	0.5% ophth soln	Ophth	Apply to affected eye.	q1–4h
Luliconazole, Luzu	1% cream	Top	≥12 y: apply to affected area.	q24h for 1–2 wk
Mafenide, Sulfamylon	8.5% cream	Top	Apply to burn.	qd–bid
	5-g pwd for reconstitution		To keep burn dressing wet	q4–8h as needed
Malathion,[a] Ovide	0.5% soln	Top	≥6 y: apply to hair and scalp.	Once
Maxitrol[a]; neomycin + polymyxin + dexamethasone	Susp, oint	Ophth	Apply to affected eye.	q4h (oint) q1–4h (susp)
Metronidazole[a]	0.75% cream, gel, lotion	Top	Adults: apply to affected area.	bid
	0.75% vag gel	Vag	Adults 1 applicatorful	qd–bid
	1% gel	Top	Adults: apply to affected area.	qd

B. TOPICAL ANTIMICROBIALS (SKIN, EYE, EAR, MUCOSA) (continued)

Generic and Trade Names	Dosage Form	Route	Dose	Interval
Noritate	1% cream	Top	Adults: apply to affected area.	qd
Nuvessa	1.3% vag gel	Vag	≥12 y: 1 applicatorful	Once
Miconazole				
Fungoid[a,b]	2% tincture	Top	Apply to affected area.	bid
Micatin[a,b] and others	2% cream, pwd, oint, spray, lotion, gel	Top	Apply to affected area.	qd–bid
Monistat-1[a,b]	1.2-g ovule + 2% cream	Vag	≥12 y: insert one ovule (plus cream to external vulva bid as needed).	Once
Monistat-3[a,b]	200-mg ovule, 4% cream			qhs for 3 days
Monistat-7[a,b]	100-mg ovule, 2% cream			qhs for 7 days
Vusion	0.25% oint	Top	To diaper dermatitis	Each diaper change for 7 days
Moxifloxacin, Vigamox	0.5% ophth soln	Ophth	Apply to affected eye.	tid
Mupirocin, Bactroban	2% oint,[a] cream[a]	Top	Apply to infected skin.	tid
Naftifine, Naftin	1%, 2% cream[a] 2% gel	Top	Apply to affected area.	qd
Natamycin, Natacyn	5% ophth soln	Ophth	Adults: apply to affected eye.	q1–4h
Neosporin[a]				
bacitracin + neomycin + polymyxin B	Ophth oint	Ophth	Apply to affected eye.	q4h
	Oint[a,b]	Top	Apply to affected area.	bid–qid
gramicidin + neomycin + polymyxin B	Ophth soln	Ophth	Apply to affected eye.	q4h

Nystatin,[a] Mycostatin	100,000 U/g cream, oint, pwd	Top	Apply to affected area.	bid–qid
Nystatin + triamcinolone,[a] Mycolog II	100,000 U/g + 0.1% cream, oint	Top	Apply to affected area.	bid
Ofloxacin,[a] Floxin Otic, Ocuflox	0.3% otic soln	Otic	5–10 drops to affected ear	qd–bid
	0.3% ophth soln	Ophth	Apply to affected eye.	q1–6h
Oxiconazole, Oxistat	1% cream,[a] lotion	Top	Apply to affected area.	qd–bid
Ozenoxacin, Xepi	1% cream		Apply to affected area.	bid for 5 days
Permethrin, Nix[a,b]	1% cream	Top	Apply to hair/scalp.	Once for 10 min
Elimite[a]	5% cream		Apply to all skin surfaces.	Once for 8–14 h
Piperonyl butoxide + pyrethrins,[a,b] Rid	4% + 0.3% shampoo, gel	Top	Apply to affected area.	Once for 10 min
Polysporin,[a] polymyxin B + bacitracin	Ophth oint	Ophth	Apply to affected eye.	qd–tid
	Oint[b]	Top	Apply to affected area.	
Polytrim,[a] polymyxin B + trimethoprim	Ophth soln	Ophth	Apply to affected eye.	q3–4h
Retapamulin, Altabax	1% oint	Top	Apply thin layer to affected area.	bid for 5 days
Selenium sulfide,[a] Selsun	2.5% lotion 2.25% shampoo	Top	Lather into scalp or affected area.	Twice weekly then every 1–2 wk
Selsun Blue[a,b]	1% shampoo			qd
Sertaconazole, Ertaczo	2% cream	Top	≥12 y: apply to affected area.	bid
Silver sulfadiazine,[a] Silvadene	1% cream	Top	Apply to affected area.	qd–bid
Spinosad,[a] Natroba	0.9% susp	Top	Apply to scalp and hair.	Once; may repeat in 7 days.
Sulconazole, Exelderm	1% soln, cream	Top	Adults: apply to affected area.	qd–bid

B. TOPICAL ANTIMICROBIALS (SKIN, EYE, EAR, MUCOSA) (continued)

Generic and Trade Names	Dosage Form	Route	Dose	Interval
Sulfacetamide sodium[a]	10% soln	Ophth	Apply to affected eye.	q1–3h
	10% ophth oint			q4–6h
	10% lotion, wash, cream	Top	≥12 y: apply to affected area.	bid–qid
Sulfacetamide sodium + prednisolone,[a] Blephamide	10% ophth oint, soln	Ophth	Apply to affected eye.	tid–qid
Tavaborole, Kerydin	5% soln	Top	Adults: apply to toenail.	qd for 48 wk
Terbinafine,[b] Lamisil-AT	1% cream,[a] spray, gel	Top	Apply to affected area.	qd–bid
Terconazole,[a] Terazol	0.4% cream	Vag	Adults 1 applicatorful or 1 suppository	qhs for 7 days
	0.8% cream 80-mg suppository			qhs for 3 days
Tioconazole[a,b]	6.5% ointment	Vag	≥12 y: 1 applicatorful	One time
Tobramycin, Tobrex	0.3% soln,[a] oint	Ophth	Apply to affected eye.	q1–4h (soln) q4–8h (oint)
Tobramycin + dexamethasone, Tobradex	0.3% soln,[a] oint	Ophth	Apply to affected eye.	q2–6h (soln) q6–8h (oint)
Tobramycin + loteprednol, Zylet	0.3% + 0.5% ophth susp	Ophth	Adults: apply to affected eye.	q4–6h
Tolnaftate,[a,b] Tinactin	1% cream, soln, pwd, spray	Top	Apply to affected area.	bid
Trifluridine,[a] Viroptic	1% ophth soln	Ophth	1 drop (max 9 drops/day)	q2h

[a] Generic available.

[b] Over the counter.

12. Antibiotic Therapy for Children Who Are Obese

When prescribing an antimicrobial for a child who is obese or overweight, selecting a dose based on milligrams per kilograms of total body weight (TBW) may overexpose the child if the drug doesn't freely distribute into fat tissue. Conversely, underexposure can occur when a dosage is reduced for obesity for drugs without distribution limitations.

The Table lists major antimicrobials classes and our suggestion on how to calculate an appropriate dose. The evidence to support these recommendations are Level II–III (pharmacokinetic studies in children, extrapolations from adult studies, and expert opinion). Whenever a dose is used that is greater than one prospectively investigated for efficacy and safety, the clinician must weigh the benefits with potential risks. Data are not available on all agents.

DOSING RECOMMENDATIONS			
DRUG CLASS	**BY EBW[a]**	**BY ADJUSTED BW**	**BY TBW[b]**
ANTIBACTERIALS			
Beta-lactams			
Piperacillin/tazobactam			X
Cephalosporins			X
Meropenem			X
Ertapenem	X		
Clindamycin			X (no max)
Vancomycin		1,500–2,000 mg/m²/day	20 mg/kg LD then 60 mg/kg/day div q6–8h
Aminoglycosides		0.7 x TBW	
Fluoroquinolones		EBW + 0.45 (TBW-EBW)	
Rifampin	X		
Miscellaneous			
TMP/SMX			X
Metronidazole			X
Linezolid			X
Daptomycin			X (see max doses in comments below)

DOSING RECOMMENDATIONS (continued)			
DRUG CLASS	**BY EBW[a]**	**BY ADJUSTED BW**	**BY TBW[b]**
ANTIFUNGALS			
Amphotericin B (all formulations)			X
Fluconazole			X (max 1,200 mg/day)
Flucytosine	X		
Anidulafungin			X (max 250 mg LD, max 125 mg/day)
Caspofungin			X (max 150 mg/day)
Micafungin			X (max 300 mg/day)
Voriconazole	X		
ANTIVIRALS (NON-HIV)			
Nucleoside analogues (acyclovir, ganciclovir)	X		
Oseltamivir	X		
ANTIMYCOBACTERIALS			
Isoniazid	X		
Rifampin			X
Pyrazinamide			X
Ethambutol			X

Abbreviations: BMI, body mass index; BW, body weight; EBW, expected body weight; HIV, human immunodeficiency virus; LD, loading dose; TBW, total body weight; TMP/SMX, trimethoprim/sulfamethoxazole.

[a] EBW (kg) = BMI 50th percentile for age × actual height (m)^2; from Le Grange D, et al. *Pediatrics*. 2012;129(2):e438–e446 PMID: 22218841.

[b] Dose up to adult max (see Chapter 11) if not otherwise specified.

For **gentamicin**, using the child's fat-free mass, an approximate 30% reduction in dosing weight, has been recommended. When performing this empiric dosing strategy with aminoglycosides in children who are obese, we recommend closely following serum concentrations.

Vancomycin is traditionally dosed based on TBW in obese adults due to increases in kidney size and glomerular filtration rate. In obese children, weight-adjusted distribution volume and clearance are slightly lower than in their nonobese counterparts. An empiric maximum dose of 60 mg/kg/day based on TBW, or dosing using body surface area, may be more appropriate. We recommend closely following serum concentrations.

In the setting of **cefazolin** for surgical prophylaxis (see Chapter 14), adult studies of obese patients have generally found that distribution to the subcutaneous fat tissue target can be subtherapeutic when standard doses are used. Although clinical data are lacking, given the wide safety margin of cephalosporins in the short-term setting of surgical prophylaxis, higher single doses are recommended in obese adults (eg, 2 g instead of the standard 1 g) with re-dosing at 4-hour intervals for longer cases. In obese children, we recommend dosing cephalosporins for surgical prophylaxis based on TBW up to the adult maximum.

In critically ill obese adults treated with **carbapenems** or **piperacillin/tazobactam**, extended infusion times (over 2–3 hours, instead of 30 minutes) have been shown to increase the likelihood of achieving therapeutic bloodstream antibiotic exposures, particularly against bacteria with higher minimum inhibitory concentrations (MICs).

Daptomycin dosing can be performed using TBW, but the maximum dose should be 500 mg for skin infections and 750 mg for bloodstream infections. Bolus administration over 2 minutes can improve the likelihood of achieving target concentrations in cases where the maximum dose is less than the calculated dose in an obese adolescent.

Adult maximum doses of **linezolid** may be inadequate to achieve target plasma concentrations to treat susceptible methicillin-resistant *Staphylococcus aureus* infections with high MICs. However, higher doses should only be attempted with the aid of concentration monitoring to avoid hematologic toxicity.

Bibliography

Camaione L, et al. *Pharmacotherapy.* 2013;33(12):1278–1287 PMID: 24019205
Chambers J, et al. *Eur J Clin Pharmacol.* 2019;75(4):511–517 PMID: 30511329
Chung EK, et al. *J Clin Pharmacol.* 2015;55(8):899–908 PMID: 25823963
Donoso F A, et al. *Arch Argent Pediatr*. 2019;117(2):e121–e130 PMID: 30869490
Hall RG. *Curr Pharm Des.* 2015;21(32):4748–4751 PMID: 26112269
Harskamp-van Ginkel MW, et al. *JAMA Pediatr.* 2015;169(7):678–685 PMID: 25961828
Meng L, et al. *Pharmacotherapy*. 2017;37(11):1415–1431 PMID: 28869666
Moffett BS, et al. *Ther Drug Monit.* 2018;40(3):322–329 PMID: 29521784
Natale S, et al. *Pharmacotherapy.* 2017;37(3):361–378 PMID: 28079262
Pai MP. *Clin Ther.* 2016;38(9):2032–2044 PMID: 27524636
Pai MP, et al. *Antimicrob Agents Chemother.* 2011;55(12):5640–5645 PMID: 21930881
Payne KD, et al. *Expert Rev Anti Infect Ther.* 2016;14(2):257–267 PMID: 26641135
Smith MJ, et al. *Antimicrob Agents Chemother*. 2017;61(4):e02014-16 PMID: 28137820
Wasmann RE, et al. *Antimicrob Agents Chemother.* 2018;62(7):e00063-18 PMID: 29712664
Wasmann RE, et al. *J Antimicrob Chemother*. 2019;74(4):978–985 PMID: 30649375
Xie F, et al. *J Antimicrob Chemother*. 2019;74(3):667–674 PMID: 30535122

13. Sequential Parenteral-Oral Antibiotic Therapy (Oral Step-down Therapy) for Serious Infections

The concept of oral *step-down* or "oral switch" therapy is not new; evidence-based recommendations from Nelson and colleagues appeared 40 years ago in the *Journal of Pediatrics.*[1,2] Bone and joint infections,[3–5] complicated bacterial pneumonia with empyema,[6] deep-tissue abscesses, and appendicitis,[7,8] as well as cellulitis or pyelonephritis,[9] may require initial parenteral therapy to control the growth and spread of pathogens and minimize injury to tissues. For abscesses in soft tissues, joints, bones, and empyema, most organisms are removed by surgical drainage and presumably, many are killed by the initial parenteral therapy. When the signs and symptoms of infection begin to resolve, often within 2 to 4 days, continuing intravenous (IV) therapy may not be required, as a normal host neutrophil response begins to assist in clearing the infection when the pathogen load drops below a certain critical density, as has been demonstrated in an animal model.[10] In addition to following the clinical response prior to oral switch, following objective laboratory markers, such as C-reactive protein (CRP) or procalcitonin (PCT), during the hospitalization may also help the clinician better assess the response to antibacterial therapy, particularly in the infant or child who is difficult to examine.[11,12] For many children who have successful drainage of their intra-abdominal abscesses and recover quickly, either short-course oral therapy (7 days total) or no additional antibiotic treatment following clinical and laboratory recovery may be appropriate.[13] However, defining those children who may benefit from oral step-down therapy (or no additional antibiotic therapy) is difficult, as the extent of a deep infection, the adequacy of source control (drainage), and the susceptibility of pathogen(s) involved are not always known.

For the beta-lactam class of antibiotics, absorption of orally administered antibiotics in *standard* dosages provides peak serum concentrations that are routinely only 5% to 20% of those achieved with IV or intramuscular administration. However, *high-dose* oral beta-lactam therapy provides the tissue antibiotic exposure thought to be required to eradicate the remaining pathogens at the infection site as the tissue perfusion improves. For beta-lactams, begin with a dosage 2 to 3 times the normal dosage (eg, 75–100 mg/kg/day of amoxicillin or 100 mg/kg/day of cephalexin). High-dose oral beta-lactam antibiotic therapy of osteoarticular infections has been associated with treatment success since 1978.[3] It is reassuring that high-quality retrospective cohort data have recently confirmed similar outcomes achieved in those treated with oral step-down therapy compared with those treated with IV.[14] High-dose prolonged oral beta-lactam therapy may be associated with reversible neutropenia; checking for hematologic toxicity every few weeks during therapy is suggested.[15]

Clindamycin and many antibiotics of the fluoroquinolone class (ciprofloxacin, levofloxacin) and oxazolidinone class (linezolid, tedizolid) have excellent absorption of their oral formulations and provide virtually the same tissue antibiotic exposure at a particular mg/kg dose, compared with that dose given intravenously. Trimethoprim/sulfamethoxazole and metronidazole are also very well absorbed.

One must also assume that the parent and child are compliant with the administration of each antibiotic dose, that the oral antibiotic will be absorbed from the gastrointestinal tract into the systemic circulation (no vomiting or diarrhea), and that the parents will seek medical care if the clinical course does not continue to improve for their child.

Monitor the child clinically for a continued response on oral therapy; follow CRP or PCT after the switch to oral therapy and if there are concerns about continued response, make sure the antibiotic and dosage you selected are appropriate and the family is compliant. In one of the first published series of oral step-down therapy for osteoarticular infection by Syrogiannopoulos and Nelson, failures caused by presumed noncompliance were reported.[16]

14. Antimicrobial Prophylaxis/Prevention of Symptomatic Infection

This chapter provides a summary of recommendations for prophylaxis of infections, defined as providing therapy prior to the onset of clinical signs or symptoms of infection. Prophylaxis can be considered in several clinical scenarios.

A. Postexposure Antimicrobial Prophylaxis to Prevent Infection

Given for a relatively short, specified period (days) after exposure to specific pathogens/organisms, where the risks of acquiring the infection are felt to justify antimicrobial treatment to eradicate a colonizing pathogen or prevent symptomatic infection in situations in which the child (healthy or with increased susceptibility to infection) is likely to have been inoculated/exposed (eg, asymptomatic child closely exposed to meningococcus; a neonate born to a mother with active genital herpes simplex virus [HSV]).

B. Long-term Antimicrobial Prophylaxis to Prevent Symptomatic New Infection

Given to a particular, defined population of children who are of relatively high risk of acquiring a severe infection from a single or multiple exposures (eg, a child postsplenectomy; a child with documented rheumatic heart disease to prevent subsequent streptococcal infection), with **prophylaxis provided during the period of risk, potentially months or years.**

C. Prophylaxis of Symptomatic Disease in Children Who Have Asymptomatic Infection/Latent Infection

Where a child has a documented but asymptomatic infection and targeted antimicrobials are given to prevent the development of symptomatic disease (eg, latent tuberculosis infection or therapy of a stem cell transplant patient with documented cytomegalovirus viremia but no symptoms of infection or rejection; to prevent reactivation of herpes simplex virus). Treatment period is usually defined, particularly in situations in which the latent infection can be cured (tuberculosis, requiring a few months of therapy), but other circumstances, such as prevention of reactivation of latent HSV, may require months or years of prophylaxis.

D. Surgical/Procedure Prophylaxis

A child receives a surgical/invasive catheter procedure, planned or unplanned, in which the risk of infection postoperatively or post-procedure may justify prophylaxis to prevent an infection from occurring (eg, prophylaxis to prevent infection following spinal rod placement). **Treatment is usually short-term (hours),** beginning just prior to the procedure and ending at the conclusion of the procedure, or within 24 hours.

E. Travel-Related Exposure Prophylaxis

Not discussed in this chapter; please refer to information on specific disease entities (eg, traveler's diarrhea, chapters 6 and 10) or specific pathogens (eg, malaria, Chapter 10). Constantly updated, current information for travelers about prophylaxis (often starting just before travel and continuing until return) and current worldwide infection risks can be found on the Centers for Disease Control and Prevention website at www.cdc.gov/travel (accessed October 9, 2019).

NOTE

- Abbreviations: AHA, American Heart Association; ALT, alanine aminotransferase; amox/clav, amoxicillin/clavulanate; ARF, acute rheumatic fever; bid, twice daily; CDC, Centers for Disease Control and Prevention; CPB, cardiopulmonary bypass; CSF, cerebrospinal fluid; div, divided; DOT, directly observed therapy; GI, gastrointestinal; HIV, human immunodeficiency virus; HSV, herpes simplex virus; IGRA, interferon-gamma release assay; IM, intramuscular; INH, isoniazid; IV, intravenous; MRSA, methicillin-resistant *Staphylococcus aureus;* N/A, not applicable; PCR, polymerase chain reaction; PO, orally; PPD, purified protein derivative; qd, once daily; qid, 4 times daily; spp, species; TB, tuberculosis; tid, 3 times daily; TIG, tetanus immune globulin; TMP/SMX, trimethoprim/sulfamethoxazole; UTI, urinary tract infection.

A. POSTEXPOSURE ANTIMICROBIAL PROPHYLAXIS TO PREVENT INFECTION

Prophylaxis Category	Therapy (evidence grade)	Comments
Bacterial		
Bites, animal and human[1–5] (*Pasteurella multocida* [animal], *Eikenella corrodens* [human], *Staphylococcus* spp, and *Streptococcus* spp)	Amox/clav 45 mg/kg/day PO div tid (amox/clav 7:1; see Chapter 1 for amox/clav description) for 3–5 days (AII) OR ampicillin and clindamycin (BII). For penicillin allergy, consider ciprofloxacin (for *Pasteurella*) plus clindamycin (BIII).	Recommended for children who (1) are immunocompromised; (2) are asplenic; (3) have moderate to severe injuries, especially to the hand or face; or (4) have injuries that may have penetrated the periosteum or joint capsule (AII).[3] Consider rabies prophylaxis for at-risk animal bites through state and local rabies consultation contacts (AI)[6]; consider tetanus prophylaxis.[7] Human bites have a very high rate of infection (do not close open wounds routinely). Cat bites have a higher rate of infection than dog bites. *Staphylococcus aureus* coverage is only fair with amox/clav and provides no coverage for MRSA.
Endocarditis prophylaxis[8,9]: Given that (1) endocarditis is rarely caused by dental/GI procedures and (2) prophylaxis for procedures prevents an exceedingly small number of cases, the risks of antibiotics most often outweigh benefits. However, some "highest risk" conditions are currently recommended for prophylaxis: (1) prosthetic heart valve (or prosthetic material used to repair a valve); (2) previous endocarditis; (3) cyanotic congenital heart disease that is unrepaired (or palliatively repaired with shunts and conduits); (4) congenital heart disease that is repaired but with defects at the site of repair adjacent to prosthetic material; (5) completely repaired congenital heart disease using prosthetic material, for the first 6 months after repair; or (6) cardiac transplant patients with valvulopathy. Routine prophylaxis no longer is required for children with native valve abnormalities. Follow-up data in children suggest that following these new guidelines, no increase in endocarditis has been detected,[10,11] but recent analyses have questioned the quality of the evidence on which the recommendations were based.[12,13]		
– In highest-risk patients: dental procedures that involve manipulation of the gingival or periodontal region of teeth	Amoxicillin 50 mg/kg PO 1 h before procedure OR ampicillin or ceftriaxone or cefazolin, all at 50 mg/kg IM/IV 30–60 min before procedure	If penicillin allergy: clindamycin 20 mg/kg PO (1 h before) or IV (30 min before) OR azithromycin 15 mg/kg or clarithromycin 15 mg/kg (1 h before)

A. POSTEXPOSURE ANTIMICROBIAL PROPHYLAXIS TO PREVENT INFECTION (continued)

Prophylaxis Category	Therapy (evidence grade)	Comments
Bacterial (continued)		
– Genitourinary and gastrointestinal procedures	None	No longer recommended
Lyme disease (*Borrelia burgdorferi*)[14]	Doxycycline 4.4 mg/kg (up to 200 mg max), once. Dental staining should not occur with a single course of doxycycline. Amoxicillin prophylaxis is not well studied, and experts recommend a full 14-day course if amoxicillin is used.	ONLY for those in highly Lyme-endemic areas AND the tick has been attached for >36 h (and is engorged) AND prophylaxis started within 72 h of tick removal.
Meningococcus (*Neisseria meningitidis*)[15,16]	For prophylaxis of close contacts, including household members, child care center contacts, and anyone directly exposed to the patient's oral secretions (eg, through kissing, mouth-to-mouth resuscitation, endotracheal intubation, endotracheal tube management) in the 7 days before symptom onset **Rifampin** Infants <1 mo: 5 mg/kg PO q12h for 4 doses Children ≥1 mo: 10 mg/kg PO q12h for 4 doses (max 600 mg/dose) OR **Ceftriaxone** Children <15 y: 125 mg IM once Children ≥16 y: 250 mg IM once OR **Ciprofloxacin** 500 mg PO once (adolescents and adults)	A single dose of ciprofloxacin should not present a significant risk of cartilage damage, but no prospective data exist in children for prophylaxis of meningococcal disease. For a child, an equivalent exposure for ciprofloxacin to that in adults would be 15–20 mg/kg as a single dose (max 500 mg). A few ciprofloxacin-resistant strains have now been reported. Insufficient data to recommend azithromycin at this time. Meningococcal vaccines that target the specific serogroup may also be recommended in case of an outbreak.
Pertussis[17,18]	Same regimen as for treatment of pertussis: azithromycin 10 mg/kg/day qd for 5 days OR clarithromycin (for infants >1 mo) 15 mg/kg/day div bid for 7 days OR erythromycin (estolate preferable) 40 mg/kg/day PO div qid for 14 days (AII)	Prophylaxis to family members; contacts defined by CDC: persons within 21 days of exposure to an infectious pertussis case, who are at high risk of severe illness or who will have close contact with a person at high risk of severe illness (including infants, pregnant women in their

	Alternative: TMP/SMX 8 mg/kg/day div bid for 14 days (BIII)	third trimester, immunocompromised persons, contacts who have close contact with infants <12 mo). Close contact can be considered as face-to-face exposure within 3 feet of a symptomatic person; direct contact with respiratory, nasal, or oral secretions; or sharing the same confined space in close proximity to an infected person for ≥1 h. Community-wide prophylaxis is not currently recommended. Azithromycin and clarithromycin are better tolerated than erythromycin (see Chapter 5); azithromycin is preferred in exposed very young infants to reduce pyloric stenosis risk.

Tetanus (*Clostridium tetani*)[7,19]

Need for Tetanus Vaccine or TIG[a]

	Clean Wound		Contaminated Wound	
Number of past tetanus vaccine doses	Need for tetanus vaccine	Need for TIG 500 U IM[a]	Need for tetanus vaccine	Need for TIG 500 U IM[a]
<3 doses	Yes	No	Yes	Yes
≥3 doses	No (if <10 y[b]) Yes (if ≥10 y[b])	No	No (if <5 y[b]) Yes (if ≥5 y[b])	No

[a] IV immune globulin should be used when TIG is not available.

[b] Years since last tetanus-containing vaccine dose.

For deep, contaminated wounds, wound debridement is essential. For wounds that cannot be fully debrided, consider metronidazole 30 mg/kg/day PO div q8h until wound healing is underway and anaerobic conditions no longer exist, as short as 3–5 days (BIII).

A. POSTEXPOSURE ANTIMICROBIAL PROPHYLAXIS TO PREVENT INFECTION (continued)

Prophylaxis Category	Therapy (evidence grade)	Comments
Bacterial (continued)		
Tuberculosis (*Mycobacterium tuberculosis*) Exposed children <4 y, or immunocompromised patient (high risk of dissemination)[20,21] For treatment of latent TB infection,[21,22] see recommendations in Section C of this chapter (Table 14C).	Scenario 1: Previously uninfected child becomes exposed to a person with active disease. Exposed children <4 y, or immunocompromised patient (high risk of dissemination): rifampin 15–20 mg/kg/dose PO qd OR INH 10–15 mg/kg PO qd; for at least 2–3 mo (AIII), at which time cellular immunity is established and the PPD/IGRA may be more accurately assessed. Children ≥4 y may also begin prophylaxis postexposure, but if exposure is questionable, can wait 2–3 mo after exposure to assess for infection; if not given prophylaxis, and PPD/IGRA at 2–3 mo is positive and child remains asymptomatic at that time, see Scenario 2.	If PPD or IGRA remains negative at 2–3 mo and child remains well, consider stopping empiric therapy. However, tests at 2–3 mo may not be reliable in immunocompromised patients. This regimen is to prevent infection in a compromised host after exposure, rather than to treat latent asymptomatic infection.
	Scenario 2: Asymptomatic child is found to have a positive skin test/IGRA test for TB, documenting latent TB infection. For children ≥2 y, once-weekly DOT for 12 wk using BOTH INH (15 mg/kg/dose, max 900 mg) AND rifapentine: 10.0–14.0 kg: 300 mg 14.1–25.0 kg: 450 mg 25.1–32.0 kg: 600 mg 32.1–49.9 kg: 750 mg ≥50.0 kg: 900 mg (max) OR Rifampin 15–20 mg/kg/dose daily, preferably the entire daily dose given once daily (max 600 mg) for 4 mo OR	Insufficient data for weekly INH AND rifapentine for children <2 y.

	INH 10–15 mg/kg PO qd for 9 mo (≥12 mo for an immunocompromised child) OR INH 20–30 mg/kg PO DOT twice weekly for 9 mo	
Viral		
Herpes simplex virus		
During pregnancy	For women with recurrent genital herpes: acyclovir 400 mg PO tid; valacyclovir 500 mg PO bid from 36-wk gestation until delivery (CII)[23]	Neonatal HSV disease after maternal suppression has been documented[24]
Neonatal: **Primary or nonprimary first clinical episode of maternal infection,** neonate exposed at delivery[25]	Asymptomatic, exposed neonate: at 24 h after birth, culture mucosal sites (see Comments), obtain CSF and whole-blood PCR for HSV DNA, obtain ALT, and start preemptive therapeutic acyclovir IV (60 mg/kg/day div q8h) for 10 days (AII). Some experts would evaluate at birth for exposure following presumed maternal primary infection and start preemptive therapy rather than wait 24 h.	Reference 25 provides a management algorithm that determines the type of maternal infection and, thus, the appropriate evaluation and preemptive therapy of the neonate. Mucosal sites for culture: conjunctivae, mouth, nasopharynx, rectum. Any symptomatic baby, at any time, requires a full evaluation for invasive infection and IV acyclovir therapy for 14–21 days, depending on extent of disease.
Neonatal: **Recurrent maternal infection,** neonate exposed at delivery[25]	Asymptomatic, exposed neonate: at 24 h after birth, culture mucosal sites (see Comments) and obtain whole-blood PCR for HSV DNA. Hold on therapy unless cultures or PCR are positive, at which time the diagnostic evaluation should be completed (CSF PCR for HSV DNA, serum ALT) and preemptive therapeutic IV acyclovir (60 mg/kg/day div q8h) should be administered for 10 days (AIII).	Reference 25 provides a management algorithm that determines the type of maternal infection and, thus, the appropriate evaluation and preemptive therapy of the neonate. Mucosal sites for culture: conjunctivae, mouth, nasopharynx, rectum. Any symptomatic baby, at any time, requires a full evaluation for invasive infection and IV acyclovir therapy for 14–21 days, depending on extent of disease.
Neonatal: Following symptomatic disease, to prevent recurrence	See recommendations in Section C of this chapter (Table 14C).	

A. POSTEXPOSURE ANTIMICROBIAL PROPHYLAXIS TO PREVENT INFECTION (continued)

Prophylaxis Category	Therapy (evidence grade)	Comments
Viral (continued)		
Keratitis (ocular) in otherwise healthy children	See recommendations in Section C of this chapter (Table 14C).	
Influenza virus (A or B)[26]	Oseltamivir prophylaxis (AI) 3–≤8 mo: 3 mg/kg/dose qd for 10 days 9–11 mo: 3.5 mg/kg/dose PO qd for 10 days[27] Based on body weight for children ≥12 mo: ≤15 kg: 30 mg qd for 10 days >15–23 kg: 45 mg qd for 10 days >23–40 kg: 60 mg qd for 10 days >40 kg: 75 mg qd for 10 days	Not routinely recommended for infants 0 to ≤3 mo unless exposure (single event or ongoing [eg, breastfeeding mother with active influenza]) judged substantial, because of limited reported data on safety/efficacy and variability of drug exposure in this age group.
	Zanamivir prophylaxis (AI) Children ≥5 y: 10 mg (two 5-mg inhalations) qd for as long as 28 days (community outbreaks) or 10 days (household settings)	
Rabies virus[28]	Rabies immune globulin, 20 IU/kg, infiltrate around wound, with remaining volume injected IM (AII) PLUS Rabies immunization (AII)	For dog, cat, or ferret bite from **symptomatic animal,** immediate rabies immune globulin and immunization; otherwise, can wait 10 days for observation of animal, if possible, prior to rabies immune globulin or vaccine. PLEASE evaluate the context of the bite. A provoked bite from a threatened or annoyed dog (especially a known dog) is not an indication for rabies prophylaxis. Bites of squirrels, hamsters, guinea pigs, gerbils, chipmunks, rats, mice and other rodents, rabbits, hares, and pikas almost never require anti-rabies prophylaxis. For bites of bats, skunks, raccoons, foxes, most other carnivores, and woodchucks, immediate rabies immune globulin and immunization (regard as rabid unless geographic area is known to be free of rabies or until animal proven negative by laboratory tests).

B. LONG-TERM ANTIMICROBIAL PROPHYLAXIS TO PREVENT SYMPTOMATIC NEW INFECTION

Prophylaxis Category	Therapy (evidence grade)	Comments
Bacterial otitis media[29,30]	Amoxicillin or other antibiotics can be used in half the therapeutic dose qd or bid to prevent infections if the benefits outweigh the risks of (1) emergence/selection of resistant organisms for that child (and contacts) and (2) antibiotic side effects.	True, recurrent acute bacterial otitis is far less common in the era of conjugate pneumococcal immunization. To prevent recurrent infections, as alternative to antibiotic prophylaxis, also consider the risks and benefits of placing tympanostomy tubes to improve middle ear ventilation. Studies have demonstrated that amoxicillin, sulfisoxazole, and TMP/SMX are effective. However, antimicrobial prophylaxis may alter the nasopharyngeal flora and foster colonization with resistant organisms, compromising long-term efficacy of the prophylactic drug. Continuous PO-administered antimicrobial prophylaxis should be reserved for control of recurrent acute otitis media, only when defined as ≥3 distinct and well-documented episodes during a period of 6 mo or ≥4 episodes during a period of 12 mo.
Rheumatic fever	For >27.3 kg (>60 lb): 1.2 million U penicillin G benzathine, q4wk (q3wk for high-risk children) For <27.3 kg: 600,000 U penicillin G benzathine, q4wk (q3wk for high-risk children) OR Penicillin V (phenoxymethyl) oral, 250 mg PO bid	AHA policy statement at http://circ.ahajournals.org/content/119/11/1541.full.pdf (accessed October 9, 2019). Doses studied many years ago, with no new data; ARF is an uncommon disease currently in the United States. Alternatives to penicillin include amoxicillin, sulfisoxazole, or macrolides, including erythromycin, azithromycin, and clarithromycin.
Urinary tract infection, recurrent[31–37]	TMP/SMX 3 mg/kg/dose TMP PO qd OR nitrofurantoin 1–2 mg/kg PO qd at bedtime; more rapid resistance may develop using beta-lactams (BII).	Only for those with grade III–V reflux or with recurrent febrile UTI: prophylaxis no longer recommended for patients with grade I–II (some also exclude grade III) reflux. Prophylaxis prevents infection but may not prevent scarring. Early treatment of new infections is recommended for children not given prophylaxis. Resistance eventually develops to every antibiotic; follow resistance patterns for each patient.

Fungal: For detailed information on prevention of candidiasis in the neonate, please see Chapter 5; for detailed information on prevention of fungal infection (*Candida* spp, *Aspergillus* spp, *Rhizopus* spp) in children undergoing chemotherapy, please see Chapter 8.

B. LONG-TERM ANTIMICROBIAL PROPHYLAXIS TO PREVENT SYMPTOMATIC NEW INFECTION (continued)

Prophylaxis Category	Therapy (evidence grade)	Comments
Pneumocystis jiroveci (previously *Pneumocystis carinii*)[38–41]	Non-HIV infection regimens TMP/SMX as 5–10 mg TMP/kg/day PO, div 2 doses, q12h, either qd or 3 times/wk on consecutive days (AI); OR TMP/SMX 5–10 mg TMP/kg/day PO as a *single dose,* qd, given 3 times/wk on consecutive days (AI) (once-weekly regimens have also been successful); OR dapsone 2 mg/kg (max 100 mg) PO qd, or 4 mg/kg (max 200 mg) once weekly; OR atovaquone 30 mg/kg/day for infants 1–3 mo; 45 mg/kg/day for infants/children 4–24 mo; and 30 mg/kg/day for children >24 mo until no longer immunocompromised, based on oncology or transplant treatment regimen	

C. PROPHYLAXIS OF SYMPTOMATIC DISEASE IN CHILDREN WHO HAVE ASYMPTOMATIC INFECTION/LATENT INFECTION

Prophylaxis Category	Therapy (evidence grade)	Comments
Herpes simplex virus		
Neonatal: Following symptomatic disease, to prevent recurrence[25]	Acyclovir 300 mg/m²/dose PO tid for 6 mo, following cessation of IV acyclovir treatment of acute disease (AI)	Follow absolute neutrophil counts at 2 and 4 wk, then monthly during prophylactic/suppressive therapy. Oral acyclovir suppression is not indicated for patients described in Section A of this chapter (Table 14A), who received IV acyclovir as postexposure antimicrobial prophylaxis to prevent infection.

Keratitis (ocular) in otherwise healthy children	Suppressive acyclovir therapy for frequent recurrence (no pediatric data): 20 mg/kg/dose bid (up to 400 mg) for ≥1 y (AIII)	Based on data from adults. Anecdotally, some children may require tid dosing to prevent recurrences. Check for acyclovir resistance for those who relapse while on appropriate therapy. Suppression oftentimes required for many years. Watch for severe recurrence at conclusion of suppression.
Tuberculosis[20–22] (latent TB infection [asymptomatic infection], defined by a positive skin test or IGRA, with no clinical or radiographic evidence of active disease)	For children ≥2 y, once-weekly DOT for 12 wk using BOTH INH 15 mg/kg/dose (max 900 mg) AND rifapentine: 10.0–14.0 kg: 300 mg 14.1–25.0 kg: 450 mg 25.1–32.0 kg: 600 mg 32.1–49.9 kg: 750 mg ≥50.0 kg: 900 mg (max) OR Rifampin (15–20 mg/kg/dose daily, preferably the entire daily dose given once daily (max 600 mg) for 4 mo OR INH 10–15 mg/kg PO qd for 9 mo (≥12 mo for an immunocompromised child) OR INH 20–30 mg/kg PO directly observed therapy twice weekly for 9 mo	Single drug therapy if no clinical or radiographic evidence of active disease. For exposure to drug-resistant strains, consult with TB specialist.

Fungal: For detailed information on prevention of fungal infection (*Candida* spp, *Aspergillus* spp, *Rhizopus* spp) in children undergoing chemotherapy, please see Chapter 8; for detailed information on prevention of candidiasis in the neonate, please see Chapter 5.

C. PROPHYLAXIS OF SYMPTOMATIC DISEASE IN CHILDREN WHO HAVE ASYMPTOMATIC INFECTION/LATENT INFECTION (continued)

Prophylaxis Category	Therapy (evidence grade)	Comments
Pneumocystis jiroveci (previously *Pneumocystis carinii*)[38–41]	Non-HIV infection regimens (stem cell transplants, solid organ transplants, many malignancies, and T-cell immune deficiencies [congenital or secondary to treatment]). Duration of prophylaxis depends on the underlying condition. TMP/SMX as 5–10 mg TMP/kg/day PO, div 2 doses, q12h, either qd or 2 times/wk or 3 times/wk, on consecutive days or alternating days (AI); OR TMP/SMX 5–10 mg TMP/kg/day PO as a *single dose,* qd, given 3 times/wk on consecutive days (AI) (once-weekly regimens have also been successful); OR dapsone 2 mg/kg (max 100 mg) PO qd, or 4 mg/kg (max 200 mg) once weekly; OR atovaquone 30 mg/kg/day for infants 1–3 mo; 45 mg/kg/day for infants/children 4–24 mo; and 30 mg/kg/day for children ≥24 mo Inhaled pentamidine only for those who cannot tolerate the regimens noted above	Prophylaxis in specific populations based on degree of immunosuppression. For children with HIV, please see the Aidsinfo.gov website for information on pediatric opportunistic infections: https://aidsinfo.nih.gov/guidelines/html/5/pediatric-oi-prevention-and-treatment-guidelines/0 (accessed October 9, 2019).

D. SURGICAL/PROCEDURE PROPHYLAXIS[42–53]

The CDC National Healthcare Safety Network uses a classification of surgical procedure-related wound infections based on an estimation of the load of bacterial contamination: Class I, clean; Class II, clean-contaminated; Class III, contaminated; and Class IV, dirty/infected.[43,49] Other major factors creating risk for postoperative surgical site infection include the duration of surgery (a longer-duration operation, defined as one that exceeded the 75th percentile for a given procedure) and the medical comorbidities of the patient, as determined by an American Society of Anesthesiologists score of III, IV, or V (presence of severe systemic disease that results in functional limitations, is life-threatening, or is expected to preclude survival from the operation). The virulence/pathogenicity of bacteria inoculated and the presence of foreign debris/devitalized tissue/surgical material in the wound are also considered risk factors for infection.

For all categories of surgical prophylaxis, dosing recommendations are derived from (1) choosing agents based on the organisms likely to be responsible for inoculation of the surgical site; (2) giving the agents at an optimal time (<60 min for cefazolin, or <60 to 120 min for vancomycin and ciprofloxacin) before starting the operation to achieve appropriate serum and tissue exposures at the time of incision; (3) providing additional doses during the procedure at times based on the standard dosing guideline for that agent; and (4) stopping the agents at the end of the procedure or for no longer than 24 h after the end of the procedure. Optimal duration of prophylaxis after delayed sternal or abdominal closure is not well defined in adults or children.

Bathing with soaps or an antiseptic agent the night before surgery is recommended, with alcohol-based presurgical skin preparation.[49]

Procedure/Operation	Recommended Agents	Preoperative Dose	Intraoperative Re-dosing Interval (h) for Prolonged Surgery
Cardiovascular			
Cardiac[53] *Staphylococcus epidermidis, Staphylococcus aureus, Corynebacterium* spp	Cefazolin	30 mg/kg	4
	Vancomycin, if MRSA likely[52]	15 mg/kg	8
	Ampicillin/sulbactam if enteric gram-negative bacilli a concern	50 mg/kg of ampicillin	3
Cardiac with cardiopulmonary bypass[54]	Cefazolin	30 mg/kg	15 mg/kg at CPB start and also at rewarming. Begin postoperative prophylaxis 30 mg/kg at 8 h after intraoperative rewarming dose.

D. SURGICAL/PROCEDURE PROPHYLAXIS[42–53] (continued)

Procedure/Operation	Recommended Agents	Preoperative Dose	Intraoperative Re-dosing Interval (h) for Prolonged Surgery
Cardiovascular (continued)			
Vascular *S epidermidis, S aureus, Corynebacterium* spp, gram-negative enteric bacilli, particularly for procedures in the groin	Cefazolin, OR	30 mg/kg	4
	Vancomycin, if MRSA likely[52]	15 mg/kg	8
Thoracic (noncardiac)			
Lobectomy, video-assisted thoracoscopic surgery, thoracotomy (but no prophylaxis needed for simple chest tube placement for pneumothorax)	Cefazolin, OR	30 mg/kg	4
	Ampicillin/sulbactam if enteric gram-negative bacilli a concern	50 mg/kg of ampicillin	3
	Vancomycin or clindamycin if drug allergy or MRSA likely[52]	15 mg/kg vancomycin	8
		10 mg/kg clindamycin	6
Gastrointestinal			
Gastroduodenal Enteric gram-negative bacilli, respiratory tract gram-positive cocci	Cefazolin	30 mg/kg	4
Biliary procedure, open Enteric gram-negative bacilli, enterococci, *Clostridia*	Cefazolin, OR	30 mg/kg	4
	Cefoxitin	40 mg/kg	2
Appendectomy, non-perforated (no prophylaxis needed post-op if appendix is intact)[55]	Cefoxitin, OR	40 mg/kg	2
	Cefazolin and metronidazole	30 mg/kg cefazolin, 10 mg/kg metronidazole	4 for cefazolin 8 for metronidazole

Complicated appendicitis or other ruptured colorectal viscus[56] Enteric gram-negative bacilli, enterococci, anaerobes. For complicated appendicitis, antibiotics provided to treat ongoing infection, rather than prophylaxis.	Cefazolin and metronidazole, OR	30 mg/kg cefazolin and 10 mg/kg metronidazole	4 for cefazolin 8 for metronidazole
	Cefoxitin, OR	40 mg/kg	2
	Ceftriaxone and metronidazole, OR	50 mg/kg ceftriaxone and 10 mg/kg metronidazole	12 for ceftriaxone 8 for metronidazole
	Ertapenem, OR	15 mg/kg (max 500 mg) for children 3 mo–12 y; 1 g for children ≥13 y	8
	Meropenem, OR	20 mg/kg	4
	Imipenem	20 mg/kg	4
Genitourinary			
Cystoscopy (only requires prophylaxis for children with suspected active UTI or those having foreign material placed) Enteric gram-negative bacilli, enterococci	Cefazolin, OR	30 mg/kg	4
	TMP/SMX (if low local resistance), OR Select a 2nd- (cefuroxime) or 3rd-generation cephalosporin or fluoroquinolone (ciprofloxacin) if the child is known to be colonized with cefazolin-resistant, TMP/SMX-resistant strains.	4–5 mg/kg	N/A
Open or laparoscopic surgery Enteric gram-negative bacilli, enterococci	Cefazolin	30 mg/kg	4

D. SURGICAL/PROCEDURE PROPHYLAXIS[42–53] (continued)

Procedure/Operation	Recommended Agents	Preoperative Dose	Intraoperative Re-dosing Interval (h) for Prolonged Surgery
Head and Neck Surgery			
Assuming incision through respiratory tract mucosa Anaerobes, enteric gram-negative bacilli, *S aureus*	Clindamycin, OR	10 mg/kg	6
	Cefazolin and metronidazole	30 mg/kg cefazolin and 10 mg/kg metronidazole	4 for cefazolin 8 for metronidazole
	Ampicillin/sulbactam if enteric gram-negative bacilli a concern	50 mg/kg of ampicillin	3
Neurosurgery			
Craniotomy, ventricular shunt placement *S epidermidis, S aureus*	Cefazolin, OR	30 mg/kg	4
	Vancomycin, if MRSA likely	15 mg/kg	8
Orthopedic			
Internal fixation of fractures, spinal rod placement, prosthetic joints *S epidermidis, S aureus*	Cefazolin, OR	30 mg/kg	4
	Vancomycin, if MRSA likely[52]	15 mg/kg	8

Trauma			
Exceptionally varied; no prospective, comparative data in children; agents should focus on skin flora (*S epidermidis, S aureus*) as well as the flora inoculated into the wound, based on the trauma exposure, that may include enteric gram-negative bacilli, anaerobes (including *Clostridia* spp), and fungi. Cultures at time of wound exploration are critical to focus therapy for potential pathogens inoculated into the wound.	Cefazolin (for skin), OR	30 mg/kg	4
	Vancomycin (for skin), if MRSA likely, OR	15 mg/kg	8
	Meropenem OR imipenem (for anaerobes, including *Clostridia* spp, and non-fermenting gram-negative bacilli), OR	20 mg/kg for either	4
	Gentamicin and metronidazole (for non-fermenting gram-negative bacilli and anaerobes, including *Clostridia* spp), OR	2.5 mg/kg gentamicin and 10 mg/kg metronidazole	6 for gentamicin 8 for metronidazole
	Piperacillin/tazobactam	100 mg/kg piperacillin component	2

Appendix

Nomogram for Determining Body Surface Area

Based on the nomogram shown below, a straight line joining the patient's height and weight will intersect the center column at the calculated body surface area (BSA). For children of normal height and weight, the child's weight in pounds is used, and then the examiner reads across to the corresponding BSA in meters. Alternatively, Mosteller's formula can be used.

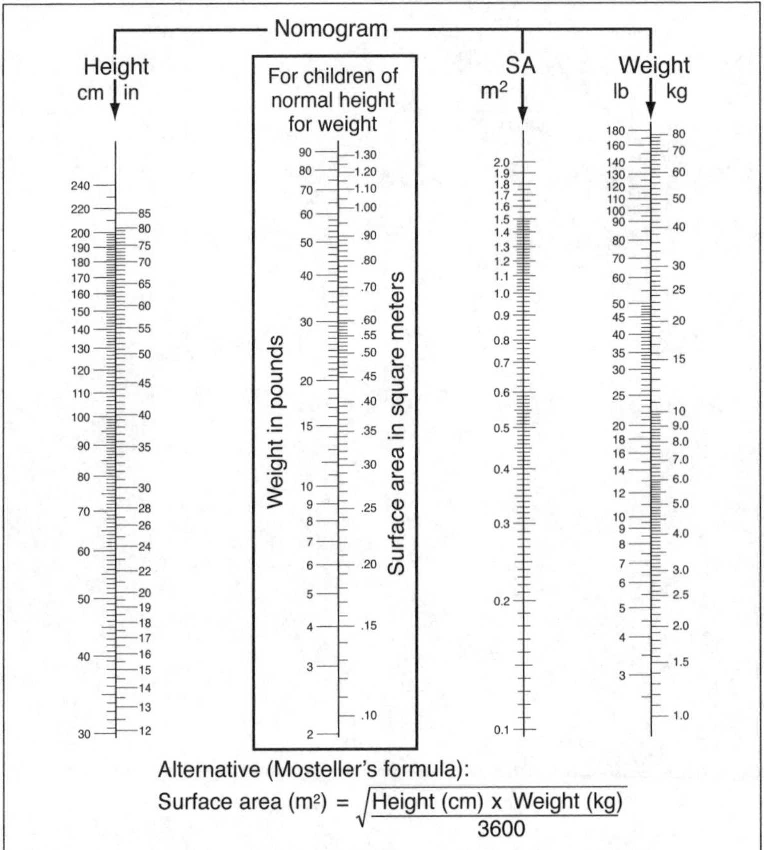

$$\text{Surface area (m}^2\text{)} = \sqrt{\frac{\text{Height (cm)} \times \text{Weight (kg)}}{3600}}$$

Nomogram and equation to determine body surface area. (From Engorn B, Flerlage J, eds. *The Harriet Lane Handbook*. 20th ed. Philadelphia, PA: Elsevier Mosby; 2015. Reprinted with permission from Elsevier.)

References

Chapter 1

1. Cannavino CR, et al. *Pediatr Infect Dis J.* 2016;35(7):752–759 PMID: 27093162
2. Smyth AR, et al. *Cochrane Database Syst Rev.* 2017;3:CD002009 PMID: 28349527
3. Wirth S, et al. *Pediatr Infect Dis J.* 2018;37(8):e207–e213 PMID: 29356761
4. Jackson MA, et al. *Pediatrics.* 2016;138(5):e20162706 PMID: 27940800
5. Bradley JS, et al. *Pediatrics.* 2014;134(1):e146–e153 PMID: 24918220

Chapter 2

1. Cornely OA, et al. *Clin Infect Dis.* 2007;44(10):1289–1297 PMID: 17443465
2. Lestner JM, et al. *Antimicrob Agents Chemother.* 2016;60(12):7340–7346 PMID: 27697762
3. Seibel NL, et al. *Antimicrob Agents Chemother.* 2017;61(2):e01477–16 PMID: 27855062
4. Azoulay E, et al. *PLoS One.* 2017;12(5):e0177093 PMID: 28531175
5. Ascher SB, et al. *Pediatr Infect Dis J.* 2012;31(5):439–443 PMID: 22189522
6. Piper L, et al. *Pediatr Infect Dis J.* 2011;30(5):375–378 PMID: 21085048
7. Gerhart JG, et al. *CPT Pharmacometrics Syst Pharmacol.* 2019;8(7):500–510 PMID: 31087536
8. Watt KM, et al. *Antimicrob Agents Chemother.* 2015;59(7):3935–3943 PMID: 25896706
9. Watt KM, et al. *CPT Pharmacometrics Syst Pharmacol.* 2018;7(10):629–637 PMID: 30033691
10. Friberg LE, et al. *Antimicrob Agents Chemother.* 2012;56(6):3032–3042 PMID: 22430956
11. Zembles TN, et al. *Pharmacotherapy.* 2016;36(10):1102–1108 PMID: 27548272
12. Moriyama B, et al. *Clin Pharmacol Ther.* 2016 PMID: 27981572
13. Maertens JA, et al. *Lancet.* 2016;387(10020):760–769 PMID: 26684607
14. Marty FM, et al. *Lancet Infect Dis.* 2016;16(7):828–837 PMID: 26969258
15. Smith PB, et al. *Pediatr Infect Dis J.* 2009;28(5):412–415 PMID: 19319022
16. Hope WW, et al. *Antimicrob Agents Chemother.* 2010;54(6):2633–2637 PMID: 20308367
17. Benjamin DK Jr, et al. *Clin Pharmacol Ther.* 2010;87(1):93–99 PMID: 19890251
18. Cohen-Wolkowiez M, et al. *Clin Pharmacol Ther.* 2011;89(5):702–707 PMID: 21412233
19. Roilides E, et al. *Pediatr Infect Dis J.* 2019;38(3):275–279 PMID: 30418357

Chapter 4

1. Hultén KG, et al. *Pediatr Infect Dis J.* 2018;37(3):235–241 PMID: 28859018
2. Liu C, et al. *Clin Infect Dis.* 2011;52(3):e18–e55 PMID: 21208910
3. Le J, et al. *Pediatr Infect Dis J.* 2013;32(4):e155–e163 PMID: 23340565
4. McNeil JC, et al. *Pediatr Infect Dis J.* 2016;35(3):263–268 PMID: 26646549
5. Sader HS, et al. *Antimicrob Agents Chemother.* 2017;61(9):e01043-17 PMID: 28630196
6. Depardieu F, et al. *Clin Microbiol Rev.* 2007;20(1):79–114 PMID: 17223624
7. Miller LG, et al. *N Engl J Med.* 2015;372(12):1093–1103 PMID: 25785967
8. Bradley J, et al. *Pediatrics.* 2017;139(3):e20162477 PMID: 28202770
9. Arrieta AC, et al. *Pediatr Infect Dis J.* 2018;37(9):890–900 PMID: 29406465
10. Korczowski B, et al. *Pediatr Infect Dis J.* 2016;35(8):e239–e247 PMID: 27164462
11. Cannavino CR, et al. *Pediatr Infect Dis J.* 2016;35(7):752–759 PMID: 27093162
12. Blumer JL, et al. *Pediatr Infect Dis J.* 2016;35(7):760–766 PMID: 27078119
13. Huang JT, et al. *Pediatrics.* 2009;123(5):e808–e814 PMID: 19403473
14. Finnell SM, et al. *Clin Pediatr (Phila).* 2015;54(5):445–450 PMID: 25385929
15. Kaplan SL, et al. *Clin Infect Dis.* 2014;58(5):679–682 PMID: 24265356
16. McNeil JC, et al. *Curr Infect Dis Rep.* 2019;21(4):12 PMID: 30859379

Chapter 5

1. Fox E, et al. Drug therapy in neonates and pediatric patients. In: Atkinson AJ, et al, eds. *Principles of Clinical Pharmacology.* 2007:359–373
2. Wagner CL, et al. *J Perinatol.* 2000;20(6):346–350 PMID: 11002871
3. Bradley JS, et al. *Pediatrics.* 2009;123(4):e609–e613 PMID: 19289450
4. Martin E, et al. *Eur J Pediatr.* 1993;152(6):530–534 PMID: 8335024
5. Zikic A, et al. *J Pediatric Infect Dis Soc.* 2018;7(3):e107–e115 PMID: 30007329
6. AAP. Chlamydial infections. In: Kimberlin DW, et al, eds. *Red Book: 2018–2021 Report of the Committee on Infectious Diseases.* 31st ed. 2018:273–274
7. Honein MA, et al. *Lancet.* 1999;354(9196):2101–2105 PMID: 10609814
8. Hammerschlag MR, et al. *Pediatr Infect Dis J.* 1998;17(11):1049–1050 PMID: 9849993
9. Abdellatif M, et al. *Eur J Pediatr.* 2019;178(3):301–314 PMID: 30470884
10. Laga M, et al. *N Engl J Med.* 1986;315(22):1382–1385 PMID: 3095641
11. Workowski KA, et al. *MMWR Recomm Rep.* 2015;64(RR-3):1–137 PMID: 26042815
12. Newman LM, et al. *Clin Infect Dis.* 2007;44(S3):S84–S101 PMID: 17342672
13. MacDonald N, et al. *Adv Exp Med Biol.* 2008;609:108–130 PMID: 18193661
14. AAP. Gonococcal infections. In: Kimberlin DW, et al, eds. *Red Book: 2018-2021 Report of the Committee on Infectious Diseases.* 31st ed. 2018:355–365
15. Cimolai N. *Am J Ophthalmol.* 2006;142(1):183–184 PMID: 16815280
16. Marangon FB, et al. *Am J Ophthalmol.* 2004;137(3):453–458 PMID: 15013867
17. AAP. Coagulase-negative staphylococcal infections. In: Kimberlin DW, et al, eds. *Red Book: 2018–2021 Report of the Committee on Infectious Diseases.* 31st ed. 2018:746–748
18. Brito DV, et al. *Braz J Infect Dis.* 2003;7(4):234–235 PMID: 14533982
19. Chen CJ, et al. *Am J Ophthalmol.* 2008;145(6):966–970 PMID: 18378213
20. Shah SS, et al. *J Perinatol.* 1999;19(6pt1):462–465 PMID: 10685281
21. Kimberlin DW, et al. *J Pediatr.* 2003;143(1):16–25 PMID: 12915819
22. Kimberlin DW, et al. *J Infect Dis.* 2008;197(6):836–845 PMID: 18279073
23. AAP. Cytomegalovirus infection. In: Kimberlin DW, et al, eds. *Red Book: 2018–2021 Report of the Committee on Infectious Diseases.* 31st ed. 2018:310–317
24. Kimberlin DW, et al. *N Engl J Med.* 2015;372(10):933–943 PMID: 25738669
25. Rawlinson WD, et al. *Lancet Infect Dis.* 2017;17(6):e177–e188 PMID: 28291720
26. Marsico C, et al. *J Infect Dis.* 2019;219(9):1398–1406 PMID: 30535363
27. AAP. Candidiasis. In: Kimberlin DW, et al, eds. *Red Book: 2018–2021 Report of the Committee on Infectious Diseases.* 31st ed. 2018:263–269
28. Hundalani S, et al. *Expert Rev Anti Infect Ther.* 2013;11(7):709–721 PMID: 23829639
29. Saez-Llorens X, et al. *Antimicrob Agents Chemother.* 2009;53(3):869–875 PMID: 19075070
30. Ericson JE, et al. *Clin Infect Dis.* 2016;63(5):604–610 PMID: 27298330
31. Smith PB, et al. *Pediatr Infect Dis J.* 2009;28(5):412–415 PMID: 19319022
32. Wurthwein G, et al. *Antimicrob Agents Chemother.* 2005;49(12):5092–5098 PMID: 16304177
33. Heresi GP, et al. *Pediatr Infect Dis J.* 2006;25(12):1110–1115 PMID: 17133155
34. Kawaguchi C, et al. *Pediatr Int.* 2009;51(2):220–224 PMID: 19405920
35. Hsieh E, et al. *Early Hum Dev.* 2012;88(S2):S6–S10 PMID: 22633516
36. Pappas PG, et al. *Clin Infect Dis.* 2016;62(4):e1–e50 PMID: 26679628
37. Hwang MF, et al. *Antimicrob Agents Chemother.* 2017;61(12):e01352-17 PMID: 28893774
38. Watt KM, et al. *Antimicrob Agents Chemother.* 2015;59(7):3935–3943 PMID: 25896706
39. Ascher SB, et al. *Pediatr Infect Dis J.* 2012;31(5):439–443 PMID: 22189522
40. Swanson JR, et al. *Pediatr Infect Dis J.* 2016;35(5):519–523 PMID: 26835970
41. Santos RP, et al. *Pediatr Infect Dis J.* 2007;26(4):364–366 PMID: 17414408
42. Frankenbusch K, et al. *J Perinatol.* 2006;26(8):511–514 PMID: 16871222
43. Thomas L, et al. *Expert Rev Anti Infect Ther.* 2009;7(4):461–472 PMID: 19400765
44. Verweij PE, et al. *Drug Resist Updat.* 2015;21–22:30–40 PMID: 26282594
45. Shah D, et al. *Cochrane Database Syst Rev.* 2012;8:CD007448 PMID: 22895960
46. Brook I. *Am J Perinatol.* 2008;25(2):111–118 PMID: 18236362
47. Denkel LA, et al. *PLoS One.* 2016;11(6):e0158136 PMID: 27332554

48. Cohen-Wolkowiez M, et al. *Clin Infect Dis.* 2012;55(11):1495–1502 PMID: 22955430
49. Jost T, et al. *PLoS One.* 2012;7(8):e44595 PMID: 22957008
50. Dilli D, et al. *J Pediatr.* 2015;166(3):545–551 PMID: 25596096
51. van den Akker CHP, et al. *J Pediatr Gastroenterol Nutr.* 2018;67(1):103–122 PMID: 29384838
52. AAP. *Salmonella* infections. In: Kimberlin DW, et al, eds. *Red Book: 2018–2021 Report of the Committee on Infectious Diseases.* 31st ed. 2018:711–718
53. Pinninti SG, et al. *Pediatr Clin North Am.* 2013;60(2):351–365 PMID: 23481105
54. AAP. Herpes simplex. In: Kimberlin DW, et al, eds. *Red Book: 2018–2021 Report of the Committee on Infectious Diseases.* 31st ed. 2018:437–449,460
55. Jones CA, et al. *Cochrane Database Syst Rev.* 2009;(3):CD004206 PMID: 19588350
56. Kimberlin DW, et al. *N Engl J Med.* 2011;365(14):1284–1292 PMID: 21991950
57. Sampson MR, et al. *Pediatr Infect Dis J.* 2014;33(1):42–49 PMID: 24346595
58. Panel on Antiretroviral Therapy and Medical Management of Children Living with HIV. Guidelines for the use of antiretroviral agents in pediatric HIV infection. http://aidsinfo.nih.gov/ContentFiles/PediatricGuidelines.pdf. Updated September 12, 2019. Accessed October 10, 2019
59. Panel on Treatment of Pregnant Women with HIV Infection and Prevention of Perinatal Transmission. Recommendations for the use of antiretroviral drugs in pregnant women with HIV infection and interventions to reduce perinatal HIV transmission in the United States. http://aidsinfo.nih.gov/guidelines/html/3/perinatal-guidelines/0. Updated December 7, 2018. Accessed October 10, 2019
60. Nielsen-Saines K, et al. *N Engl J Med.* 2012;366(25):2368–2379 PMID: 22716975
61. Luzuriaga K, et al. *N Engl J Med.* 2015;372(8):786–788 PMID: 25693029
62. AAP Committee on Infectious Diseases. *Pediatrics.* 2019;144(4):e20192478 PMID: 31477606
63. Acosta EP, et al. *J Infect Dis.* 2010;202(4):563–566 PMID: 20594104
64. McPherson C, et al. *J Infect Dis.* 2012;206(6):847–850 PMID: 22807525
65. Kamal MA, et al. *Clin Pharmacol Ther.* 2014;96(3):380–389 PMID: 24865390
66. Kimberlin DW, et al. *J Infect Dis.* 2013;207(5):709–720 PMID: 23230059
67. Bradley JS, et al. *Pediatrics.* 2017;140(5):e20162727 PMID: 29051331
68. Hayden FG, et al. *N Engl J Med.* 2018;379(10):913–923 PMID: 30184455
69. Fraser N, et al. *Acta Paediatr.*2006;95(5):519–522 PMID: 16825129
70. Ulloa-Gutierrez R, et al. *Pediatr Emerg Care.* 2005;21(9):600–602 PMID: 16160666
71. Sawardekar KP. *Pediatr Infect Dis J.* 2004;23(1):22–26 PMID: 14743041
72. Bingol-Kologlu M, et al. *J Pediatr Surg.* 2007;42(11):1892–1897 PMID: 18022442
73. Brook I. *J Perinat Med.* 2002;30(3):197–208 PMID: 12122901
74. Kaplan SL. *Adv Exp Med Biol.* 2009;634:111–120 PMID: 19280853
75. Korakaki E, et al. *Jpn J Infect Dis.* 2007;60(2-3):129–131 PMID: 17515648
76. Dessi A, et al. *J Chemother.* 2008;20(5):542–550 PMID: 19028615
77. Berkun Y, et al. *Arch Dis Child.* 2008;93(8):690–694 PMID: 18337275
78. Greenberg D, et al. *Paediatr Drugs.* 2008;10(2):75–83 PMID: 18345717
79. Ismail EA, et al. *Pediatr Int.* 2013;55(1):60–64 PMID: 23039834
80. Megged O, et al. *J Pediatr.* 2018;196:319 PMID: 29428272
81. Engle WD, et al. *J Perinatol.* 2000;20(7):421–426 PMID: 11076325
82. Brook I. *Microbes Infect.* 2002;4(12):1271–1280 PMID: 12467770
83. Darville T. *Semin Pediatr Infect Dis.* 2005;16(4):235–244 PMID: 16210104
84. Eberly MD, et al. *Pediatrics.* 2015;135(3):483–488 PMID: 25687145
85. Waites KB, et al. *Semin Fetal Neonatal Med.* 2009;14(4):190–199 PMID: 19109084
86. Morrison W. *Pediatr Infect Dis J.* 2007;26(2):186–188 PMID: 17259889
87. AAP. Pertussis. In: Kimberlin DW, et al, eds. *Red Book: 2018–2021 Report of the Committee on Infectious Diseases.* 31st ed. 2018:620–634
88. Foca MD. *Semin Perinatol.* 2002;26(5):332–339 PMID: 12452505
89. AAP Committee on Infectious Diseases and Bronchiolitis Guidelines Committee. *Pediatrics.* 2014;134(2):e620–e638 PMID: 25070304
90. Banerji A, et al. *CMAJ Open.* 2016;4(4):E623–E633 PMID: 28443266
91. Borse RH, et al. *J Pediatric Infec Dis Soc.* 2014;3(3):201–212 PMID: 26625383
92. Vergnano S, et al. *Pediatr Infect Dis J.* 2011;30(10):850–854 PMID: 21654546

93. Nelson MU, et al. *Semin Perinatol.* 2012;36(6):424–430 PMID: 23177801
94. Lyseng-Williamson KA, et al. *Paediatr Drugs.* 2003;5(6):419–431 PMID: 12765493
95. AAP. Group B streptococcal infections. In: Kimberlin DW, et al, eds. *Red Book: 2018–2021 Report of the Committee on Infectious Diseases.* 31st ed. 2018:762–768,908
96. Schrag S, et al. *MMWR Recomm Rep.* 2002;51(RR-11):1–22 PMID: 12211284
97. AAP. *Ureaplasma urealyticum* infections. In: Kimberlin DW, et al, eds. *Red Book: 2018–2021 Report of the Committee on Infectious Diseases.* 31st ed. 2018:240,867–869
98. AAP. *Ureaplasma parvum* infections. In: Kimberlin DW, et al, eds. *Red Book: 2018–2021 Report of the Committee on Infectious Diseases.* 31st ed. 2018:240,867–869
99. Merchan LM, et al. *Antimicrob Agents Chemother.* 2015;59(1):570–578 PMID: 25385115
100. AAP. *Escherichia coli* and other gram-negative bacilli. In: Kimberlin DW, et al, eds. *Red Book: 2018–2021 Report of the Committee on Infectious Diseases.* 31st ed. 2018:338–344
101. Venkatesh MP, et al. *Expert Rev Anti Infect Ther.* 2008;6(6):929–938 PMID: 19053905
102. Abzug MJ, et al. *J Pediatric Infect Dis Soc.* 2016;5(1):53–62 PMID: 26407253
103. AAP. *Listeria monocytogenes* infections. In: Kimberlin DW, et al, eds. *Red Book: 2018–2021 Report of the Committee on Infectious Diseases.* 31st ed. 2018:511–515
104. Fortunov RM, et al. *Pediatrics.* 2006;118(3):874–881 PMID: 16950976
105. Fortunov RM, et al. *Pediatrics.* 2007;120(5):937–945 PMID: 17974729
106. Riccobene TA, et al. *J Clin Pharmacol.* 2017;57(3):345–355 PMID: 27510635
107. van der Lugt NM, et al. *BMC Pediatr.* 2010;10:84 PMID: 21092087
108. Stauffer WM, et al. *Pediatr Emerg Care.* 2003;19(3):165–166 PMID: 12813301
109. Kaufman DA, et al. *Clin Infect Dis.* 2017;64(10):1387–1395 PMID: 28158439
110. Dehority W, et al. *Pediatr Infect Dis J.* 2006;25(11):1080–1081 PMID: 17072137
111. AAP. Syphilis. In: Kimberlin DW, et al, eds. *Red Book: 2018–2021 Report of the Committee on Infectious Diseases.* 31st ed. 2018:773–778
112. AAP. Tetanus. In: Kimberlin DW, et al, eds. *Red Book: 2018–2021 Report of the Committee on Infectious Diseases.* 31st ed. 2018:793–798
113. AAP. *Toxoplasma gondii* infections. In: Kimberlin DW, et al, eds. *Red Book: 2018–2021 Report of the Committee on Infectious Diseases.* 31st ed. 2018:809–819,1018–1019
114. Petersen E. *Semin Fetal Neonatal Med.* 2007;12(3):214–223 PMID: 17321812
115. Beetz R. *Curr Opin Pediatr.* 2012;24(2):205–211 PMID: 22227782
116. RIVUR Trial Investigators, et al. *N Engl J Med.* 2014;370(25):2367–2376 PMID: 24795142
117. Williams G, et al. *Cochrane Database Syst Rev.* 2019;4:CD001534 PMID: 30932167
118. van Donge T, et al. *Antimicrob Agents Chemother.* 2018;62(4):e02004-17 PMID: 29358294
119. Sahin L, et al. *Clin Pharmacol Ther.* 2016;100(1):23–25 PMID: 27082701
120. Roberts SW, et al. Placental transmission of antibiotics. In: *Glob Libr Women's Med.* https://www.glowm.com/section_view/heading/Placental%20Transmission%20of%20Antibiotics/item/174. Updated June 2008. Accessed October 10, 2019
121. Zhang Z, et al. *Drug Metab Dispos.* 2017;45(8):939–946 PMID: 28049636
122. Pacifici GM. *Int J Clin Pharmacol Ther.* 2006;44(2):57–63 PMID: 16502764
123. Sachs HC, et al. *Pediatrics.* 2013;132(3):e796–e809 PMID: 23979084
124. Hale TW. *Medication and Mothers' Milk 2019: A Manual of Lactational Pharmacology.* 18th ed.
125. Briggs GG, et al. *Drugs in Pregnancy and Lactation.* 11th ed. 2017
126. Ito S, et al. *Am J Obstet Gynecol.* 1993;168(5):1393–1399 PMID: 8498418

Chapter 6

1. Hultén KG, et al. *Pediatr Infect Dis J.* 2018;37(3):235–241 PMID: 28859018
2. Spaulding AB, et al. *Infect Control Hosp Epidemiol.* 2018;39(12):1487–1490 PMID: 30370879
3. Stevens DL, et al. *Clin Infect Dis.* 2014;59(2):147–159 PMID: 24947530
4. Liu C, et al. *Clin Infect Dis.* 2011;52(3):e18–e55 PMID: 21208910
5. Elliott DJ, et al. *Pediatrics.* 2009;123(6):e959–e966 PMID: 19470525
6. Walker PC, et al. *Laryngoscope.* 2013;123(1):249–252 PMID: 22952027
7. Shorbatli LA, et al. *Int J Clin Pharm.* 2018;40(6):1458–1461 PMID: 30446895

8. AAP. *Staphylococcus aureus*. In: Kimberlin DW, et al, eds. *Red Book: 2018–2021 Report of the Committee on Infectious Diseases.* 31st ed. 2018:733–746
9. AAP. Group A streptococcal infections. In: Kimberlin DW, et al, eds. *Red Book: 2018–2021 Report of the Committee on Infectious Diseases.* 31st ed. 2018:748–762
10. Bass JW, et al. *Pediatr Infect Dis J.* 1998;17(6):447–452 PMID: 9655532
11. Hatzenbuehler LA, et al. *Pediatr Infect Dis J.* 2014;33(1):89–91 PMID: 24346597
12. Lindeboom JA. *J Oral Maxillofac Surg.* 2012;70(2):345–348 PMID: 21741739
13. Zimmermann P, et al. *J Infect.* 2017;74(Suppl1):S136–S142 PMID: 28646953
14. Tebruegge M, et al. *PLoS One.* 2016;26;11(1):e0147513 PMID: 26812154
15. Nahid P, et al. *Clin Infect Dis.* 2016;63(7):e147–e195 PMID: 27516382
16. AAP. Tuberculosis. In: Kimberlin DW, et al, eds. *Red Book: 2018–2021 Report of the Committee on Infectious Diseases.* 31st ed. 2018:829–853
17. Bradley JS, et al. *Pediatrics.* 2014;133(5):e1411–e1436 PMID: 24777226
18. Oehler RL, et al. *Lancet Infect Dis.* 2009;9(7):439–447 PMID: 19555903
19. Thomas N, et al. *Expert Rev Anti Infect Ther.* 2011;9(2):215–226 PMID: 21342069
20. Bula-Rudas FJ, et al. *Pediatr Rev.* 2018;39(10):490–500 PMID: 30275032
21. Aziz H, et al. *J Trauma Acute Care Surg.* 2015;78(3):641–648 PMID: 25710440
22. Talan DA, et al. *N Engl J Med.* 1999;340(2):85–92 PMID: 9887159
23. Goldstein EJ, et al. *Antimicrob Agents Chemother.* 2012;56(12):6319–6323 PMID: 23027193
24. AAP. Rabies. In: Kimberlin DW, et al, eds. *Red Book: 2018–2021 Report of the Committee on Infectious Diseases.* 31st ed. 2018:673–680
25. Talan DA, et al. *Clin Infect Dis.* 2003;37(11):1481–1489 PMID: 14614671
26. Miller LG, et al. *N Engl J Med.* 2015;372(12):1093–1103 PMID: 25785967
27. Talan DA, et al. *N Engl J Med.* 2016;374(9):823–832 PMID: 26962903
28. Moran GJ, et al. *JAMA.* 2017;317(20):2088–2096 PMID: 28535235
29. AAP. *Haemophilus influenzae* infections. In: Kimberlin DW, et al, eds. *Red Book: 2018–2021 Report of the Committee on Infectious Diseases.* 31st ed. 2018:367–375,615,628,646
30. Ferreira A, et al. *Infection.* 2016;44(5):607–615 PMID: 27085865
31. Koning S, et al. *Cochrane Database Syst Rev.* 2012;1:CD003261 PMID: 22258953
32. George A, et al. *Br J Gen Pract.* 2003;53(491):480–487 PMID: 12939895
33. Lin HW, et al. *Clin Pediatr (Phila).* 2009;48(6):583–587 PMID: 19286617
34. Pannaraj PS, et al. *Clin Infect Dis.* 2006;43(8):953–960 PMID: 16983604
35. Young BC, et al. *Elife.* 2019;8:e42486 PMID: 30794157
36. Jamal N, et al. *Pediatr Emerg Care.* 2011;27(12):1195–1199 PMID: 22158285
37. Zundel S, et al. *Eur J Pediatr Surg.* 2017;27(2):127–137 PMID: 27380058
38. Totapally BR. *Pediatr Infect Dis J.* 2017;36(7):641–644 PMID: 28005689
39. Levett D, et al. *Cochrane Database Syst Rev.* 2015;1:CD007937 PMID: 25879088
40. Daum RS. *N Engl J Med.* 2007;357(4):380–390 PMID: 17652653
41. Lee MC, et al. *Pediatr Infect Dis J.* 2004;23(2):123–127 PMID: 14872177
42. Karamatsu ML, et al. *Pediatr Emerg Care.* 2012;28(2):131–135 PMID: 22270497
43. Creech CB, et al. *Infect Dis Clin North Am.* 2015;29(3):429–464 PMID: 26311356
44. Elliott SP. *Clin Microbiol Rev.* 2007;20(1):13–22 PMID: 17223620
45. Berk DR, et al. *Pediatr Ann.* 2010;39(10):627–633 PMID: 20954609
46. Braunstein I, et al. *Pediatr Dermatol.* 2014;31(3):305–308 PMID: 24033633
47. Kaplan SL. *Adv Exp Med Biol.* 2009;634:111–120 PMID: 19280853
48. Branson J, et al. *Pediatr Infect Dis J.* 2017;36(3):267–273 PMID: 27870814
49. Keren R, et al. *JAMA Pediatr.* 2015;169(2):120–128 PMID: 25506733
50. McNeil JC, et al. *Pediatr Infect Dis J.* 2017;36(6):572–577 PMID: 28027279
51. Pääkkönen M, et al. *Expert Rev Anti Infect Ther.* 2011;9(12):1125–1131 PMID: 22114963
52. Montgomery NI, et al. *Orthop Clin North Am.* 2017;48(2):209–216 PMID: 28336043
53. Arnold JC, et al. *Pediatrics.* 2012;130(4):e821–e828 PMID: 22966033
54. Chou AC, et al. *J Pediatr Orthop.* 2016;36(2):173–177 PMID: 25929777
55. Delgado-Noguera MF, et al. *Cochrane Database Syst Rev.* 2018;11:CD012125 PMID: 30480764

56. Farrow L. *BMC Musculoskelet Disord.* 2015;16:241 PMID: 26342736
57. Workowski KA, et al. *MMWR Recomm Rep.* 2015;64(RR-03):1–137 PMID: 26042815
58. AAP. Gonococcal infections. In: Kimberlin DW, et al, eds. *Red Book: 2018–2021 Report of the Committee on Infectious Diseases.* 31st ed. 2018:355–365
59. Peltola H, et al. *N Engl J Med.* 2014;370(4):352–360 PMID: 24450893
60. Funk SS, et al. *Orthop Clin North Am.* 2017;48(2):199–208 PMID: 28336042
61. Messina AF, et al. *Pediatr Infect Dis J.* 2011;30(12):1019–1021 PMID: 21817950
62. Howard-Jones AR, et al. *J Paediatr Child Health.* 2013;49(9):760–768 PMID: 23745943
63. Jacqueline C, et al. *J Antimicrob Chemother.* 2014;69(Suppl1):i37–i40 PMID: 25135088
64. Ceroni D, et al. *J Pediatr Orthop.* 2010;30(3):301–304 PMID: 20357599
65. Kok EY, et al. *Antimicrob Agents Chemother*. 2018;62(5):e00084-18 PMID: 29530845
66. Chen CJ, et al. *Pediatr Infect Dis J.* 2007;26(11):985–988 PMID: 17984803
67. Chachad S, et al. *Clin Pediatr (Phila).* 2004;43(3):213–216 PMID: 15094944
68. Volk A, et al. *Pediatr Emerg Care.* 2017;33(11):724–729 PMID: 26785095
69. Jackson MA, et al. *Pediatrics.* 2016;138(5):e20162706 PMID: 27940800
70. McKenna D, et al. *Clin Case Rep.* 2019;7(3):593–594 PMID: 30899507
71. Seltz LB, et al. *Pediatrics.* 2011;127(3):e566–e572 PMID: 21321025
72. Peña MT, et al. *JAMA Otolaryngol Head Neck Surg.* 2013;139(3):223–227 PMID: 23429877
73. Smith JM, et al. *Am J Ophthalmol.* 2014;158(2):387–394 PMID: 24794092
74. Wald ER. *Pediatr Rev.* 2004;25(9):312–320 PMID: 15342822
75. Sheikh A, et al. *Cochrane Database Syst Rev.* 2012;9:CD001211 PMID: 22972049
76. Williams L, et al. *J Pediatr.* 2013;162(4):857–861 PMID: 23092529
77. Pichichero ME. *Clin Pediatr (Phila).* 2011;50(1):7–13 PMID: 20724317
78. Wilhelmus KR. *Cochrane Database Syst Rev.* 2015;1:CD002898 PMID: 25879115
79. Liu S, et al. *Ophthalmology.* 2012;119(10):2003–2008 PMID: 22796308
80. Young RC, et al. *Arch Ophthalmol.* 2010;128(9):1178–1183 PMID: 20837803
81. Azher TN, et al. *Clin Opthalmol.* 2017;11:185–191 PMID: 28176902
82. Khan S, et al. *J Pediatr Ophthalmol Strabismus.* 2014;51(3):140–153 PMID: 24877526
83. Schwartz SG, et al. *Expert Rev Ophthalmol.* 2014;9(5):425–430 PMID: 26609317
84. Pappas PG, et al. *Clin Infect Dis.* 2016;62(4):e1–e50 PMID: 26679628
85. Vishnevskia-Dai V, et al. *Ophthalmology.* 2015;122(4):866–868.e3 PMID: 25556113
86. Nassetta L, et al. *J Antimicrob Chemother.* 2009;63(5):862–867 PMID: 19287011
87. James SH, et al. *Curr Opin Pediatr*. 2016;28(1):81–85 PMID: 26709686
88. Groth A, et al. *Int J Pediatr Otorhinolaryngol.* 2012;76(10):1494–1500 PMID: 22832239
89. Loh R, et al. *J Laryngol Otol.* 2018;132(2):96–104 PMID: 28879826
90. Laulajainen-Hongisto A, et al. *Int J Pediatr Otorhinolaryngol.* 2014;78(12):2072–2078 PMID: 25281339
91. Rosenfeld RM, et al. *Otolaryngol Head Neck Surg.* 2014;150(1Suppl):S1–S24 PMID: 24491310
92. Kaushik V, et al. *Cochrane Database Syst Rev.* 2010;(1):CD004740 PMID: 20091565
93. Prentice P. *Arch Dis Child Educ Pract Ed.* 2015;100(4):197 PMID: 26187983
94. Hoberman A, et al. *N Engl J Med.* 2011;364(2):105–115 PMID: 21226576
95. Tähtinen PA, et al. *N Engl J Med.* 2011;364(2):116–126 PMID: 21226577
96. Lieberthal AS, et al. *Pediatrics.* 2013;131(3):e964–e999 PMID: 23439909
97. Venekamp RP, et al. *Cochrane Database Syst Rev*. 2015;(6):CD000219 PMID: 26099233
98. Shaikh N, et al. *J Pediatr*. 2017;189:54–60.e3 PMID: 28666536
99. Wald ER, et al. *Pediatr Infect Dis J*. 2018;37(12):1255–1257 PMID: 29570583
100. Van Dyke MK, et al. *Pediatr Infect Dis J.* 2017;36(3):274–281 PMID: 27918383
101. Levy C, et al. *PLoS One.* 2019;14(2):e0211712 PMID: 30707730
102. Olarte L, et al. *J Clin Microbiol.* 2017;55(3):724–734 PMID: 27847379
103. Sader HS, et al. *Open Forum Infect Dis.* 2019;6(Suppl1):S14–S23 PMID: 30895211
104. Kutz JW Jr, et al. *Expert Opin Pharmacother.* 2013;14(17):2399–2405 PMID: 24093464
105. Haynes DS, et al. *Otolaryngol Clin North Am.* 2007;40(3):669–683 PMID: 17544701
106. Wald ER, et al. *Pediatrics.* 2009;124(1):9–15 PMID: 19564277
107. Wald ER, et al. *Pediatrics.* 2013;132(1):e262–e280 PMID: 23796742
108. Shaikh N, et al. *Cochrane Database Syst Rev*. 2014;(10):CD007909 PMID: 25347280

109. Chow AW, et al. *Clin Infect Dis.* 2012;54(8):e72–e112 PMID: 22438350
110. Brook I. *Int J Pediatr Otorhinolaryngol.* 2016;84:21–26 PMID: 27063747
111. Ogle OE. *Dent Clin North Am.* 2017;61(2):235–252 PMID: 28317564
112. Cope AL, et al. *Cochrane Database Syst Rev.* 2018;9:CD010136 PMID: 30259968
113. AAP. Diphtheria. In: Kimberlin DW, et al, eds. *Red Book: 2018–2021 Report of the Committee on Infectious Diseases.* 31st ed. 2018:319–323
114. Wheeler DS, et al. *Pediatr Emerg Care.* 2008;24(1):46–49 PMID: 18212612
115. Sobol SE, et al. *Otolaryngol Clin North Am.* 2008;41(3):551–566 PMID: 18435998
116. Nasser M, et al. *Cochrane Database Syst Rev.* 2008;(4):CD006700 PMID: 18843726
117. Amir J, et al. *BMJ.* 1997;314(7097):1800–1803 PMID: 9224082
118. Kimberlin DW, et al. *Clin Infect Dis.* 2010;50(2):221–228 PMID: 20014952
119. Riordan T. *Clin Microbiol Rev.* 2007;20(4):622–659 PMID: 17934077
120. Jariwala RH, et al. *Pediatr Infect Dis J.* 2017;36(4):429–431 PMID: 27977559
121. Ridgway JM, et al. *Am J Otolaryngol.* 2010;31(1):38–45 PMID: 19944898
122. Osowicki J, et al. *J Infect.* 2017;74(Suppl1):S47–S53 PMID: 28646962
123. Agrafiotis M, et al. *Am J Emerg Med.* 2015;33(5):733.e3–733.e4 PMID: 25455045
124. Baldassari CM, et al. *Otolaryngol Head Neck Surg.* 2011;144(4):592–595 PMID: 21493241
125. Hur K, et al. *Laryngoscope.* 2018;128(1):72–77 PMID: 28561258
126. Shulman ST, et al. *Clin Infect Dis.* 2012;55(10):e86–e102 PMID: 22965026
127. Gerber MA, et al. *Circulation.* 2009;119(11):1541–1551 PMID: 19246689
128. AAP. Group A streptococcal infections. In: Kimberlin DW, et al, eds. *Red Book: 2018–2021 Report of the Committee on Infectious Diseases.* 31st ed. 2018:754–755
129. Casey JR, et al. *Diagn Microbiol Infect Dis.* 2007;57(3Suppl):39S–45S PMID: 17292576
130. Altamimi S, et al. *Cochrane Database Syst Rev.* 2012;8:CD004872 PMID: 22895944
131. Abdel-Haq N, et al. *Pediatr Infect Dis J.* 2012;31(7):696–699 PMID: 22481424
132. Cheng J, et al. *Otolaryngol Head Neck Surg.* 2013;148(6):1037–1042 PMID: 23520072
133. Brown NK, et al. *Pediatr Infect Dis J.* 2015;34(4):454–456 PMID: 25760568
134. Shargorodsky J, et al. *Laryngoscope.* 2010;120(12):2498–2501 PMID: 21108480
135. Casazza G, et al. *Otolaryngol Head Neck Surg.* 2019;160(3):546–549 PMID: 30348058
136. Lemaître C, et al. *Pediatr Infect Dis J.* 2013;32(10):1146–1149 PMID: 23722529
137. Bender JM, et al. *Clin Infect Dis.* 2008;46(9):1346–1352 PMID: 18419434
138. Ramgopal S, et al. *Pediatr Emerg Care.* 2017;33(2):112–115 PMID: 26785088
139. Brook I. *J Chemother.* 2016;28(3):143–150 PMID: 26365224
140. Agarwal R, et al. *Expert Rev Respir Med.* 2016;10(12):1317–1334 PMID: 27744712
141. Agarwal R, et al. *Eur Respir J.* 2018;52(3):1801159 PMID: 30049743
142. Agarwal R, et al. *Chest.* 2018;153(3):656–664 PMID: 29331473
143. Meissner HC. *N Engl J Med.* 2016;374(1):62–72 PMID: 26735994
144. Zobell JT, et al. *Pediatr Pulmonol.* 2013;48(2):107–122 PMID: 22949297
145. Hahn A, et al. *J Pediatr Pharmacol Ther.* 2018;23(5):379–389 PMID: 30429692
146. Chmiel JF, et al. *Ann Am Thorac Soc.* 2014;11(7):1120–1129 PMID: 25102221
147. Flume PA, et al. *Am J Respir Crit Care Med.* 2009;180(9):802–808 PMID: 19729669
148. Cogen JD, et al. *Pediatrics.* 2017;139(2):e20162642 PMID: 28126911
149. Mayer-Hamblett N, et al. *Pediatr Pulmonol.* 2013;48(10):943–953 PMID: 23818295
150. Chmiel JF, et al. *Ann Am Thorac Soc.* 2014;11(8):1298–1306 PMID: 25167882
151. Waters V, et al. *Cochrane Database Syst Rev.* 2016;12:CD010004 PMID: 28000919
152. Smith S, et al. *Cochrane Database Syst Rev.* 2018;10:CD008319 PMID: 30376155
153. Lahiri T, et al. *Pediatrics.* 2016;137(4):e20151784 PMID: 27009033
154. Waters V, et al. *Cochrane Database Syst Rev.* 2017;6:CD006961 PMID: 28628280
155. Langton Hewer SC, et al. *Cochrane Database Syst Rev.* 2017;4:CD004197 PMID: 28440853
156. Smith S, et al. *Cochrane Database Syst Rev.* 2018;3:CD001021 PMID: 29607494
157. Flume PA, et al. *J Cyst Fibros.* 2016;15(6):809–815 PMID: 27233377
158. Mogayzel PJ Jr, et al. *Am J Respir Crit Care Med.* 2013;187(7):680–689 PMID: 23540878
159. Southern KW, et al. *Cochrane Database Syst Rev.* 2012;11:CD002203 PMID: 23152214
160. Conole D, et al. *Drugs.* 2014;74(3):377–387 PMID: 24510624

161. AAP. Pertussis. In: Kimberlin DW, et al, eds. *Red Book: 2018–2021 Report of the Committee on Infectious Diseases*. 31st ed. 2018:620–634
162. Altunaiji S, et al. *Cochrane Database Syst Rev.* 2007;(3):CD004404 PMID: 17636756
163. Kilgore PE, et al. *Clin Microbiol Rev.* 2016;29(3):449–486 PMID: 27029594
164. Wang K, et al. *Cochrane Database Syst Rev.* 2014;(9):CD003257 PMID: 25243777
165. Jain S, et al. *N Engl J Med.* 2015;372(9):835–845 PMID: 25714161
166. Bradley JS, et al. *Clin Infect Dis.* 2011;53(7):e25–e76 PMID: 21880587
167. Blumer JL, et al. *Pediatr Infect Dis J.* 2016;35(7):760–766 PMID: 27078119
168. Queen MA, et al. *Pediatrics.* 2014;133(1):e23–e29 PMID: 24324001
169. Williams DJ, et al. *JAMA Pediatr.* 2017;171(12):1184–1191 PMID: 29084336
170. Leyenaar JK, et al. *Pediatr Infect Dis J.* 2014;33(4):387–392 PMID: 24168982
171. Bradley JS, et al. *Pediatr Infect Dis J.* 2007;26(10):868–878 PMID: 17901791
172. Hidron AI, et al. *Lancet Infect Dis.* 2009;9(6):384–392 PMID: 19467478
173. Frush JM, et al. *J Hosp Med.* 2018;13(12):848–852 PMID: 30379141
174. Wunderink RG, et al. *Clin Infect Dis.* 2012;54(5):621–629 PMID: 22247123
175. Freifeld AG, et al. *Clin Infect Dis.* 2011;52(4):e56–e93 PMID: 21258094
176. Kalil AC, et al. *Clin Infect Dis.* 2016;63(5):e61–e111 PMID: 27418577
177. Foglia E, et al. *Clin Microbiol Rev.* 2007;20(3):409–425 PMID: 17630332
178. Srinivasan R, et al. *Pediatrics.* 2009;123(4):1108–1115 PMID: 19336369
179. Wood GC, et al. *Ann Pharmacother.* 2017;51(12):1112–1121 PMID: 28778127
180. Gasior AC, et al. *J Pediatr Surg.* 2013;48(6):1312–1315 PMID: 23845624
181. Islam S, et al. *J Pediatr Surg.* 2012;47(11):2101–2110 PMID: 23164006
182. Redden MD, et al. *Cochrane Database Syst Rev.* 2017;3:CD010651 PMID: 28304084
183. Randolph AG, et al. *Clin Infect Dis.* 2019;68(3):365–372 PMID: 29893805
184. AAP. Chlamydial infections. In: Kimberlin DW, et al, eds. *Red Book: 2018–2021 Report of the Committee on Infectious Diseases.* 31st ed. 2018:273–274
185. AAP. Cytomegalovirus infection. In: Kimberlin DW, et al, eds. *Red Book: 2018–2021 Report of the Committee on Infectious Diseases.* 31st ed. 2018:310–317
186. Kotton CN, et al. *Transplantation.* 2018;102(6):900–931 PMID: 29596116
187. Erard V, et al. *Clin Infect Dis.* 2015;61(1):31–39 PMID: 25778751
188. Travi G, et al. *J Intensive Care Med.* 2014;29(4):200–212 PMID: 23753231
189. Danziger-Isakov L, et al. *J Pediatric Infect Dis Soc.* 2018;7(Suppl2):S72–S74 PMID: 30590625
190. AAP. Tularemia. In: Kimberlin DW, et al, eds. *Red Book: 2018–2021 Report of the Committee on Infectious Diseases.* 31st ed. 2018:861–864
191. Galgiani JN, et al. *Clin Infect Dis.* 2016;63(6):e112–e146 PMID: 27470238
192. AAP. Coccidioidomycosis. In: Kimberlin DW, et al, eds. *Red Book: 2018–2021 Report of the Committee on Infectious Diseases.* 31st ed. 2018:294–297
193. AAP. Histoplasmosis. In: Kimberlin DW, et al, eds. *Red Book: 2018–2021 Report of the Committee on Infectious Diseases.* 31st ed. 2018:449–453
194. Wheat LJ, et al. *Clin Infect Dis.* 2007;45(7):807–825 PMID: 17806045
195. Uyeki TM, et al. *Clin Infect Dis.* 2019;68(6):895–902 PMID: 30834445
196. AAP Committee on Infectious Diseases. *Pediatrics.* 2019;144(4):e20192478 PMID: 31477606
197. Kimberlin DW, et al. *J Infect Dis.* 2013;207(5):709–720 PMID: 23230059
198. Ng TM, et al. *PLoS One.* 2016;11(4):e0153696 PMID: 27104951
199. Harris PNA, et al. *JAMA.* 2018;320(10):984–994 PMID: 30208454
200. Johnson MM, et al. *J Thorac Dis.* 2014;6(3):210–220 PMID: 24624285
201. Gardiner SJ. *Cochrane Database Syst Rev.* 2015;1:CD004875 PMID: 25566754
202. Cardinale F, et al. *J Clin Microbiol.* 2013;51(2):723–724 PMID: 23224091
203. Panel on Opportunistic Infections in HIV-Exposed and HIV-Infected Children. Guidelines for the prevention and treatment of opportunistic infections in HIV-exposed and HIV-infected children. https://aidsinfo.nih.gov/contentfiles/lvguidelines/oi_guidelines_pediatrics.pdf. Updated November 5, 2018. Accessed October 10, 2019
204. Caselli D, et al. *J Pediatr.* 2014;164(2):389–392.e1 PMID: 24252793
205. Rafailidis PI, et al. *Curr Opin Infect Dis.* 2014;27(6):479–483 PMID: 25259809

206. Micek ST, et al. *Medicine (Baltimore)*. 2011;90(6):390–395 PMID: 22033455
207. Micek ST, et al. *Crit Care*. 2015;19:219 PMID: 25944081
208. AAP. Respiratory syncytial virus. In: Kimberlin DW, et al, eds. *Red Book: 2018–2021 Report of the Committee on Infectious Diseases*. 31st ed. 2018:682–692
209. Villarino ME, et al. *JAMA Pediatr*. 2015;169(3):247–255 PMID: 25580725
210. Scarfone R, et al. *J Pediatr*. 2017;187:200–205.e1 PMID: 28526220
211. Aronson PL, et al. *Pediatrics*. 2018;142(6):e20181879 PMID: 30425130
212. Aronson PL, et al. *Pediatrics*. 2019;144(1):e20183604 PMID: 31167938
213. Greenhow TL, et al. *Pediatrics*. 2017;139(4):e20162098 PMID: 28283611
214. Pantell RH, et al. *Adv Pediatr*. 2018;65(1):173–208 PMID: 30053923
215. Kuppermann N, et al. *JAMA Pediatr*. 2019;173(4):342–351 PMID: 30776077
216. McMullan BJ, et al. *JAMA Pediatr*. 2016;170(10):979–986 PMID: 27533601
217. Ruiz J, et al. *Minerva Pediatr*. 2018 PMID: 29651827
218. Russell CD, et al. *J Med Microbiol*. 2014;63(Pt6):841–848 PMID: 24623637
219. Ligon J, et al. *Pediatr Infect Dis J*. 2014;33(5):e132–e134 PMID: 24732394
220. Baddour LM, et al. *Circulation*. 2015;132(15):1435–1486 [Erratum: *Circulation*. 2015;132(17):e215. Erratum: *Circulation*. 2016;134(8):e113] PMID: 26373316
221. Baltimore RS, et al. *Circulation*. 2015;132(15):1487–1515 PMID: 26373317
222. Russell HM, et al. *Ann Thorac Surg*. 2013;96(1):171–174 PMID: 23602067
223. Sharma A, et al. *JACC Cardiovasc Interv*. 2017;10(14):1449–1458 PMID: 28728659
224. Dixon G, et al. *Curr Opin Infect Dis*. 2017;30(3):257–267 PMID: 28319472
225. Pappas PG, et al. *Clin Infect Dis*. 2016;62(4):e1–e50 PMID: 26679628
226. Wilson W, et al. *Circulation*. 2007;116(15):1736–1754 PMID: 17446442
227. Sakai Bizmark R, et al. *Am Heart J*. 2017;189:110–119 PMID: 28625367
228. Lutmer JE, et al. *Ann Am Thorac Soc*. 2013;10(3):235–238 PMID: 23802820
229. Abdel-Haq N, et al. *Int J Pediatr*. 2018;2018:5450697 PMID: 30532791
230. Shane AL, et al. *Clin Infect Dis*. 2017;65(12):1963–1973 PMID: 29194529
231. Denno DM, et al. *Clin Infect Dis*. 2012;55(7):897–904 PMID: 22700832
232. Butler T. *Trans R Soc Trop Med Hyg*. 2012;106(7):395–399 PMID: 22579556
233. Freedman SB, et al. *Clin Infect Dis*. 2016;62(10):1251–1258 PMID: 26917812
234. Bennish ML, et al. *Clin Infect Dis*. 2006;42(3):356–362 PMID: 16392080
235. Smith KE, et al. *Pediatr Infect Dis J*. 2012;31(1):37–41 PMID: 21892124
236. Bruyand M, et al. *Med Mal Infect*. 2018;48(3):167–174 PMID: 29054297
237. Tribble DR, et al. *Clin Infect Dis*. 2007;44(3):338–346 PMID: 17205438
238. Ashkenazi S, et al. *Pediatr Infect Dis J*. 2016;35(6):698–700 PMID: 26986771
239. Taylor DN, et al. *J Travel Med*. 2017;24(Suppl1):S17–S22 PMID: 28520998
240. Riddle MS, et al. *J Travel Med*. 2017;24(Suppl1):S57–S74 PMID: 28521004
241. Williams PCM, et al. *Paediatr Int Child Health*. 2018;38(Supp1):S50–S65 PMID: 29790845
242. O'Ryan M, et al. *Expert Rev Anti Infect Ther*. 2010;8(6):671–682 PMID: 20521895
243. Steffen R, et al. *J Travel Med*. 2018;25(1) PMID: 30462260
244. Advice for travelers. *Med Lett Drugs Ther*. 2015;57(1466):52–58 PMID: 25853663
245. Kantele A, et al. *Clin Infect Dis*. 2015;60(6):837–846 PMID: 25613287
246. Riddle MS, et al. *Clin Infect Dis*. 2008;47(8):1007–1014 PMID: 18781873
247. Butler T. *Clin Infect Dis*. 2008;47(8):1015–1016 PMID: 18781871
248. Janda JM, et al. *Clin Microbiol Rev*. 2010;23(1):35–73 PMID: 20065325
249. AAP. *Campylobacter* infections. In: Kimberlin DW, et al, eds. *Red Book: 2018–2021 Report of the Committee on Infectious Diseases*. 31st ed. 2018:260–263,1094
250. Fullerton KE, et al. *Pediatr Infect Dis J*. 2007;26(1):19–24 PMID: 17195700
251. Kirkpatrick BD, et al. *Curr Opin Gastroenterol*. 2011;27(1):1–7 PMID: 21124212
252. Leibovici-Weissman Y, et al. *Cochrane Database Syst Rev*. 2014;6:CD008625 PMID: 24944120
253. Sammons JS, et al. *JAMA Pediatr*. 2013;167(6):567–573 PMID: 23460123
254. AAP. *Clostridium difficile*. In: Kimberlin DW, et al, eds. *Red Book: 2018–2021 Report of the Committee on Infectious Diseases*. 31st ed. 2018:288–292
255. McDonald LC, et al. *Clin Infect Dis*. 2018;66(7):987–994 PMID: 29562266

256. Adams DJ, et al. *J Pediatr*. 2017;186:105–109 PMID: 28396027
257. O'Gorman MA, et al. *J Pediatric Infect Dis Soc*. 2018;7(3):210–218 PMID: 28575523
258. Weng MK, et al. *Epidemiol Infect*. 2019;147:e172 PMID: 31063097
259. Jones NL, et al. *J Pediatr Gastroenterol Nutr*. 2017;64(6):991–1003 PMID: 28541262
260. McColl KE. *N Engl J Med*. 2010;362(17):1597–1604 PMID: 20427808
261. Kalach N, et al. *Ann Gastroenterol*. 2015;28(1):10–18 PMID: 25608573
262. AAP. *Helicobacter pylori* infections. In: Kimberlin DW, et al, eds. *Red Book: 2018–2021 Report of the Committee on Infectious Diseases*. 31st ed. 2018:378–381
263. Fallone CA, et al. *Gastroenterology*. 2016;151(1):51–69.e14 PMID: 27102658
264. Kalach N, et al. *Helicobacter*. 2017;22(Suppl1) PMID: 28891139
265. AAP. *Giardia intestinalis* (formerly *Giardia lamblia* and *Giardia duodenalis*) infections. In: Kimberlin DW, et al, eds. *Red Book: 2018–2021 Report of the Committee on Infectious Diseases*. 31st ed. 2018:249,352–355
266. Bula-Rudas FJ, et al. *Adv Pediatr*. 2015;62(1):29–58 PMID: 26205108
267. Wen SC, et al. *J Paediatr Child Health*. 2017;53(10):936–941 PMID: 28556448
268. AAP. *Salmonella* infections. In: Kimberlin DW, et al, eds. *Red Book: 2018–2021 Report of the Committee on Infectious Diseases*. 31st ed. 2018:711–718
269. Frenck RW Jr, et al. *Clin Infect Dis*. 2004;38(7):951–957 PMID: 15034826
270. Trivedi NA, et al. *J Postgrad Med*. 2012;58(2):112–118 PMID: 22718054
271. Effa EE, et al. *Cochrane Database Syst Rev*. 2011;(10):CD004530 PMID: 21975746
272. Begum B, et al. *Mymensingh Med J*. 2014;23(3):441–448 PMID: 25178594
273. Centers for Disease Control and Prevention. National Antimicrobial Resistance Monitoring System for Enteric Bacteria (NARMS). http://www.cdc.gov/narms/reports/index.html. Reviewed March 15, 2019. Accessed October 10, 2019
274. Christopher PR, et al. *Cochrane Database Syst Rev*. 2010;(8):CD006784 PMID: 20687081
275. AAP. *Shigella* infections. In: Kimberlin DW, et al, eds. *Red Book: 2018–2021 Report of the Committee on Infectious Diseases*. 31st ed. 2018:723–727
276. Abdel-Haq NM, et al. *Pediatr Infect Dis J*. 2000;19(10):954–958 PMID: 11055595
277. Abdel-Haq NM, et al. *Int J Antimicrob Agents*. 2006;27(5):449–452 PMID: 16621458
278. El Qouqa IA, et al. *Int J Infect Dis*. 2011;15(1):e48–e53 PMID: 21131221
279. Yousef Y, et al. *J Pediatr Surg*. 2018;53(2):250–255 PMID: 29223673
280. Marino NE, et al. *Surg Infect (Larchmt)*. 2017;18(8):894–903 PMID: 29064344
281. Chen CY, et al. *Surg Infect (Larchmt)*. 2012;13(6):383–390 PMID: 23231389
282. Solomkin JS, et al. *Clin Infect Dis*. 2010;50(2):133–164 PMID: 20034345
283. Sawyer RG, et al. *N Engl J Med*. 2015;372(21):1996–2005 PMID: 25992746
284. Fraser JD, et al. *J Pediatr Surg*. 2010;45(6):1198–1202 PMID: 20620320
285. Bradley JS, et al. *Pediatr Infect Dis J*. 2001;20(1):19–24 PMID: 11176562
286. Lee JY, et al. *J Pediatr Pharmacol Ther*. 2016;21(2):140–145 PMID: 27199621
287. Hurst AL, et al. *J Pediatric Infect Dis Soc*. 2017;6(1):57–64 PMID: 26703242
288. Kronman MP, et al. *Pediatrics*. 2016;138(1):e20154547 PMID: 27354453
289. Cruz AT, et al. *Int J Tuberc Lung Dis*. 2013;17(2):169–174 PMID: 23317951
290. Hlavsa MC, et al. *Clin Infect Dis*. 2008;47(2):168–175 PMID: 18532886
291. Alrajhi AA, et al. *Clin Infect Dis*. 1998;27(1):52–56 PMID: 9675450
292. Arditi M, et al. *Pediatr Infect Dis J*. 1990;9(6):411–415 PMID: 2367163
293. Sethna CB, et al. *Clin J Am Soc Nephrol*. 2016;11(9):1590–1596 PMID: 27340282
294. Warady BA, et al. *Perit Dial Int*. 2012;32(Suppl2):S32–S86 PMID: 22851742
295. Preece ER, et al. *ANZ J Surg*. 2012;82(4):283–284 PMID: 22510192
296. Workowski K. *Ann Intern Med*. 2013;158(3):ITC2–1 PMID: 23381058
297. Santillanes G, et al. *Pediatr Emerg Care*. 2011;27(3):174–178 PMID: 21346680
298. Gkentzis A, et al. *Ann R Coll Surg Engl*. 2014;96(3):181–183 PMID: 24780779
299. George CRR, et al. *PLoS One*. 2019;14(4):e0213312 PMID: 30943199
300. Wi T, et al. *PLoS Med*. 2017;14(7):e1002344 PMID: 28686231
301. Kirkcaldy RD, et al. *MMWR Surveill Summ*. 2016;65(7):1–19 PMID: 27414503
302. James SH, et al. *Clin Pharmacol Ther*. 2010;88(5):720–724 PMID: 20881952

303. Fife KH, et al. *Sex Transm Dis.* 2008;35(7):668–673 PMID: 18461016
304. Stephenson-Famy A, et al. *Obstet Gynecol Clin North Am.* 2014;41(4):601–614 PMID: 25454993
305. Le Cleach L, et al. *Cochrane Database Syst Rev.* 2014;(8):CD009036 PMID: 25086573
306. Savaris RF, et al. *Sex Transm Infect.* 2019;95(1):21–27 PMID: 30341232
307. Peeling RW, et al. *Nat Rev Dis Primers.* 2017;3:17073 PMID: 29022569
308. Manhart LE, et al. *Clin Infect Dis.* 2015;61(Suppl8):S802–S817 PMID: 26602619
309. Bradshaw CS, et al. *J Infect Dis.* 2016;214(Suppl1):S14–S20 PMID: 27449869
310. Matheson A, et al. *Aust N Z J Obstet Gynaecol.* 2017;57(2):139–145 PMID: 28299777
311. Brander EPA, et al. *CMAJ.* 2018;190(26):E800 PMID: 29970369
312. Jasper JM, et al. *Pediatr Emerg Care.* 2006;22(8):585–586 PMID: 16912629
313. Hansen MT, et al. *J Pediatr Adolesc Gynecol.* 2007;20(5):315–317 PMID: 17868900
314. Brouwer MC, et al. *N Engl J Med.* 2014;371(5):447–456 PMID: 25075836
315. Bonfield CM, et al. *J Infect.* 2015;71(Suppl1):S42–S46 PMID: 25917804
316. Boucher A, et al. *Med Mal Infect.* 2017;47(3):221–235 PMID: 28341533
317. Dalmau J, et al. *N Engl J Med.* 2018;378(9):840–851 PMID: 29490181
318. Abzug MJ, et al. *J Pediatr Infect Dis Soc.* 2016;5(1):53–62 PMID: 26407253
319. Doja A, et al. *J Child Neurol.* 2006;21(5):384–391 PMID: 16901443
320. Gnann JW Jr, et al. *Curr Infect Dis Rep.* 2017;19(3):13 PMID: 28251511
321. Brouwer MC, et al. *Cochrane Database Syst Rev.* 2015;(9):CD004405 PMID: 26362566
322. Fritz D, et al. *Neurology.* 2012;79(22):2177–2179 PMID: 23152589
323. Tunkel AR, et al. *Clin Infect Dis.* 2004;39(9):1267–1284 PMID: 15494903
324. Prasad K, et al. *Cochrane Database Syst Rev.* 2016;4:CD002244 PMID: 27121755
325. James G, et al. *J Neurosurg Pediatr.* 2014;13(1):101–106 PMID: 24206346
326. Tunkel AR, et al. *Clin Infect Dis.* 2017 PMID: 28203777
327. National Institute for Health and Care Excellence. Urinary tract infection in under 16s: diagnosis and management. http://www.nice.org.uk/guidance/CG54. Updated October 2018. Accessed October 10, 2019
328. Montini G, et al. *N Engl J Med.* 2011;365(3):239–250 PMID: 21774712
329. Meesters K, et al. *Antimicrob Agents Chemother.* 2018;62(9):e00517-18 PMID: 29987142
330. Chen WL, et al. *Pediatr Neonatal.* 2015;56(3):176–182 PMID: 25459491
331. Conley SP, et al. *J Emerg Med.* 2014;46(5):624–626 PMID: 24286715
332. Strohmeier Y, et al. *Cochrane Database Syst Rev.* 2014;7:CD003772 PMID: 25066627
333. Perez F, et al. *Clin Infect Dis.* 2015;60(9):1326–1329 PMID: 25586684
334. Tamma PD, et al. *Clin Infect Dis.* 2015;60(9):1319–1325 PMID: 25586681
335. Bocquet N, et al. *Pediatrics.* 2012;129(2):e269–e275 PMID: 22291112
336. AAP Subcommittee on Urinary Tract Infection, Steering Committee on Quality Improvement and Management. *Pediatrics.* 2011;128(3):595–610 PMID: 21873693
337. Craig JC, et al. *N Engl J Med.* 2009;361(18):1748–1759 PMID: 19864673
338. Williams G, et al. *Cochrane Database Syst Rev.* 2019;4:CD001534 PMID: 30932167
339. Hoberman A, et al. *N Engl J Med.* 2014;370(25):2367–2376 PMID: 24795142
340. Craig JC. *J Pediatr.* 2015;166(3):778 PMID: 25722276
341. AAP. Actinomycosis. In: Kimberlin DW, et al, eds. *Red Book: 2018–2021 Report of the Committee on Infectious Diseases.* 31st ed. 2018:205–206
342. Brook I. *South Med J.* 2008;101(10):1019–1023 PMID: 18791528
343. Wacharachaisurapol N, et al. *Pediatr Infect Dis J.* 2017;36(3):e76–e79 PMID: 27870811
344. Biggs HM, et al. *MMWR Recomm Rep.* 2016;65(2):1–44 PMID: 27172113
345. Dahlgren FS, et al. *Am J Trop Med Hyg.* 2015;93(1):66–72 PMID: 25870428
346. AAP. Brucellosis. In: Kimberlin DW, et al, eds. *Red Book: 2018–2021 Report of the Committee on Infectious Diseases.* 31st ed. 2018:255–257
347. Shen MW. *Pediatrics.* 2008;121(5):e1178–e1183 PMID: 18450861
348. Bukhari EE. *Saudi Med J.* 2018;39(4):336–341 PMID: 29619483
349. Yagupsky P. *Adv Exp Med Biol.* 2011;719:123–132 PMID: 22125040
350. Shorbatli LA, et al. *Int J Clin Pharm.* 2018;40(6):1458–1461 PMID: 30446895
351. Zangwill KM. *Adv Exp Med Biol.* 2013;764:159–166 PMID: 23654065

352. Chang CC, et al. *Paediatr Int Child Health*. 2016;36(3):232–234 PMID: 25940800
353. Nichols Heitman K, et al. *Am J Trop Med Hyg*. 2016;94(1):52–60 PMID: 26621561
354. Schutze GE, et al. *Pediatr Infect Dis J*. 2007;26(6):475–479 PMID: 17529862
355. Mukkada S, et al. *Infect Dis Clin North Am*. 2015;29(3):539–555 PMID: 26188606
356. Lehrnbecher T, et al. *J Clin Oncol*. 2017;35(18):2082–2094 PMID: 28459614
357. Freifeld AG, et al. *Clin Infect Dis*. 2011;52(4):e56–e93 PMID: 21258094
358. Miedema KG, et al. *Eur J Cancer*. 2016;53:16–24 PMID: 26700076
359. Payne JR, et al. *J Pediatr*. 2018;193:172–177 PMID: 29229452
360. Son MBF, et al. *Pediatr Rev*. 2018;39(2):78–90 PMID: 29437127
361. Wardle AJ, et al. *Cochrane Database Syst Rev*. 2017;1:CD011188 PMID: 28129459
362. Jone PN, et al. *Pediatr Infect Dis J*. 2018;37(10):976–980 PMID: 29461447
363. McCrindle BW, et al. *Circulation*. 2017;135(17):e927–e999 PMID: 28356445
364. AAP. Leprosy. In: Kimberlin DW, et al, eds. *Red Book: 2018–2021 Report of the Committee on Infectious Diseases*. 31st ed. 2018:504–508
365. Haake DA, et al. *Curr Top Microbiol Immunol*. 2015;387:65–97 PMID: 25388133
366. AAP. Leptospirosis. In: Kimberlin DW, et al, eds. *Red Book: 2018–2021 Report of the Committee on Infectious Diseases*. 31st ed. 2018:508–511
367. AAP. Lyme disease. In: Kimberlin DW, et al, eds. *Red Book: 2018–2021 Report of the Committee on Infectious Diseases*. 31st ed. 2018:195,515–523
368. Shapiro ED. *N Engl J Med*. 2014;370(18):1724–1731 PMID: 24785207
369. Shapiro ED, et al. *JAMA*. 2018;320(7):635–636 PMID: 30073279
370. Wiersinga WJ, et al. *Nat Rev Dis Primers*. 2018;4:17107 PMID: 29388572
371. Chetchotisakd P, et al. *Lancet*. 2014;383(9919):807–814 PMID: 24284287
372. Griffith DE, et al. *Am J Respir Crit Care Med*. 2007;175(4):367–416 [Erratum: *Am J Respir Crit Care Med*. 2007;175(7):744–745] PMID: 17277290
373. Philley JV, et al. *Thorac Surg Clin*. 2019;29(1):65–76 PMID: 30454923
374. Kasperbauer SH, et al. *Clin Chest Med*. 2015;36(1):67–78 PMID: 25676520
375. Kang YA, et al. *Expert Rev Respir Med*. 2016;10(5):557–568 PMID: 26967761
376. Pasipanodya JG, et al. *Antimicrob Agents Chemother*. 2017;61(11):e01206-17 PMID: 28807911
377. Wilson JW. *Mayo Clin Proc*. 2012;87(4):403–407 PMID: 22469352
378. AAP. Nocardiosis. In: Kimberlin DW, et al, eds. *Red Book: 2018–2021 Report of the Committee on Infectious Diseases*. 31st ed. 2018:575–577
379. Butler T. *Clin Infect Dis*. 2009;49(5):736–742 PMID: 19606935
380. Yang R. *J Clin Microbiol*. 2017;56(1):e01519-17 PMID: 29070654
381. Apangu T, et al. *Emerg Infect Dis*. 2017;23(3) PMID: 28125398
382. Kersh GJ. *Expert Rev Anti Infect Ther*. 2013;11(11):1207–1214 PMID: 24073941
383. Anderson A, et al. *MMWR Recomm Rep*. 2013;62(RR-03):1–30 PMID: 23535757
384. Woods CR. *Pediatr Clin North Am*. 2013;60(2):455–470 PMID: 23481111
385. AAP. Rocky Mountain spotted fever. In: Kimberlin DW, et al, eds. *Red Book: 2018–2021 Report of the Committee on Infectious Diseases*. 31st ed. 2018:697–700
386. AAP. Tetanus. In: Kimberlin DW, et al, eds. *Red Book: 2018–2021 Report of the Committee on Infectious Diseases*. 31st ed. 2018:793–798
387. Brook I. *Expert Rev Anti Infect Ther*. 2008;6(3):327–336 PMID: 18588497
388. Adalat S, et al. *Arch Dis Child*. 2014;99(12):1078–1082 PMID: 24790135
389. Low DE. *Crit Care Clin*. 2013;29(3):651–675 PMID: 23830657
390. Harik NS. *Pediatr Ann*. 2013;42(7):288–292 PMID: 23805970

Chapter 7

1. Sáez-Llorens X, et al. *Pediatr Infect Dis J*. 2001;20(3):356–361 PMID: 11303850
2. Rodriguez WJ, et al. *Pediatr Infect Dis*. 1986;5(4):408–415 PMID: 3523457
3. Qureshi ZA, et al. *Clin Infect Dis*. 2015;60(9):1295–1303 PMID: 25632010
4. Hsu AJ, et al. *Clin Infect Dis*. 2014;58(10):1439–1448 PMID: 24501388
5. Shin B, et al. *J Microbiol*. 2017;55(11):837–849 PMID: 29076065
6. Menegucci TC, et al. *Microb Drug Resist*. 2019 PMID: 31216222

7. Wacharachaisurapol N, et al. *Pediatr Infect Dis J*. 2017;36(3):e76–e79 PMID: 27870811
8. Janda JM, et al. *Clin Microbiol Rev*. 2010;23(1):35–73 PMID: 20065325
9. Sharma K, et al. *Ann Clin Microbiol Antimicrob*. 2017;16(1):12 PMID: 28288638
10. Sigurjonsdottir VK, et al. *Diagn Microbiol Infect Dis*. 2017;89(3):230–234 PMID: 29050793
11. Ismail N, et al. *Clin Lab Med*. 2017;37(2):317–340 PMID: 28457353
12. Therriault BL, et al. *Ann Pharmacother*. 2008;42(11):1697–1702 PMID: 18812563
13. Bradley JS, et al. *Pediatrics*. 2014;133(5):e1411–e1436 PMID: 24777226
14. AAP. *Bacillus cereus* infections. In: Kimberlin DW, et al, eds. *Red Book: 2018–2021 Report of the Committee on Infectious Diseases*. 31st ed. 2018:215–220
15. Bottone EJ. *Clin Microbiol Rev*. 2010;23(2):382–398 PMID: 20375358
16. Wexler HM. *Clin Microbiol Rev*. 2007;20(4):593–621 PMID: 17934076
17. Snydman DR, et al. *Anaerobe*. 2017;43:21–26 PMID: 27867083
18. Shorbatli LA, et al. *Int J Clin Pharm*. 2018;40(6):1458–1461 PMID: 30446895
19. Zangwill KM. *Adv Exp Med Biol*. 2013;764:159–166 PMID: 23654065
20. Angelakis E, et al. *Int J Antimicrob Agents*. 2014;44(1):16–25 PMID: 24933445
21. Kilgore PE, et al. *Clin Microbiol Rev*. 2016;29(3):449–486 PMID: 27029594
22. AAP. Pertussis. In: Kimberlin DW, et al, eds. *Red Book: 2018–2021 Report of the Committee on Infectious Diseases*. 31st ed. 2018:620–634
23. Shapiro ED. *N Engl J Med*. 2014;370(18):1724–1731 PMID: 24785207
24. AAP. Lyme disease. In: Kimberlin DW, et al, eds. *Red Book: 2018–2021 Report of the Committee on Infectious Diseases*. 31st ed. 2018:195,515–523
25. Sanchez E, et al. *JAMA*. 2016;315(16):1767–1777 PMID: 27115378
26. AAP. *Borrelia* infections other than Lyme disease. In: Kimberlin DW, et al, eds. *Red Book: 2018–2021 Report of the Committee on Infectious Diseases*. 31st ed. 2018:252–255,1095
27. Dworkin MS, et al. *Infect Dis Clin North Am*. 2008;22(3):449–468 PMID: 18755384
28. AAP. Brucellosis. In: Kimberlin DW, et al, eds. *Red Book: 2018–2021 Report of the Committee on Infectious Diseases*. 31st ed. 2018:255–257
29. Bukhari EE. *Saudi Med J*. 2018;39(4):336–341 PMID: 29619483
30. Yagupsky P. *Adv Exp Med Biol*. 2011;719:123–132 PMID: 22125040
31. AAP. *Burkholderia* infections. In: Kimberlin DW, et al, eds. *Red Book: 2018–2021 Report of the Committee on Infectious Diseases*. 31st ed. 2018:258–260
32. Waters V. *Curr Pharm Des*. 2012;18(5):696–725 PMID: 22229574
33. Mazer DM, et al. *Antimicrob Agents Chemother*. 2017;61(9):e00766-17 PMID: 28674053
34. Horsley A, et al. *Cochrane Database Syst Rev*. 2016;(1):CD009529 PMID: 26789750
35. Wiersinga WJ, et al. *N Engl J Med*. 2012;367(11):1035–1044 PMID: 22970946
36. Wiersinga WJ, et al. *Nat Rev Dis Primers*. 2018;4:17107 PMID: 29388572
37. Chetchotisakd P, et al. *Lancet*. 2014;383(9919):807–814 PMID: 24284287
38. Fujihara N, et al. *J Infect*. 2006;53(5):e199–e202 PMID: 16542730
39. Wagenaar JA, et al. *Clin Infect Dis*. 2014;58(11):1579–1586 PMID: 24550377
40. AAP. *Campylobacter* infections. In: Kimberlin DW, et al, eds. *Red Book: 2018–2021 Report of the Committee on Infectious Diseases*. 31st ed. 2018:260–263,1094
41. Schiaffino F, et al. *Antimicrob Agents Chemother*. 2019;63(2):e01911-18 PMID: 30420482
42. Bula-Rudas FJ, et al. *Pediatr Rev*. 2018;39(10):490–500 PMID: 30275032
43. Jolivet-Gougeon A, et al. *Int J Antimicrob Agents*. 2007;29(4):367–373 PMID: 17250994
44. Wang HK, et al. *J Clin Microbiol*. 2007;45(2):645–647 PMID: 17135428
45. Magro-Checa C, et al. *J Clin Microbiol*. 2011;49(12):4391–4393 PMID: 21998421
46. Kohlhoff SA, et al. *Expert Opin Pharmacother*. 2015;16(2):205–212 PMID: 25579069
47. AAP. Chlamydial infections. In: Kimberlin DW, et al, eds. *Red Book: 2018–2021 Report of the Committee on Infectious Diseases*. 31st ed. 2018:273–274
48. Workowski KA, et al. *MMWR Recomm Rep*. 2015;64(RR-03):1–137 PMID: 26042815
49. Blasi F, et al. *Clin Microbiol Infect*. 2009;15(1):29–35 PMID: 19220337
50. Sharma L, et al. *Clin Chest Med*. 2017;38(1):45–58 PMID: 28159161
51. Knittler MR, et al. *Pathog Dis*. 2015;73(1):1–15 PMID: 25853998
52. Campbell JI, et al. *BMC Infect Dis*. 2013;13:4 PMID: 23286235

53. Sirinavin S, et al. *Pediatr Infect Dis J.* 2005;24(6):559–561 PMID: 15933571
54. Deveci A, et al. *Expert Rev Anti Infect Ther.* 2014;12(9):1137–1142 PMID: 25088467
55. Harris PN, et al. *J Antimicrob Chemother.* 2016;71(2):296–306 PMID: 26542304
56. Carrillo-Marquez MA. *Pediatr Rev.* 2016;37(5):183–192 PMID: 27139326
57. AAP. Botulism and infant botulism. In: Kimberlin DW, et al, eds. *Red Book: 2018–2021 Report of the Committee on Infectious Diseases.* 31st ed. 2018:283–286
58. Hill SE, et al. *Ann Pharmacother.* 2013;47(2):e12 PMID: 23362041
59. Sammons JS, et al. *JAMA Pediatr.* 2013;167(6):567–573 PMID: 23460123
60. AAP. *Clostridium difficile.* In: Kimberlin DW, et al, eds. *Red Book: 2018–2021 Report of the Committee on Infectious Diseases.* 31st ed. 2018:288–292
61. McDonald LC, et al. *Clin Infect Dis.* 2018;66(7):987–994 PMID: 29562266
62. O'Gorman MA, et al. *J Pediatric Infect Dis Soc.* 2018;7(3):210–218 PMID: 28575523
63. AAP. Clostridial myonecrosis. In: Kimberlin DW, et al, eds. *Red Book: 2018–2021 Report of the Committee on Infectious Diseases.* 31st ed. 2018:286–288
64. AAP. *Clostridium perfringens* food poisoning. In: Kimberlin DW, et al, eds. *Red Book: 2018–2021 Report of the Committee on Infectious Diseases.* 31st ed. 2018:292–294
65. AAP. Tetanus. In: Kimberlin DW, et al, eds. *Red Book: 2018-2021 Report of the Committee on Infectious Diseases.* 31st ed. 2018:793–798
66. Yen LM, et al. *Lancet.* 2019;393(10181):1657–1668 PMID: 30935736
67. AAP. Diphtheria. In: Kimberlin DW, et al, eds. *Red Book: 2018–2021 Report of the Committee on Infectious Diseases.* 31st ed. 2018:319–323
68. Fernandez-Roblas R, et al. *Int J Antimicrob Agents.* 2009;33(5):453–455 PMID: 19153032
69. Mookadam F, et al. *Eur J Clin Microbiol Infect Dis.* 2006;25(6):349–353 PMID: 16767481
70. Holdiness MR. *Drugs.* 2002;62(8):1131–1141 PMID: 12010076
71. Dalal A, et al. *J Infect.* 2008;56(1):77–79 PMID: 18036665
72. Eldin C, et al. *Clin Microbiol Rev.* 2017;30(1):115–190 PMID: 27856520
73. Kersh GJ. *Expert Rev Anti Infect Ther.* 2013;11(11):1207–1214 PMID: 24073941
74. Pritt BS, et al. *N Engl J Med.* 2011;365(5):422–429 PMID: 21812671
75. Xu G, et al. *Emerg Infect Dis.* 2018;24(6):1143–1144 PMID: 29774863
76. Paul K, et al. *Clin Infect Dis.* 2001;33(1):54–61 PMID: 11389495
77. Tricard T, et al. *Arch Pediatr.* 2016;23(11):1146–1149 PMID: 27663465
78. Ceyhan M, et al. *Int J Pediatr.* 2011;2011:215–237 PMID: 22046191
79. Huang YC, et al. *Int J Antimicrob Agents.* 2018;51(1):47–51 PMID: 28668676
80. Siedner MJ, et al. *Clin Infect Dis.* 2014;58(11):1554–1563 PMID: 24647022
81. Tamma PD, et al. *Clin Infect Dis.* 2013;57(6):781–788 PMID: 23759352
82. Doi Y, et al. *Semin Respir Crit Care Med.* 2015;36(1):74–84 PMID: 25643272
83. Arias CA, et al. *Nat Rev Microbiol.* 2012;10(4):266–278 PMID: 22421879
84. Yim J, et al. *Pharmacotherapy.* 2017;37(5):579–592 PMID: 28273381
85. Beganovic M, et al. *Clin Infect Dis.* 2018;67(2):303–309 PMID: 29390132
86. Veraldi S, et al. *Clin Exp Dermatol.* 2009;34(8):859–862 PMID: 19663854
87. Principe L, et al. *Infect Dis Rep.* 2016;8(1):6368 PMID: 27103974
88. AAP. Tularemia. In: Kimberlin DW, et al, eds. *Red Book: 2018–2021 Report of the Committee on Infectious Diseases.* 31st ed. 2018:861–864
89. Mittal S, et al. *Pediatr Rev.* 2019;40(4):197–201 PMID: 30936402
90. Van TT, et al. *J Clin Microbiol.* 2018;56(12):e00487-18 PMID: 30482869
91. Riordan T. *Clin Microbiol Rev.* 2007;20(4):622–659 PMID: 17934077
92. Bradshaw CS, et al. *J Infect Dis.* 2016;214(Suppl1):S14–S20 PMID: 27449869
93. Maraki S, et al. *J Microbiol Immunol Infect.* 2016;49(1):119–122 PMID: 24529567
94. Butler DF, et al. *Infect Dis Clin North Am.* 2018;32(1):119–128 PMID: 29233576
95. AAP. *Helicobacter pylori* infections. In: Kimberlin DW, et al, eds. *Red Book: 2018–2021 Report of the Committee on Infectious Diseases.* 31st ed. 2018:378–381
96. Jones NL, et al. *J Pediatr Gastroenterol Nutr.* 2017;64(6):991–1003 PMID: 28541262
97. Kalach N, et al. *Helicobacter.* 2017;22(Suppl1) PMID: 28891139
98. Yagupsky P. *Clin Microbiol Rev.* 2015;28(1):54–79 PMID: 25567222

99. Hernández-Rupérez MB, et al. *Pediatr Infect Dis J.* 2018 PMID: 29620718
100. Petrosillo N, et al. *Expert Rev Anti Infect Ther.* 2013;11(2):159–177 PMID: 23409822
101. Doi Y, et al. *Semin Respir Crit Care Med.* 2015;36(1):74–84 PMID: 25643272
102. Mesini A, et al. *Clin Infect Dis.* 2018;66(5):808–809 PMID: 29020309
103. Nation RL. *Clin Infect Dis.* 2018;66(5):810–811 PMID: 29211826
104. van Duin D, et al. *Clin Infect Dis.* 2018;66(2):163–171 PMID: 29020404
105. Cunha CB, et al. *Infect Dis Clin North Am.* 2017;31(1):1–5 PMID: 27979687
106. Jiménez JIS, et al. *J Crit Care.* 2018;43:361–365 PMID: 29129539
107. Florescu D, et al. *Pediatr Infect Dis J.* 2008;27(11):1013–1019 PMID: 18833028
108. Bortolussi R. *CMAJ.* 2008;179(8):795–797 PMID: 18787096
109. Murphy TF, et al. *Clin Infect Dis.* 2009;49(1):124–131 PMID: 19480579
110. Liu H, et al. *Int J Infect Dis.* 2016;50:10–17 PMID: 27421818
111. Milligan KL, et al. *Clin Pediatr (Phila).* 2013;52(5):462–464 PMID: 22267858
112. AAP. Nontuberculous mycobacteria. In: Kimberlin DW, et al, eds. *Red Book: 2018–2021 Report of the Committee on Infectious Diseases.* 31st ed. 2018:853–861
113. Lee MR, et al. *Emerg Infect Dis.* 2015;21(9):1638–1646 PMID: 26295364
114. Mougari F, et al. *Expert Rev Anti Infect Ther.* 2016;14(12):1139–1154 PMID: 27690688
115. Koh WJ, et al. *Clin Infect Dis.* 2017;64(3):309–316 PMID: 28011608
116. Adelman MH, et al. *Curr Opin Pulm Med.* 2018;24(3):212–219 PMID: 29470253
117. Philley JV, et al. *Curr Treat Options Infect Dis.* 2016;8(4):275–296 PMID: 28529461
118. AAP. Tuberculosis. In: Kimberlin DW, et al, eds. *Red Book: 2018–2021 Report of the Committee on Infectious Diseases.* 31st ed. 2018:829–853
119. Hlavsa MC, et al. *Clin Infect Dis.* 2008;47(2):168–175 PMID: 18532886
120. Brown-Elliott BA, et al. *Microbiol Spectr.* 2017;5(1) PMID: 28084211
121. Kasperbauer SH, et al. *Clin Chest Med.* 2015;36(1):67–78 PMID: 25676520
122. Centers for Disease Control and Prevention. Hansen's disease (leprosy). https://www.cdc.gov/leprosy/health-care-workers/treatment.html. Reviewed February 10, 2017. Accessed October 10, 2019
123. Johnson MG, et al. *Infection.* 2015;43(6):655–662 PMID: 25869820
124. Nahid P, et al. *Clin Infect Dis.* 2016;63(7):e147–e195 PMID: 27516382
125. Scaggs Huang FA, et al. *Pediatr Infect Dis J.* 2019;38(7):749–751 PMID: 30985508
126. Watt KM, et al. *Pediatr Infect Dis J.* 2012;31(2):197–199 PMID: 22016080
127. Waites KB, et al. *Clin Microbiol Rev.* 2017;30(3):747–809 PMID: 28539503
128. Gardiner SJ, et al. *Cochrane Database Syst Rev.* 2015;1:CD004875 PMID: 25566754
129. Lee H, et al. *Expert Rev Anti Infect Ther.* 2018;16(1):23–34 PMID: 29212389
130. Centers for Disease Control and Prevention. *MMWR Morb Mortal Wkly Rep.* 2012;61(31):590–594 PMID: 22874837
131. van de Beek D, et al. *Clin Microbiol Infect.* 2016;22(Suppl3):S37–S62 PMID: 27062097
132. Nadel S, et al. *Front Pediatr.* 2018;6:321 PMID: 30474022
133. Wilson JW. *Mayo Clin Proc.* 2012;87(4):403–407 PMID: 22469352
134. AAP. Nocardiosis. In: Kimberlin DW, et al, eds. *Red Book: 2018–2021 Report of the Committee on Infectious Diseases.* 31st ed. 2018:575–577
135. Magro-Checa C, et al. *J Clin Microbiol.* 2011;49(12):4391–4393 PMID: 21998421
136. Wilson BA, et al. *Clin Microbiol Rev.* 2013;26(3):631–655 PMID: 23824375
137. Mogilner L, et al. *Pediatr Rev.* 2019;40(2):90–92 PMID: 30709978
138. Murphy EC, et al. *FEMS Microbiol Rev.* 2013;37(4):520–553 PMID: 23030831
139. Ozdemir O, et al. *J Microbiol Immunol Infect.* 2010;43(4):344–346 PMID: 20688296
140. Janda JM, et al. *Clin Microbiol Rev.* 2016;29(2):349–374 PMID: 26960939
141. Brook I, et al. *Clin Microbiol Rev.* 2013;26(3):526–546 PMID: 23824372
142. Perry A, et al. *Expert Rev Anti Infect Ther.* 2011;9(12):1149–1156 PMID: 22114965
143. Tunkel AR, et al. *Clin Infect Dis.* 2017 PMID: 28203777
144. Schaffer JN, et al. *Microbiol Spectr.* 2015;3(5) PMID: 26542036
145. Abdallah M, et al. *New Microbes New Infect.* 2018;25:16–23 PMID: 29983987
146. Fish DN, et al. *Pharmacotherapy.* 2013;33(10):1022–1034 PMID: 23744833
147. Tennant SJ, et al. *Antibiotics (Basel).* 2015;4(4):643–652 PMID: 27025644

148. Kalil AC, et al. *Clin Infect Dis.* 2016;63(5):e61–e111 PMID: 27418577
149. Nguyen L, et al. *Curr Infect Dis Rep.* 2018;20(8):23 PMID: 29876674
150. Freifeld AG, et al. *Clin Infect Dis.* 2011;52(4):e56–e93 PMID: 21258094
151. Tran TB, et al. *Int J Antimicrob Agents.* 2016;48(6):592–597 PMID: 27793510
152. McCarthy KL, et al. *Infect Dis (Lond).* 2018;50(5):403–406 PMID: 29205079
153. Kim HS, et al. *BMC Infect Dis.* 2017;17(1):500 PMID: 28716109
154. Döring G, et al. *J Cyst Fibros.* 2012;11(6):461–479 PMID: 23137712
155. Mogayzel PJ Jr, et al. *Am J Respir Crit Care Med.* 2013;187(7):680–689 PMID: 23540878
156. Langton Hewer SC, et al. *Cochrane Database Syst Rev.* 2017;4:CD004197 PMID: 28440853
157. Mogayzel PJ Jr, et al. *Ann Am Thorac Soc.* 2014;11(10):1640–1650 PMID: 25549030
158. Lin WV, et al. *Clin Microbiol Infect.* 2019;25(3):310–315 PMID: 29777923
159. AAP. Rickettsial diseases. In: Kimberlin DW, et al, eds. *Red Book: 2018–2021 Report of the Committee on Infectious Diseases.* 31st ed. 2018:693–696
160. Woods CR. *Pediatr Clin North Am.* 2013;60(2):455–470 PMID: 23481111
161. AAP. *Salmonella* infections. In: Kimberlin DW, et al, eds. *Red Book: 2018–2021 Report of the Committee on Infectious Diseases.* 31st ed. 2018:711–718
162. Haeusler GM, et al. *Adv Exp Med Biol.* 2013;764:13–26 PMID: 23654054
163. Onwuezobe IA, et al. *Cochrane Database Syst Rev.* 2012;11:CD001167 PMID: 23152205
164. Effa EE, et al. *Cochrane Database Syst Rev.* 2008;(4):CD006083 PMID: 18843701
165. Yousfi K, et al. *Eur J Clin Microbiol Infect Dis.* 2017;36(8):1353–1362 PMID: 28299457
166. Janda JM, et al. *Crit Rev Microbiol.* 2014;40(4):293–312 PMID: 23043419
167. Klontz KC, et al. *Expert Rev Anti Infect Ther.* 2015;13(1):69–80 PMID: 25399653
168. AAP. *Shigella* infections. In: Kimberlin DW, et al, eds. *Red Book: 2018–2021 Report of the Committee on Infectious Diseases.* 31st ed. 2018:723–727
169. Sjölund Karlsson M, et al. *Antimicrob Agents Chemother.* 2013;57(3):1559–1560 PMID: 23274665
170. Holmes LC. *Pediatr Rev.* 2014;35(6):261–262 PMID: 24891600
171. AAP. Rat-bite fever. In: Kimberlin DW, et al, eds. *Red Book: 2018–2021 Report of the Committee on Infectious Diseases.* 31st ed. 2018:680–682,1095
172. Kullar R, et al. *J Antimicrob Chemother.* 2016;71(3):576–586 PMID: 26565015
173. Long CB, et al. *Expert Rev Anti Infect Ther.* 2010;8(2):183–195 PMID: 20109048
174. Korczowski B, et al. *Pediatr Infect Dis J.* 2016;35(8):e239–e247 PMID: 27164462
175. Bradley J, et al. *Pediatrics.* 2017;139(3):e20162477 PMID: 28202770
176. Arrieta AC, et al. *Pediatr Infect Dis J.* 2018;37(9):893–900 PMID: 29406465
177. Blanchard AC, et al. *Clin Perinatol.* 2015;42(1):119–132 PMID: 25678000
178. Becker K, et al. *Clin Microbiol Rev.* 2014;27(4):870–926 PMID: 25278577
179. Samonis G, et al. *PLoS One.* 2012;7(5):e37375 PMID: 22624022
180. Anđelković MV, et al. *J Chemother.* 2019:1–10 PMID: 31130079
181. Crews JD, et al. *JAMA Pediatr.* 2014;168(12):1165–1166 PMID: 25436846
182. Gerber MA, et al. *Circulation.* 2009;119(11):1541–1551 PMID: 19246689
183. AAP. Group B streptococcal infections. In: Kimberlin DW, et al, eds. *Red Book: 2018–2021 Report of the Committee on Infectious Diseases.* 31st ed. 2018:762–768,908
184. Faden H, et al. *Pediatr Infect Dis J.* 2017;36(11):1099–1100 PMID: 28640003
185. Broyles LN, et al. *Clin Infect Dis.* 2009;48(6):706–712 PMID: 19187026
186. Stelzmueller I, et al. *Eur J Pediatr Surg.* 2009;19(1):21–24 PMID: 19221948
187. Fazili T, et al. *Am J Med Sci.* 2017;354(3):257–261 PMID: 28918832
188. Deutschmann MW, et al. *JAMA Otolaryngol Head Neck Surg.* 2013;139(2):157–160 PMID: 23429946
189. Pichichero ME. *Pediatr Clin North Am.* 2013;60(2):391–407 PMID: 23481107
190. Olarte L, et al. *Pediatr Infect Dis J.* 2017;36(12):1201–1204 PMID: 28723870
191. Mendes RE, et al. *Diagn Microbiol Infect Dis.* 2014;80(1):19–25 PMID: 24974272
192. Kaplan SL, et al. *Pediatrics.* 2019;144(3):e20190567 PMID: 31420369
193. Baltimore RS, et al. *Circulation.* 2015;132(13):1487–1515 PMID: 26373317
194. AAP. Syphilis. In: Kimberlin DW, et al, eds. *Red Book: 2018–2021 Report of the Committee on Infectious Diseases.* 31st ed. 2018:773–788
195. Merchan LM, et al. *Antimicrob Agents Chemother.* 2015;59(1):570–578 PMID: 25385115

196. Centers for Disease Control and Prevention. Cholera – *Vibrio cholerae* infection. https://www.cdc.gov/cholera/treatment/antibiotic-treatment.html. Reviewed January 20, 2015. Accessed October 10, 2019
197. Clemens JD, et al. *Lancet.* 2017;390(10101):1539–1549 PMID: 28302312
198. Heng SP, et al. *Front Microbiol.* 2017;8:997 PMID: 28620366
199. Daniels NA. *Clin Infect Dis.* 2011;52(6):788–792 PMID: 21367733
200. AAP. *Yersinia enterocolitica.* In: Kimberlin DW, et al, eds. *Red Book: 2018–2021 Report of the Committee on Infectious Diseases.* 31st ed. 2018:256,891–894
201. Kato H, et al. *Medicine (Baltimore).* 2016;95(26):e3988 PMID: 27368001
202. Yang R. *J Clin Microbiol.* 2017;56(1):e01519-17 PMID: 29070654
203. Butler T. *Clin Infect Dis.* 2009;49(5):736–742 PMID: 19606935
204. Centers for Disease Control and Prevention. Plague. https://www.cdc.gov/plague/healthcare/clinicians.html. Reviewed November 27, 2018. Accessed October 10, 2019
205. Bertelli L, et al. *J Pediatr.* 2014;165(2):411 PMID: 24793203
206. AAP. *Yersinia pseudotuberculosis.* In: Kimberlin DW, et al, eds. *Red Book: 2018–2021 Report of the Committee on Infectious Diseases.* 31st ed. 2018:891–894

Chapter 8

1. Groll AH, et al. *Lancet Oncol.* 2014;15(8):e327–e340 PMID: 24988936
2. Wingard JR, et al. *Blood.* 2010;116(24):5111–5118 PMID: 20826719
3. Van Burik JA, et al. *Clin Infect Dis.* 2004;39(10):1407–1416 PMID: 15546073
4. Cornely OA, et al. *N Engl J Med.* 2007;356(4):348–359 PMID: 17251531
5. Kung HC, et al. *Cancer Med.* 2014;3(3):667–673 PMID: 24644249
6. Science M, et al. *Pediatr Blood Cancer.* 2014;61(3):393–400 PMID: 24424789
7. Bow EJ, et al. *BMC Infect Dis.* 2015;15:128 PMID: 25887385
8. Tacke D, et al. *Ann Hematol.* 2014;93(9):1449–1456 PMID: 24951122
9. Almyroudis NG, et al. *Curr Opin Infect Dis.* 2009;22(4):385–393 PMID: 19506476
10. Maschmeyer G. *J Antimicrob Chemother.* 2009;63(Suppl1):i27–i30 PMID: 19372178
11. Freifeld AG, et al. *Clin Infect Dis.* 2011;52(4):e56–e93 PMID: 21258094
12. De Pauw BE, et al. *N Engl J Med.* 2007;356(4):409–411 PMID: 17251538
13. Salavert M. *Int J Antimicrob Agents.* 2008;32(Suppl2):S149–S153 PMID: 19013340
14. Eschenauer GA, et al. *Liver Transpl.* 2009;15(8):842–858 PMID: 19642130
15. Winston DJ, et al. *Am J Transplant.* 2014;14(12):2758–2764 PMID: 25376267
16. Sun HY, et al. *Transplantation.* 2013;96(6):573–578 PMID: 23842191
17. Radack KP, et al. *Curr Infect Dis Rep.* 2009;11(6):427–434 PMID: 19857381
18. Patterson TF, et al. *Clin Infect Dis.* 2016;63(4):e1–e60 PMID: 27365388
19. Thomas L, et al. *Expert Rev Anti Infect Ther.* 2009;7(4):461–472 PMID: 19400765
20. Friberg LE, et al. *Antimicrob Agents Chemother.* 2012;56(6):3032–3042 PMID: 22430956
21. Burgos A, et al. *Pediatrics.* 2008;121(5):e1286–e1294 PMID: 18450871
22. Herbrecht R, et al. *N Engl J Med.* 2002;347(6):408–415 PMID: 12167683
23. Mousset S, et al. *Ann Hematol.* 2014;93(1):13–32 PMID: 24026426
24. Blyth CC, et al. *Intern Med J.* 2014;44(12b):1333–1349 PMID: 25482744
25. Denning DW, et al. *Eur Respir J.* 2016;47(1):45–68 PMID: 26699723
26. Cornely OA, et al. *Clin Infect Dis.* 2007;44(10):1289–1297 PMID: 17443465
27. Maertens JA, et al. *Lancet.* 2016;387(10020):760–769 PMID: 26684607
28. Tissot F, et al. *Haematologica.* 2017;102(3):433–444 PMID: 28011902
29. Ullmann AJ, et al. *Clin Microbiol Infect.* 2018;24(Suppl1):e1–e38 PMID: 29544767
30. Walsh TJ, et al. *Antimicrob Agents Chemother.* 2010;54(10):4116–4123 PMID: 20660687
31. Bartelink IH, et al. *Antimicrob Agents Chemother.* 2013;57(1):235–240 PMID: 23114771
32. Marr KA, et al. *Ann Intern Med.* 2015;162(2):81–89 PMID: 25599346
33. Verweij PE, et al. *Drug Resist Updat.* 2015;21-22:30–40 PMID: 26282594
34. Kohno S, et al. *Eur J Clin Microbiol Infect Dis.* 2013;32(3):387–397 PMID: 23052987
35. Naggie S, et al. *Clin Chest Med.* 2009;30(2):337–353 PMID: 19375639
36. Revankar SG, et al. *Clin Microbiol Rev.* 2010;23(4):884–928 PMID: 20930077
37. Wong EH, et al. *Infect Dis Clin North Am.* 2016;30(1):165–178 PMID: 26897066

38. Revankar SG, et al. *Clin Infect Dis.* 2004;38(2):206–216 PMID: 14699452
39. Li DM, et al. *Lancet Infect Dis.* 2009;9(6):376–383 PMID: 19467477
40. Chowdhary A, et al. *Clin Microbiol Infect.* 2014;20(Suppl3):47–75 PMID: 24483780
41. McCarty TP, et al. *Med Mycol.* 2015;53(5):440–446 PMID: 25908651
42. Schieffelin JS, et al. *Transplant Infect Dis.* 2014;16(2):270–278 PMID: 24628809
43. Chapman SW, et al. *Clin Infect Dis.* 2008;46(12):1801–1812 PMID: 18462107
44. McKinnell JA, et al. *Clin Chest Med.* 2009;30(2):227–239 PMID: 19375630
45. Walsh CM, et al. *Pediatr Infect Dis J.* 2006;25(7):656–658 PMID: 16804444
46. Fanella S, et al. *Med Mycol.* 2011;49(6):627–632 PMID: 21208027
47. Smith JA, et al. *Proc Am Thorac Soc.* 2010;7(3):173–180 PMID: 20463245
48. Bariola JR, et al. *Clin Infect Dis.* 2010;50(6):797–804 PMID: 20166817
49. Limper AH, et al. *Am J Respir Crit Care Med.* 2011;183(1):96–128 PMID: 21193785
50. Pappas PG, et al. *Clin Infect Dis.* 2016;62(4):e1–e50 PMID: 26679628
51. Lortholary O, et al. *Clin Microbiol Infect.* 2012;18(Suppl7):68–77 PMID: 23137138
52. Ullman AJ, et al. *Clin Microbiol Infect.* 2012;18(Suppl7):53–67 PMID: 23137137
53. Hope WW, et al. *Clin Microbiol Infect.* 2012;18(Suppl7):38–52 PMID: 23137136
54. Cornely OA, et al. *Clin Microbiol Infect.* 2012;18(Suppl7):19–37 PMID: 23137135
55. Hope WW, et al. *Antimicrob Agents Chemother.* 2015;59(2):905–913 PMID: 25421470
56. Piper L, et al. *Pediatr Infect Dis J.* 2011;30(5):375–378 PMID: 21085048
57. Watt KM, et al. *Antimicrob Agents Chemother.* 2015;59(7):3935–3943 PMID: 25896706
58. Ascher SB, et al. *Pediatr Infect Dis J.* 2012;31(5):439–443 PMID: 22189522
59. Sobel JD. *Lancet.* 2007;369(9577):1961–1971 PMID: 17560449
60. Lopez Martinez R, et al. *Clin Dermatol.* 2007;25(2):188–194 PMID: 17350498
61. Ameen M. *Clin Exp Dermatol.* 2009;34(8):849–854 PMID: 19575735
62. Chowdhary A, et al. *Clin Microbiol Infect.* 2014;20(Suppl3):47–75 PMID: 24483780
63. Queiroz-Telles F. *Rev Inst Med Trop Sao Paulo.* 2015;57(Suppl19):46–50 PMID: 26465369
64. Queiroz-Telles F, et al. *Clin Microbiol Rev.* 2017;30(1):233–276 PMID: 27856522
65. Galgiani JN, et al. *Clin Infect Dis.* 2016;63(6):717–722 PMID: 27559032
66. Anstead GM, et al. *Infect Dis Clin North Am.* 2006;20(3):621–643 PMID: 16984872
67. Williams PL. *Ann N Y Acad Sci.* 2007;1111:377–384 PMID: 17363442
68. Homans JD, et al. *Pediatr Infect Dis J.* 2010;29(1):65–67 PMID: 19884875
69. Kauffman CA, et al. *Transplant Infectious Diseases.* 2014;16(2):213–224 PMID: 24589027
70. McCarty JM, et al. *Clin Infect Dis.* 2013;56(11):1579–1585 PMID: 23463637
71. Bravo R, et al. *J Pediatr Hematol Oncol.* 2012;34(5):389–394 PMID: 22510771
72. Catanzaro A, et al. *Clin Infect Dis.* 2007;45(5):562–568 PMID: 17682989
73. Thompson GR, et al. *Clin Infect Dis.* 2016;63(3):356–362 PMID: 27169478
74. Thompson GR 3rd, et al. *Clin Infect Dis.* 2017;65(2):338–341 PMID: 28419259
75. Chayakulkeeree M, et al. *Infect Dis Clin North Am.* 2006;20(3):507–544 PMID: 16984867
76. Jarvis JN, et al. *Semin Respir Crit Care Med.* 2008;29(2):141–150 PMID: 18365996
77. Perfect JR, et al. *Clin Infect Dis.* 2010;50(3):291–322 PMID: 20047480
78. Joshi NS, et al. *Pediatr Infect Dis J.* 2010;29(12):e91–e95 PMID: 20935590
79. Day JN, et al. *N Engl J Med.* 2013;368(14):1291–1302 PMID: 23550668
80. Cortez KJ, et al. *Clin Microbiol Rev.* 2008;21(1):157–197 PMID: 18202441
81. Tortorano AM, et al. *Clin Microbiol Infect.* 2014;20(Suppl3):27–46 PMID: 24548001
82. Horn DL, et al. *Mycoses.* 2014;57(11):652–658 PMID: 24943384
83. Muhammed M, et al. *Medicine (Baltimore).* 2013;92(6):305–316 PMID: 24145697
84. Rodriguez-Tudela JL, et al. *Med Mycol.* 2009;47(4):359–370 PMID: 19031336
85. Wheat LJ, et al. *Clin Infect Dis.* 2007;45(7):807–825 PMID: 17806045
86. Myint T, et al. *Medicine (Baltimore).* 2014;93(1):11–18 PMID: 24378739
87. Assi M, et al. *Clin Infect Dis.* 2013;57(11):1542–1549 PMID: 24046304
88. Chayakulkeeree M, et al. *Eur J Clin Microbiol Infect Dis.* 2006;25(4):215–229 PMID: 16568297
89. Spellberg B, et al. *Clin Infect Dis.* 2009;48(12):1743–1751 PMID: 19435437
90. Reed C, et al. *Clin Infect Dis.* 2008;47(3):364–371 PMID: 18558882
91. Cornely OA, et al. *Clin Microbiol Infect.* 2014;20(Suppl3):5–26 PMID: 24479848

92. Spellberg B, et al. *Clin Infect Dis.* 2012;54(Suppl1):S73–S78 PMID: 22247449
93. Chitasombat MN, et al. *Curr Opin Infect Dis.* 2016;29(4):340–345 PMID: 27191199
94. Pana ZD, et al. *BMC Infect Dis.* 2016;16(1):667 PMID: 27832748
95. Kyvernitakis A, et al. *Clin Microbiol Infect.* 2016;22(9):811.e1–811.e8 PMID: 27085727
96. Pagano L, et al. *Haematologica.* 2013;98(10):e127–e130 PMID: 23716556
97. Marty FM, et al. *Lancet Infect Dis.* 2016;16(7):828–837 PMID: 26969258
98. Queiroz-Telles F, et al. *Clin Infect Dis.* 2007;45(11):1462–1469 PMID: 17990229
99. Menezes VM, et al. *Cochrane Database Syst Rev.* 2006;(2):CD004967 PMID: 16625617
100. Marques SA. *An Bras Dermatol.* 2013;88(5):700–711 PMID: 24173174
101. Borges SR, et al. *Med Mycol.* 2014;52(3):303–310 PMID: 24577007
102. Panel on Opportunistic Infections in HIV-Exposed and HIV-Infected Children. Guidelines for the prevention and treatment of opportunistic infections in HIV-exposed and HIV-infected children. http://aidsinfo.nih.gov/contentfiles/lvguidelines/oi_guidelines_pediatrics.pdf. Updated November 5, 2018. Accessed October 10, 2019
103. Siberry GK, et al. *Pediatr Infect Dis J.* 2013;32(Suppl2):i–KK4 PMID: 24569199
104. Maschmeyer G, et al. *J Antimicrob Chemother.* 2016;71(9):2405–2413 PMID: 27550993
105. Kauffman CA, et al. *Clin Infect Dis.* 2007;45(10):1255–1265 PMID: 17968818
106. Aung AK, et al. *Med Mycol.* 2013;51(5):534–544 PMID: 23286352
107. Ali S, et al. *Pediatr Emerg Care.* 2007;23(9):662–668 PMID: 17876261
108. Shy R. *Pediatr Rev.* 2007;28(5):164–174 PMID: 17473121
109. Andrews MD, et al. *Am Fam Physician.* 2008;77(10):1415–1420 PMID: 18533375
110. Kakourou T, et al. *Pediatr Dermatol.* 2010;27(3):226–228 PMID: 20609140
111. Gupta AK, et al. *Pediatr Dermatol.* 2013;30(1):1–6 PMID: 22994156
112. Chen X, et al. *J Am Acad Dermatol.* 2017;76(2):368–374 PMID: 27816294
113. de Berker D. *N Engl J Med.* 2009;360(20):2108–2116 PMID: 19439745
114. Ameen M, et al. *Br J Dermatol.* 2014;171(5):937–958 PMID: 25409999
115. Pantazidou A, et al. *Arch Dis Child.* 2007;92(11):1040–1042 PMID: 17954488
116. Gupta AK, et al. *J Cutan Med Surg.* 2014;18(2):79–90 PMID: 24636433

Chapter 9

1. Lenaerts L, et al. *Rev Med Virol.* 2008;18(6):357–374 PMID: 18655013
2. Michaels MG. *Expert Rev Anti Infect Ther.* 2007;5(3):441–448 PMID: 17547508
3. Biron KK. *Antiviral Res.* 2006;71(2–3):154–163 PMID: 16765457
4. Boeckh M, et al. *Blood.* 2009;113(23):5711–5719 PMID: 19299333
5. Vaudry W, et al. *Am J Transplant.* 2009;9(3):636–643 PMID: 19260840
6. Emanuel D, et al. *Ann Intern Med.* 1988;109(10):777–782 PMID: 2847609
7. Reed EC, et al. *Ann Intern Med.* 1988;109(10):783–788 PMID: 2847610
8. *Ophthalmology.* 1994;101(7):1250–1261 PMID: 8035989
9. Singh N, et al. *N Engl J Med.* 2019. In press
10. Martin DF, et al. *N Engl J Med.* 2002;346(15):1119–1126 PMID: 11948271
11. Kempen JH, et al. *Arch Ophthalmol.* 2003;121(4):466–476 PMID: 12695243
12. Studies of Ocular Complications of AIDS Research Group. The AIDS Clinical Trials Group. *Am J Ophthalmol.* 2001;131(4):457–467 PMID: 11292409
13. Dieterich DT, et al. *J Infect Dis.* 1993;167(2):278–282 PMID: 8380610
14. Gerna G, et al. *Antiviral Res.* 1997;34(1):39–50 PMID: 9107384
15. Markham A, et al. *Drugs.* 1994;48(3):455–484 PMID: 7527763
16. Kimberlin DW, et al. *J Infect Dis.* 2008;197(6):836–845 PMID: 18279073
17. Kimberlin DW, et al. *N Engl J Med.* 2015;372(10):933–943 PMID: 25738669
18. Griffiths P, et al. *Herpes.* 2008;15(1):4–12 PMID: 18983762
19. Panel on Opportunistic Infections in HIV-Exposed and HIV-Infected Children. Guidelines for the prevention and treatment of opportunistic infections in HIV-exposed and HIV-infected children. http://aidsinfo.nih.gov/contentfiles/lvguidelines/oi_guidelines_pediatrics.pdf. Updated November 5, 2018. Accessed October 10, 2019
20. Marty FM, et al. *N Engl J Med.* 2017;377(25):2433–2444 PMID: 29211658

21. Abzug MJ, et al. *J Pediatr Infect Dis Soc.* 2016;5(1):53–62 PMID: 26407253
22. Biebl A, et al. *Nat Clin Pract Neurol.* 2009;5(3):171–174 PMID: 19262593
23. Chadaide Z, et al. *J Med Virol.* 2008;80(11):1930–1932 PMID: 18814244
24. AAP. Epstein-Barr virus infections. In: Kimberlin DW, et al, eds. *Red Book: 2018–2021 Report of the Committee on Infectious Diseases.* 31st ed. 2018:334–338,458,460
25. Gross TG. *Herpes.* 2009;15(3):64–67 PMID: 19306606
26. Styczynski J, et al. *Bone Marrow Transplant.* 2009;43(10):757–770 PMID: 19043458
27. Jonas MM, et al. *Hepatology.* 2016;63(2):377–387 PMID: 26223345
28. Marcellin P, et al. *Gastroenterology.* 2016;150(1):134–144.e10 PMID: 26453773
29. Chen HL, et al. *Hepatology.* 2015;62(2):375–386 PMID: 25851052
30. Wu Q, et al. *Clin Gastroenterol Hepatol.* 2015;13(6):1170–1176 PMID: 25251571
31. Hou JL, et al. *J Viral Hepat.* 2015;22(2):85–93 PMID: 25243325
32. Kurbegov AC, et al. *Expert Rev Gastroenterol Hepatol.* 2009;3(1):39–49 PMID: 19210112
33. Jonas MM, et al. *Hepatology.* 2008;47(6):1863–1871 PMID: 18433023
34. Lai CL, et al. *Gastroenterology.* 2002;123(6):1831–1838 PMID: 12454840
35. Honkoop P, et al. *Expert Opin Investig Drugs.* 2003;12(4):683–688 PMID: 12665423
36. Shaw T, et al. *Expert Rev Anti Infect Ther.* 2004;2(6):853–871 PMID: 15566330
37. Elisofon SA, et al. *Clin Liver Dis.* 2006;10(1):133–148 PMID: 16376798
38. Jonas MM, et al. *Hepatology.* 2010;52(6):2192–2205 PMID: 20890947
39. Haber BA, et al. *Pediatrics.* 2009;124(5):e1007–e1013 PMID: 19805457
40. Shneider BL, et al. *Hepatology.* 2006;44(5):1344–1354 PMID: 17058223
41. Jain MK, et al. *J Viral Hepat.* 2007;14(3):176–182 PMID: 17305883
42. Sokal EM, et al. *Gastroenterology.* 1998;114(5):988–995 PMID: 9558288
43. Jonas MM, et al. *N Engl J Med.* 2002;346(22):1706–1713 PMID: 12037150
44. Chang TT, et al. *N Engl J Med.* 2006;354(10):1001–1010 PMID: 16525137
45. Liaw YF, et al. *Gastroenterology.* 2009;136(2):486–495 PMID: 19027013
46. Terrault NA, et al. *Hepatology*. 2018;67(4):1560–1599 PMID: 29405329
47. Keam SJ, et al. *Drugs.* 2008;68(9):1273–1317 PMID: 18547135
48. Marcellin P, et al. *Gastroenterology.* 2011;140(2):459–468 PMID: 21034744
49. Poordad F, et al. *N Engl J Med.* 2011;364(13):1195–1206 PMID: 21449783
50. Schwarz KB, et al. *Gastroenterology.* 2011;140(2):450–458 PMID: 21036173
51. Nelson DR. *Liver Int.* 2011;31(Suppl1):53–57 PMID: 21205138
52. Strader DB, et al. *Hepatology.* 2004;39(4):1147–1171 PMID: 15057920
53. Soriano V, et al. *AIDS.* 2007;21(9):1073–1089 PMID: 17502718
54. Murray KF, et al. *Hepatology*. 2018;68(6):2158–2166 PMID: 30070726
55. Feld JJ, et al. *N Engl J Med.* 2014;370(17):1594–1603 PMID: 24720703
56. Zeuzem S, et al. *N Engl J Med.* 2014;370(17):1604–1614 PMID: 24720679
57. Andreone P, et al. *Gastroenterology.* 2014;147(2):359–365.e1 PMID: 24818763
58. Ferenci P, et al. *N Engl J Med.* 2014;370(21):1983–1992 PMID: 24795200
59. Poordad F, et al. *N Engl J Med.* 2014;370(21):1973–1982 PMID: 24725237
60. Jacobson IM, et al. *Lancet.* 2014;384(9941):403–413 PMID: 24907225
61. Manns M, et al. *Lancet.* 2014;384(9941):414–426 PMID: 24907224
62. Forns X, et al. *Gastroenterology.* 2014;146(7):1669–1679.e3 PMID: 24602923
63. Zeuzem S, et al. *Gastroenterology.* 2014;146(2):430–441.e6 PMID: 24184810
64. Lawitz E, et al. *Lancet.* 2014;384(9956):1756–1765 PMID: 25078309
65. Afdhal N, et al. *N Engl J Med.* 2014;370(20):1889–1898 PMID: 24725239
66. Afdhal N, et al. *N Engl J Med.* 2014;370(16):1483–1493 PMID: 24725238
67. Kowdley KV, et al. *N Engl J Med.* 2014;370(20):1879–1888 PMID: 24720702
68. Lawitz E, et al. *N Engl J Med.* 2013;368(20):1878–1887 PMID: 23607594
69. Jacobson IM, et al. *N Engl J Med.* 2013;368(20):1867–1877 PMID: 23607593
70. Zeuzem S, et al. *N Engl J Med.* 2014;370(21):1993–2001 PMID: 24795201
71. American Association for the Study of Liver Diseases, Infectious Diseases Society of America. HCV in children. https://www.hcvguidelines.org/unique-populations/children. Updated May 24, 2018. Accessed October 10, 2019

72. Hollier LM, et al. *Cochrane Database Syst Rev.* 2008;(1):CD004946 PMID: 18254066
73. Pinninti SG, et al. *J Pediatr.* 2012;161(1):134–138 PMID: 22336576
74. ACOG Committee on Practice Bulletins. *Obstet Gynecol.* 2007;109(6):1489–1498 PMID: 17569194
75. Kimberlin DW, et al. *Clin Infect Dis.* 2010;50(2):221–228 PMID: 20014952
76. Abdel Massih RC, et al. *World J Gastroenterol.* 2009;15(21):2561–2569 PMID: 19496184
77. Mofenson LM, et al. *MMWR Recomm Rep.* 2009;58(RR-11):1–166 PMID: 19730409
78. Kuhar DT, et al. *Infect Control Hosp Epidemiol.* 2013;34(9):875–892 PMID: 23917901
79. Acosta EP, et al. *J Infect Dis.* 2010;202(4):563–566 PMID: 20594104
80. Kimberlin DW, et al. *J Infect Dis.* 2013;207(5):709–720 PMID: 23230059
81. McPherson C, et al. *J Infect Dis.* 2012;206(6):847–850 PMID: 22807525
82. Bradley JS, et al. *Pediatrics.* 2017;140(5):e20162727 PMID: 29051331
83. AAP. Measles. In: Kimberlin DW, et al, eds. *Red Book: 2018–2021 Report of the Committee on Infectious Diseases.* 31st ed. 2018:537–550
84. AAP Committee on Infectious Diseases and Bronchiolitis Guidelines Committee. *Pediatrics.* 2014;134(2):415–420 PMID: 25070315
85. AAP Committee on Infectious Diseases and Bronchiolitis Guidelines Committee. *Pediatrics.* 2014;134(2):e620–e638 PMID: 25070304
86. Whitley RJ. *Adv Exp Med Biol.* 2008;609:216–232 PMID: 18193668

Chapter 10

1. Blessmann J, et al. *J Clin Microbiol.* 2003;41(10):4745–4750 PMID: 14532214
2. Haque R, et al. *N Engl J Med.* 2003;348(16):1565–1573 PMID: 1270037
3. Rossignol JF, et al. *Trans R Soc Trop Med Hyg.* 2007;101(10):1025–1031 PMID: 17658567
4. Mackey-Lawrence NM, et al. *BMJ Clin Evid.* 2011;pii:0918 PMID: 21477391
5. Fox LM, et al. *Clin Infect Dis.* 2005;40(8):1173–1180 PMID: 15791519
6. Cope JR, et al. *Clin Infect Dis.* 2016;62(6):774–776 PMID: 26679626
7. Vargas-Zepeda J, et al. *Arch Med Res.* 2005;36(1):83–86 PMID: 15900627
8. Linam WM, et al. *Pediatrics.* 2015;135(3):e744–e748 PMID: 25667249
9. Visvesvara GS, et al. *FEMS Immunol Med Microbiol.* 2007;50(1):1–26 PMID: 17428307
10. Deetz TR, et al. *Clin Infect Dis.* 2003;37(10):1304–1312 PMID: 14583863
11. Chotmongkol V, et al. *Am J Trop Med Hyg.* 2009;81(3):443–445 PMID: 19706911
12. Lo Re V III, et al. *Am J Med.* 2003;114(3):217–223 PMID: 12637136
13. Jitpimolmard S, et al. *Parasitol Res.* 2007;100(6):1293–1296 PMID: 17177056
14. Checkley AM, et al. *J Infect.* 2010;60(1):1–20 PMID: 19931558
15. Bethony J, et al. *Lancet.* 2006;367(9521):1521–1532 PMID: 16679166
16. Krause PJ, et al. *N Engl J Med.* 2000;343(20):1454–1458 PMID: 11078770
17. Vannier E, et al. *Infect Dis Clin North Am.* 2008;22(3):469–488 PMID: 18755385
18. Wormser GP, et al. *Clin Infect Dis.* 2006;43(9):1089–1134 PMID: 17029130
19. Sanchez E, et al. *JAMA.* 2016;315(16):1767–1777 PMID: 27115378
20. Kletsova EA, et al. *Ann Clin Microbiol Antimicrob.* 2017;16(1):26 PMID: 28399851
21. Schuster FL, et al. *Clin Microbiol Rev.* 2008;21(4):626–638 PMID: 18854484
22. Murray WJ, et al. *Clin Infect Dis.* 2004;39(10):1484–1492 PMID: 15546085
23. Sircar AD, et al. *MMWR Morb Mortal Wkly Rep.* 2016;65(35):930–933 PMID: 27608169
24. Rossignol JF, et al. *Clin Gastroenterol Hepatol.* 2005;3(10):987–991 PMID: 16234044
25. Nigro L, et al. *J Travel Med.* 2003;10(2):128–130 PMID: 12650658
26. Bern C, et al. *JAMA.* 2007;298(18):2171–2181 PMID: 18000201
27. Salvador F, et al. *Clin Infect Dis.* 2015;61(11):1688–1694 PMID: 26265500
28. Miller DA, et al. *Clin Infect Dis.* 2015;60(8):1237–1240 PMID: 25601454
29. Smith HV, et al. *Curr Opin Infect Dis.* 2004;17(6):557–564 PMID: 15640710
30. Davies AP, et al. *BMJ.* 2009;339:b4168 PMID: 19841008
31. Krause I, et al. *Pediatr Infect Dis J.* 2012;31(11):1135–1138 PMID: 22810017
32. Abubakar I, et al. *Cochrane Database Syst Rev.* 2007;(1):CD004932 PMID: 17253532
33. Jelinek T, et al. *Clin Infect Dis.* 1994;19(6):1062–1066 PMID: 7534125
34. Schuster A, et al. *Clin Infect Dis.* 2013;57(8):1155–1157 PMID: 23811416

35. Hoge CW, et al. *Lancet.* 1995;345(8951):691–693 PMID: 7885125
36. Ortega YR, et al. *Clin Microbiol Rev.* 2010;23(1):218–234 PMID: 20065331
37. Nash TE, et al. *Neurology.* 2006;67(7):1120–1127 PMID: 17030744
38. Garcia HH, et al. *Lancet Neurol.* 2014;13(12):1202–1215 PMID: 25453460
39. Lillie P, et al. *J Infect.* 2010;60(5):403–404 PMID: 20153773
40. White AC Jr, et al. *Clin Infect Dis.* 2018;66(8):1159–1163 PMID: 29617787
41. Verdier RI, et al. *Ann Intern Med.* 2000;132(11):885–888 PMID: 10836915
42. Stark DJ, et al. *Trends Parasitol.* 2006;22(2):92–96 PMID: 16380293
43. Röser D, et al. *Clin Infect Dis.* 2014;58(12):1692–1699 PMID: 24647023
44. Smego RA Jr, et al. *Clin Infect Dis.* 2003;37(8):1073–1083 PMID: 14523772
45. Brunetti E, et al. *Acta Trop.* 2010;114(1):1–16 PMID: 19931502
46. Fernando SD, et al. *J Trop Med.* 2011;2011:175941 PMID: 21234244
47. Walker M, et al. *Clin Infect Dis.* 2015;60(8):1199–2017 PMID: 25537873
48. Debrah AY, et al. *Clin Infect Dis.* 2015;61(4):517–526 PMID: 25948064
49. Mand S, et al. *Clin Infect Dis.* 2012;55(5):621–630 PMID: 22610930
50. Ottesen EA, et al. *Annu Rev Med.* 1992;43:417–424 PMID: 1580599
51. Jong EC, et al. *J Infect Dis.* 1985;152(3):637–640 PMID: 3897401
52. Sayasone S, et al. *Clin Infect Dis.* 2017;64(4):451–458 PMID: 28174906
53. Calvopina M, et al. *Trans R Soc Trop Med Hyg.* 1998;92(5):566–569 PMID: 9861383
54. Johnson RJ, et al. *Rev Infect Dis.* 1985;7(2):200–206 PMID: 4001715
55. Graham CS, et al. *Clin Infect Dis.* 2001;33(1):1–5 PMID: 11389487
56. Granados CE, et al. *Cochrane Database Syst Rev.* 2012;12:CD007787 PMID: 23235648
57. Ross AG, et al. *N Engl J Med.* 2013;368(19):1817–1825 PMID: 23656647
58. Requena-Mendez A, et al. *J Infect Dis.* 2017;215(6):946–953 PMID: 28453841
59. Hotez PJ, et al. *N Engl J Med.* 2004;351(8):799–807 PMID: 15317893
60. Keiser J, et al. *JAMA.* 2008;299(16):1937–1948 PMID: 18430913
61. Steinmann P, et al. *PLoS One.* 2011;6(9):e25003 PMID: 21980373
62. Aronson N, et al. *Clin Infect Dis.* 2016;63(12):e202–e264 PMID: 27941151
63. World Health Organization, Technical Report Series 949. Control of the leishmaniases. Report of a meeting of the WHO Expert Committee on the Control of Leishmaniases, Geneva, 22–26 March 2010
64. Alrajhi AA, et al. *N Engl J Med.* 2002;346(12):891–895 PMID: 11907288
65. Bern C, et al. *Clin Infect Dis.* 2006;43(7):917–924 PMID: 16941377
66. Ritmeijer K, et al. *Clin Infect Dis.* 2006;43(3):357–364 PMID: 16804852
67. Monge-Maillo B, et al. *Clin Infect Dis.* 2015;60(9):1398–1404 PMID: 25601455
68. Sundar S, et al. *N Engl J Med.* 2002;347(22):1739–1746 PMID: 12456849
69. Sundar S, et al. *N Engl J Med.* 2007;356(25):2571–2581 PMID: 17582067
70. Drugs for head lice. *JAMA.* 2017;317(19):2010–2011
71. Foucault C, et al. *J Infect Dis.* 2006;193(3):474–476 PMID: 16388498
72. Fischer PR, et al. *Clin Infect Dis.* 2002;34(4):493–498 PMID: 11797176
73. Tan KR, et al. Malaria. In: Brunette GW, Nemhauser JB, eds. *Yellow Book 2020: CDC Health Information for International Travel.* 2019:267–287
74. Usha V, et al. *J Am Acad Dermatol.* 2000;42(2pt1):236–240 PMID: 10642678
75. Brodine SK, et al. *Am J Trop Med Hyg.* 2009;80(3):425–430 PMID: 19270293
76. Doenhoff MJ, et al. *Expert Rev Anti Infect Ther.* 2006;4(2):199–210 PMID: 16597202
77. Fenwick A, et al. *Curr Opin Infect Dis.* 2006;19(6):577–582 PMID: 17075334
78. Marti H, et al. *Am J Trop Med Hyg.* 1996;55(5):477–481 PMID: 8940976
79. Segarra-Newnham M. *Ann Pharmacother.* 2007;41(12):1992–2001 PMID: 17940124
80. Barisani-Asenbauer T, et al. *J Ocul Pharmacol Ther.* 2001;17(3):287–294 PMID: 11436948
81. McAuley JB. *Pediatr Infect Dis J.* 2008;27(2):161–162 PMID: 18227714
82. McLeod R, et al. *Clin Infect Dis.* 2006;42(10):1383–1394 PMID: 16619149
83. Petersen E. *Expert Rev Anti Infect Ther.* 2007;5(2):285–293 PMID: 17402843
84. Shane AL, et al. *Clin Infect Dis.* 2017;65(12):e45–e80 PMID: 29053792
85. Steffen R, et al. *J Travel Med.* 2018;25(1) PMID: 30462260

86. DuPont HL. *Clin Infect Dis.* 2007;45(Suppl1):S78–S84 PMID: 17582576
87. Riddle MS, et al. *J Travel Med.* 2017;24(Suppl1):S57–S74 PMID: 28521004
88. Gottstein B, et al. *Clin Microbiol Rev.* 2009;22(1):127–145 PMID: 19136437
89. Workowski KA, et al. *MMWR Recomm Rep.* 2015;64(RR-03):1–137 PMID: 26042815
90. Fairlamb AH. *Trends Parasitol.* 2003;19(11):488–494 PMID: 14580959
91. Schmid C, et al. *Lancet.* 2004;364(9436):789–790 PMID: 15337407
92. Bisser S, et al. *J Infect Dis.* 2007;195(3):322–329 PMID: 17205469
93. Priotto G, et al. *Lancet.* 2009;374(9683):56–64 PMID: 19559476

Chapter 13

1. Nelson JD. *J Pediatr.* 1978;92(1):175–176 PMID: 619073
2. Nelson JD, et al. *J Pediatr.* 1978;92(1):131–134 PMID: 619055
3. Tetzlaff TR, et al. *J Pediatr.* 1978;92(3):485–490 PMID: 632997
4. Ballock RT, et al. *J Pediatr Orthop.* 2009;29(6):636–642 PMID: 19700997
5. Peltola H, et al. *N Engl J Med.* 2014;370(4):352–360 PMID: 24450893
6. Bradley JS, et al. *Pediatrics.* 2011;128(4):e1034–e1045 PMID: 21949152
7. Rice HE, et al. *Arch Surg.* 2001;136(12):1391–1395 PMID: 11735866
8. Fraser JD, et al. *J Pediatr Surg.* 2010;45(6):1198–1202 PMID: 20620320
9. Strohmeier Y, et al. *Cochrane Database Syst Rev.* 2014;7:CD003772 PMID: 25066627
10. Drusano GL, et al. *J Infect Dis.* 2014;210(8):1319–1324 PMID: 24760199
11. Arnold JC, et al. *Pediatrics.* 2012;130(4):e821–e828 PMID: 22966033
12. Zaoutis T, et al. *Pediatrics.* 2009;123(2):636–642 PMID: 19171632
13. Desai AA, et al. *J Pediatr Surg.* 2015;50(6):912–914 PMID: 25812441
14. Keren R, et al. *JAMA Pediatr.* 2015;169(2):120–128 PMID: 25506733
15. Liu C, et al. *Clin Infect Dis.* 2011;52(3):e18–e55 [Erratum: *Clin Infect Dis.* 2011;53(3):319] PMID: 21208910
16. Syrogiannopoulos GA, et al. *Lancet.* 1988;1(8575–8576):37–40 PMID: 2891899

Chapter 14

1. Oehler RL, et al. *Lancet Infect Dis.* 2009;9(7):439–447 PMID: 19555903
2. Bula-Rudas FJ, et al. *Pediatr Rev.* 2018;39(10):490–500 PMID: 30275032
3. Stevens DL, et al. *Clin Infect Dis.* 2014;59(2):147–159 PMID: 24947530
4. Talan DA, et al. *Clin Infect Dis.* 2003;37(11):1481–1489 PMID: 14614671
5. Aziz H, et al. *J Trauma Acute Care Surg.* 2015;78(3):641–648 PMID: 25710440
6. Centers for Disease Control and Prevention. Rabies. State and local rabies consultation contacts. http://www.cdc.gov/rabies/resources/contacts.html. Reviewed August 7, 2019. Accessed October 10, 2019
7. AAP. Tetanus. In: Kimberlin DW, et al, eds. *Red Book: 2018–2021 Report of the Committee on Infectious Diseases.* 31st ed. 2018:793–798
8. Wilson W, et al. *Circulation.* 2007;116(15):1736–1754 PMID: 17446442
9. Baltimore RS, et al. *Circulation.* 2015;132(15):1487–1515 PMID: 26373317
10. Sakai Bizmark R, et al. *Am Heart J.* 2017;189:110–119 PMID: 28625367
11. Gupta S, et al. *Congenit Heart Dis.* 2017;12(2):196–201 PMID: 27885814
12. Cahill TJ, et al. *Heart.* 2017;103(12):937–944 PMID: 28213367
13. Dayer M, et al. *J Infect Chemother.* 2018;24(1):18–24 PMID: 29107651
14. AAP. Lyme disease. In: Kimberlin DW, et al, eds. *Red Book: 2018–2021 Report of the Committee on Infectious Diseases.* 31st ed. 2018:195,515–523
15. Cohn AC, et al. *MMWR Recomm Rep.* 2013;62(RR-2):1–28 PMID: 23515099
16. McNamara LA, et al. *Lancet Infect Dis.* 2018;18(9):e272–e281 PMID: 29858150
17. AAP. Pertussis. In: Kimberlin DW, et al, eds. *Red Book: 2018–2021 Report of the Committee on Infectious Diseases.* 31st ed. 2018:620–634
18. Centers for Disease Control and Prevention. Pertussis (whooping cough). Postexposure antimicrobial prophylaxis. http://www.cdc.gov/pertussis/outbreaks/PEP.html. Reviewed August 7, 2017. Accessed October 10, 2019

19. Brook I. *Expert Rev Anti Infect Ther.* 2008;6(3):327–336 PMID: 18588497
20. Centers for Disease Control and Prevention. Tuberculosis (TB). Treatment regimens for latent TB infection (LBTI). http://www.cdc.gov/tb/topic/treatment/ltbi.htm. Reviewed April 5, 2016. Accessed October 10, 2019
21. AAP. Tuberculosis. In: Kimberlin DW, et al, eds. *Red Book: 2018–2021 Report of the Committee on Infectious Diseases*. 31st ed. 2018:829–853
22. Borisov AS, et al. *MMWR Morb Mortal Wkly Rep*. 2018;67(25):723–726 PMID: 29953429
23. ACOG Committee on Practice Bulletins. *Obstet Gynecol.* 2007;109(6):1489–1498 PMID: 17569194
24. Pinninti SG, et al. *Semin Perinatol.* 2018;42(3):168–175 PMID: 29544668
25. Kimberlin DW, et al. *N Engl J Med.* 2011;365(14):1284–1292 PMID: 21991950
26. AAP Committee on Infectious Diseases. *Pediatrics.* 2019;144(4):e20192478 PMID: 31477606
27. Kimberlin DW, et al. *J Infect Dis.* 2013;207(5):709–720 PMID: 23230059
28. AAP. Rabies. In: Kimberlin DW, et al, eds. *Red Book: 2018–2021 Report of the Committee on Infectious Diseases*. 31st ed. 2018:673–680
29. Leach AJ, et al. *Cochrane Database Syst Rev.* 2006;(4):CD004401 PMID: 17054203
30. Venekamp RP, et al. *Cochrane Database Syst Rev*. 2018;5:CD012017 PMID: 29741289
31. Williams GJ, et al. *Adv Exp Med Biol.* 2013;764:211–218 PMID: 23654070
32. Craig JC, et al. *N Engl J Med.* 2009;361(18):1748–1759 PMID: 19864673
33. RIVUR Trial Investigators, et al. *N Engl J Med.* 2014;370(25):2367–2376 PMID: 24795142
34. AAP Subcommittee on Urinary Tract Infection, Steering Committee on Quality Improvement and Management. *Pediatrics.* 2011;128(3):595–610 PMID: 21873693
35. Craig JC. *J Pediatr*. 2015;166(3):778 PMID: 25722276
36. National Institute for Health and Care Excellence. Urinary tract infection in under 16s: diagnosis and management. http://www.nice.org.uk/guidance/CG54. Updated October 2018. Accessed October 10, 2019
37. Williams G, et al. *Cochrane Database Syst Rev.* 2019;4:CD001534 PMID: 30932167
38. AAP. *Pneumocystis jirovecii* infections. In: Kimberlin DW, et al, eds. *Red Book: 2018–2021 Report of the Committee on Infectious Diseases*. 31st ed. 2018:651–657
39. Caselli D, et al. *J Pediatr*. 2014;164(2):389–392.e1 PMID: 24252793
40. Proudfoot R, et al. *J Pediatr Hematol Oncol.* 2017;39(3):194–202 PMID: 28267082
41. Stern A, et al. *Cochrane Database Syst Rev*. 2014;(10):CD005590 PMID: 25269391
42. *Med Lett Drugs Ther.* 2016;58(1495):63–68 PMID: 27192618
43. Mangram AJ, et al. *Infect Control Hosp Epidemiol.* 1999;20(4):250–280 PMID: 10219875
44. Engelman R, et al. *Ann Thorac Surg*. 2007;83(4):1569–1576 PMID: 17383396
45. Paruk F, et al. *Int J Antimicrob Agents*. 2017;49(4):395–402 PMID: 28254373
46. Hansen E, et al. *J Orthop Res.* 2014;32(Suppl1):S31–S59 PMID: 24464896
47. Branch-Elliman W, et al. *PLoS Med.* 2017;14(7):e1002340 PMID: 28692690
48. Branch-Elliman W, et al. *JAMA Surg*. 2019;154(7):590–598 PMID: 31017647
49. Berríos-Torres SI, et al. *JAMA Surg*. 2017;152(8):784–791 PMID: 28467526
50. Hawn MT, et al. *JAMA Surg*. 2013;148(7):649–657 PMID: 23552769
51. Shaffer WO, et al. *Spine J.* 2013;13(10):1387–1392 PMID: 23988461
52. Bratzler DW, et al. *Am J Health Syst Pharm.* 2013;70(3):195–283 PMID: 23327981
53. Lador A, et al. *J Antimicrob Chemother*. 2012;67(3):541–550 PMID: 22083832
54. De Cock PA, et al. *J Antimicrob Chemother.* 2017;72(3):791–800 PMID: 27999040
55. Marino NE, et al. *Surg Infect (Larchmt).* 2017;18(8):894–903 PMID: 29064344
56. Nelson RL, et al. *Tech Coloproctol*. 2018;22(8):573–587 PMID: 30019145

Index

B

D

E

F

M

Index

N

O

Index

P

Index

Q

R

Index

U

Index

Index